The Balanced Body

A Guide to Deep Tissue and Neuromuscular Therapy

THIRD EDITION

The Balanced Body

A Guide to Deep Tissue and Neuromuscular Therapy

THIRD EDITION

Donald W. Scheumann

 Lippincott Williams & Wilkins
a Wolters Kluwer business
Philadelphia · Baltimore · New York · London
Buenos Aires · Hong Kong · Sydney · Tokyo

Acquisitions Editor: John Goucher
Managing Editor: Karen M. Ruppert
Marketing Manager: Hilary Henderson
Production Editor: Sirkka E.H. Bertling
Designer: Risa J. Clow
Illustrator: David R. Rini
Compositor: Maryland Composition, Inc.
Printer: Courier Corporation—Kendallville

351 West Camden Street
Baltimore, MD 21201

530 Walnut Street
Philadelphia, PA 19106

The publisher is not responsible (as a matter of product liability, negligence, or otherwise) for any injury resulting from any material contained herein. This publication contains information relating to general principles of medical care that should not be construed as specific instructions for individual patients. Manufacturers' product information and package inserts should be reviewed for current information, including contraindications, dosages, and precautions.

Printed in the United States of America

First Edition, 1997
Second Edition, 2002

Library of Congress Cataloging-in-Publication Data

Scheumann, Donald W.
     The balanced body : a guide to deep tissue and neuromuscular therapy
 / Donald W. Scheumann. — 3rd ed.
        p. ; cm.
     Includes bibliographical references and index.
     ISBN 0-7817-6308-8
     1. Massage therapy.   I. Title.
     [DNLM: 1. Massage—methods.   2. Physical Therapy Techniques.
 WB 537 S328b 2007]
 RM721.S326 2007
 615.8′22—dc22

                                                                    2005030173

The publishers have made every effort to trace the copyright holders for borrowed material. If they have inadvertently overlooked any, they will be pleased to make the necessary arrangements at the first opportunity.

To purchase additional copies of this book, call our customer service department at **(800) 638-3030** or fax orders to **(301) 223-2320.** International customers should call **(301) 223-2300.**

Visit Lippincott Williams & Wilkins on the Internet: http://www.LWW.com. Lippincott Williams & Wilkins customer service representatives are available from 8:30 am to 6:00 pm, EST.

06 07 08 09
1 2 3 4 5 6 7 8 9 10

To Jeanne Aland,
who always believed in me.
—DS

About the Author

Don Scheumann has been a massage practitioner and instructor for more than 20 years. For much of that time, he taught at the Atlanta School of Massage, where he was a major contributor to curriculum development, having created many of the classes for the Integrated Massage and Deep Tissue Program as well as classes in the Wellness and Spa Therapies Program, including the original shiatsu course. He co-authored his first deep tissue training manual for the school in 1985 and has also designed and taught many continuing education courses, including Rocking Techniques for the Massage Therapist, Yoga for Body-workers, Introduction to the Meridians, and Upper Body Disorders.

Don's education in personal growth and transformation began as a teenager, when he commenced yoga studies at the Yoga Society of New York. After graduating from SUNY at Purchase with a BFA in dance, he pursued a career in modern dance in New York City. During this period, he undertook an internship at a major holistic health center, where he studied with many of the premier educators in the human potential movement. This experience led him to move away from the performing arts and devote his career to the exploration of the body as a tool for healing. In 1980, he became a certified yoga instructor, and in 1982, he graduated from massage school. His other certifications in bodywork modalities include polarity, neuromuscular therapy, reiki, Pfrimmer deep muscle therapy, acupressure, and zen therapy.

As a yoga instructor and former dancer, movement has always played a major role in Don's approach to teaching massage therapy. He imparts to his students the importance of understanding and being comfortable in one's own body as the foundation for performing any type of somatic-based healing modality. His proudest achievement to date has been the recognition of his passion for teaching by the American Massage Therapy Association, which honored him with the 2001 Jerome Perlinski Teacher of the Year Award.

Preface

The Balanced Body: A Guide to Deep Tissue and Neuromuscular Therapy is a comprehensive course in deep tissue–style massage therapy. It contains all the elements necessary for a student to become competent in performing this goal-oriented approach to full-body muscle tension release.

Many styles of massage have emerged over the past few decades and have been categorized as deep tissue therapy. These methods expand upon the effects of Swedish massage, in that they target chronically contracted muscle groups in a more specific manner than primarily circulatory system–based modalities. Whereas Swedish techniques tend to cover broad surfaces of the body, deep tissue strokes pinpoint dysfunctional conditions within individual muscles. This focused approach to body therapy allows for manual alteration of muscular, fascial, and skeletal relationships, often producing dramatic changes in structural alignment and reduction of muscular tension.

The style of deep tissue therapy presented in this book evolved initially from concepts introduced during my training in massage therapy at the Atlanta School of Massage more than 20 years ago. The first edition of this book was written in 1997 as the primary textbook for the deep tissue course taught there. It was a less complete text than the second edition, having been designed to supplement the curriculum taught in classes at the school. In preparing the second edition for widespread publication, the book was greatly expanded, making it more of a self-contained teaching aid.

The success of the second edition has led to the release of the current third edition, which includes more visual reinforcement of the learning material. Forty new illustrations have been added to this edition. An important new feature is the inclusion of a CD-ROM containing videotaped demonstrations of 20 massage techniques from the book and 10 segments from the Acland DVD Atlas of Human Anatomy series. Look for CD icons (⊙ for massage techniques, ⊙ for Acland anatomy clips) throughout the book that refer you to corresponding materials on the CD-ROM. An expanded section on ethics is also part of this new edition.

FORMAT

The book is divided into two parts. The first part presents an overview of the integrated deep tissue therapy approach to massage along with important foundational information for students. The philosophy and background for this method of progressive deep muscle release is described in this part of the book. The second part consists of the deep tissue lessons, which are divided into two segments. The first segment of each lesson provides essential supplementary material about the region of the body being studied, including kinesiology, musculoskeletal anatomy, supplementary exercises, common conditions, and a perspective on the mind/body interface. The second segment is the deep tissue therapy routine for that particular area of the body.

The lessons are arranged in a precise order that combines a regional approach to deep tissue therapy with a structural realignment orientation. The progression through the body moves from the central axis to the upper extremity, followed by the lower extremity, the core, and the neck and head. These particular areas are addressed over a period of time through a series of deep tissue sessions.

I developed this sequence of deep muscle release after studying the Rolfing plan of methodical fascial manipulation formulated to align the body's personal axis of gravity with the gravitational axis of the earth. Adherence to a logical order of deep muscle release based on the structural integration model is a distinct characteristic of this system of integrated deep tissue therapy. Working with this sequence over the past several years, both in my personal practice and in teaching massage students, has convinced me of its effectiveness in guiding the body to states of equipoise and stress-free movement.

Complementary Modalities

Another unique feature of the deep tissue therapy approach taught in this book is the use of several complementary modalities to enhance the results of the bodywork. Many forms of myofascial manipulation have evolved within various cultures, with each emphasizing different characteristics of the body's tissues and physiological systems. Combining elements from these diverse systems creates a synergistic effect that greatly intensifies the transformative capability of deep tissue therapy.

The other bodywork systems incorporated into the deep tissue routines are neuromuscular therapy, Swedish massage, connective tissue release, cross fiber therapy, assisted stretching, shiatsu, and polarity. Although these styles are not examined to the same degree as deep tissue therapy, their use is explained sufficiently to allow students to incorporate them effectively within the context of the deep tissue sessions. Students who learn this integrated approach to bodywork are extremely well rounded and adaptable in their application of massage therapy.

The Art of Effective Touch

Providing a complete educational foundation in integrated deep tissue therapy was given foremost consideration when deciding which topics to include in this book. Subtle concepts like teaching proper quality of touch are difficult to convey in written materials and are often neglected in massage teaching manuals. To provide assistance in this crucial area of learning, topics such as characteristics of different muscle types, palpation skills, and body mechanics are covered.

Perhaps the most important contribution to learning the art of effective touch is provided in the section titled *Principles of Conscious Bodywork* in Chapter 3. I have formulated 10 guidelines that succinctly state the theory and proper application of deep tissue therapy to achieve the most beneficial outcome. Regular study of these concepts will ensure that students are employing the proper attitude and methodology to perform superior deep tissue massage consistently.

LESSON STRUCTURE

The chapters in *The Balanced Body* are formatted to be used as the curriculum for classes in learning deep tissue therapy. These lessons should be taught in the same order as they are presented in the book. The foundational information covered in the first four chapters may be incorporated into massage theory and history classes. Chapter 5 begins the hands-on training with a discussion of the role of fascia, followed by a full-body routine of connective tissue

techniques. These strokes are utilized in the succeeding deep tissue routines in Chapters 6 through 10.

Beginning with Chapter 6, the progressive deep tissue therapy protocol is introduced. Although within the lessons the body is necessarily divided into segments for learning purposes, there is an overlying theme expressed throughout the book of viewing the body as a functional whole. In accordance with a structural integration perspective, emphasis is placed on the concept that altering any part of the body through myofascial manipulation changes relationships throughout the entire structure that may resonate on many levels of a person's being. This viewpoint finds voice in the introductory portion of each lesson.

Special Features

The *General Concepts* section describes the functions that the particular part of the body being studied serves and how it interacts with and affects the body as a whole. The *Musculoskeletal Anatomy and Function* section emphasizes the kinesiological role of the body part through descriptions of the interrelationships of muscles and the bones they move. It is extremely important for massage therapists to have detailed knowledge of the skeleton, including the shapes of bones and the actions of joints. Muscles and bones are inextricably related, a concept that often is not adequately emphasized in massage textbooks.

A number of crucial topics are covered in easy-to-follow chart and list form. These include indications/contraindications, essential anatomy, common conditions, range of motion for joints and associated muscles, and common postural distortions. The *Exercises and Self-Treatment* section is extremely beneficial in providing the therapist with simple exercises he or she can teach clients to perform at home to reinforce the neuromuscular changes brought about by the deep tissue sessions.

The *Mind/Body Connection* introduces students to concepts that are integral to somatic psychology, wherein the role of beliefs and emotions in determining the shapes and tension states of areas of the body is explored. Because of the more subjective nature of this material, it is a distinguished feature in the text. Depending on the viewpoint of a particular school or teacher, this material may be incorporated to a greater or lesser degree in a student's training.

The deep tissue routines are presented in a linear fashion, listing accessory techniques, muscles to be massaged, and strokes to be practiced. As discussed in the body of the text, this orderly method of practice serves more as a learning tool than as a blueprint for actual deep tissue sessions. Although the overall format of each deep tissue routine may be retained as an organizational guide, each therapy session must be shaped to the unique distribution of muscle tension in the individual client.

To aid in this endeavor, postural evaluation procedures are listed in the lessons for each area of the body. Body reading the clients in this manner greatly assists students in determining the crucial muscle groups to address to unlock a client's pattern of distortion and stress. The ability to assess a client on this level is the most important skill a deep tissue therapist can acquire. Correct postural evaluation allows a therapist to be accurate and efficient in determining the proper application of deep tissue therapy for a client. The information and guidance provided in *The Balanced Body* will accelerate a student's mastery of skillful body reading.

Within the deep tissue routines, deep tissue strokes and neuromuscular therapy techniques are combined. Before the deep tissue strokes for each muscle are described, the attachment sites and actions for that muscle are listed. A brief description of the locations of common trigger points for that muscle is also included. This information is derived from the work of Janet Travell, MD, and David Simons, MD. Being aware of these sites of possible trigger points greatly assists students in finding and treating them while applying deep tissue techniques to a muscle.

CONCLUSION

A new era is dawning in the field of bodywork with the proliferation of textbooks designed specifically to educate students in professional massage therapy training programs. For many years, practically no widespread publications described actual deep tissue therapy procedures. Most articles and books written on the subject focused on the theory and philosophy of the work but offered little or no practical instruction for how to perform deep tissue techniques. To see and learn actual deep tissue strokes, students were required to enroll in a workshop or a full course.

Hands-on training under the supervision of a qualified instructor is the only way to learn massage therapy skills properly. Having high-quality written materials available to reinforce and even guide classroom instruction, however, is revolutionizing massage therapy training throughout the world. New communication technologies, like the Internet and digital audio-video resources, are further hastening the dissemination of leading-edge massage therapy training tools.

To my knowledge, *The Balanced Body* is one of the only commercially published books that outlines a complete course in an integrated application of deep tissue therapy. The comprehensive blending of structural realignment methodology with deep tissue tension release and trigger point treatment in a lesson format, as detailed in this book, is unique in the massage therapy field.

In this age of specialization, many people are finding great benefit in the exploration of traditional approaches to health care, like Ayurvedic and Chinese medicine, that view all aspects of a person's being and lifestyle as important health-determining factors. *The Balanced Body* represents my contribution to this holistic perspective within the realm of hands-on bodywork. I hope that the audience this book reaches will find the study of this system of massage as rewarding as I have in the many years I have devoted to practicing and teaching it.

Don Scheumann

User's Guide

The Balanced Body: A Guide to Deep Tissue and Neuromuscular Therapy provides a complete program for integrated deep tissue therapy, presented in an easy-to-use format. This User's Guide shows you how to put the book's features to work for you.

Section One provides a solid knowledge base and foundation for students to build upon before moving on to the second section. **Section Two**, which comprises most of the book, focuses on hands-on techniques and routines for providing safe and effective deep tissue therapy to massage clients.

You'll find these helpful learning features throughout the text:

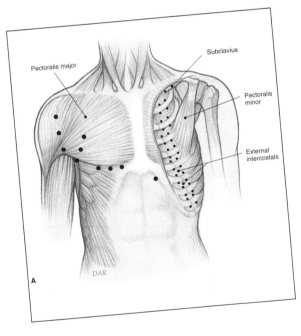

DETAILED ILLUSTRATIONS AND PHOTOGRAPHS (with 40 new illustrations in this edition) bring the techniques to life and clearly demonstrate anatomy and physiology.

INDICATIONS/CONTRAINDICATIONS

Boxes list the conditions affecting massage of a particular body region.

THE MIND/BODY CONNECTION boxes

detail the connection between the scientific functioning of the body and the mind, and achieving a balance between the two.

ROUTINES for massage practice that focus on the

particular body region are outlined in detailed format in each chapter. A variety of techniques are presented. Each routine outlines a sequence, with detailed steps for each muscle set in the sequence.

CASE STUDIES in each chapter present students with clinical scenarios.

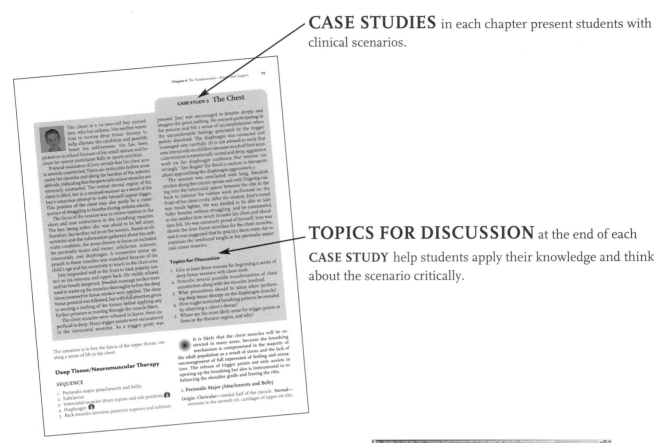

TOPICS FOR DISCUSSION at the end of each **CASE STUDY** help students apply their knowledge and think about the scenario critically.

ICONS in the text refer students to video clips of demonstrations of massage routines and real-life anatomy footage .

A BONUS CD packaged with every book brings the book content to life by presenting video demonstrations of routines and real-life anatomy footage.

Acknowledgments

I would like to thank the following people for their participation in the creation of the third edition of *The Balanced Body: A Guide to Deep Tissue and Neuromuscular Therapy*:

Peter Darcy, acquisitions editor at LWW, for having the vision to foresee the success of this book;

Karen Ruppert, managing editor at LWW, for her meticulous guidance throughout the editorial phase of the book;

David Rini, for his exquisite execution of all the illustrations created for the book;

Chris MacHarg, for contributing his time to model and for turning my visions into pictorial realities through his artistic talent.

The reviewers of the second edition for their helpful suggestions.

All the people who granted permission for the use of photographs, illustrations, and written materials for the third edition.

Brief Contents

Expanded Contents

Introduction to the Integrated Deep Tissue Therapy System

Overview of the Integrated Deep Tissue System

This is a training manual for learning an integrated approach to massage therapy, emphasizing deep tissue and neuromuscular therapy. It is designed for students who have completed an introductory program of basic massage procedures. This course will incorporate and expand on techniques used in Swedish and other forms of circulatory massage and introduce many other methods of addressing soft tissue dysfunction.

Integrated deep tissue therapy is a highly effective method of soft tissue treatment in that it combines several modalities that emphasize different aspects and qualities of the myofascial system. When combined, these techniques provide a comprehensive protocol for reducing or eliminating many different manifestations of restriction in muscles and fascia and the means to return the body to a healthy, strong, and vital condition.

The integrated deep tissue approach to massage therapy aligns with the Wellness Model proposed by Dr. John Travis in the 1970s.[1] This model has served as a prototype for many complementary healthcare treatment protocols and holistic health centers that have been created since that time.

Travis and his coauthor, Regina Sara Ryan, viewed wellness as an ongoing, dynamic process of self-activated participation in the health and welfare of one's being. According to this perspective, humans are composed of a series of integrated systems that all work synergistically toward optimal health and well-being. This means that our physical, mental, emotional, and spiritual states are vital factors in determining the condition of our bodies and our outlooks on life.

According to Ilya Prigogene's Nobel prize-winning theory of dissipative structures,[2] human beings, as well as all living organisms, are examples of an organizing principle known as the open system (Fig. 1-1) An open system operates by taking in energy, metabolizing or converting energy for use, and then releasing or dissipating energy back into the environment. All our vital processes depend on the smooth and efficient transfor-

mation of energy for the health and integrity of the human system to remain intact.

The three primary ways that we receive energy are through the air we breathe, the food we eat, and the sensory input we receive through the nervous system and sense organs. In a state of health, the physiologic pathways provided for conduction and transformation of energy throughout the body operate effectively and efficiently. When our biologic conduits falter, the stage is set for disease and breakdown to occur.

Massage therapy provides excellent assistance in the maintenance of high-level wellness, because it directly or indirectly affects many of the systems that transport and transform energy within the body. The circulatory, respiratory, muscular, endocrine, and nervous system functions can all be improved through the application of manual massage techniques.

As the flow of energy through the body is improved, psychological and physiologic activities are affected. When the body is performing at peak levels, our ability to interact with our environment is vastly improved. This can have a direct effect on the quality of our relationships and on our mental and emotional outlooks in general.

Dr. Travis' Wellness Model depicts the process of achieving wellness as a journey along a continuum (Fig. 1-2). The midpoint of the scale, labeled neutral, represents a condition of moderate well-being in which the individual is capable of functioning in everyday life without too much difficulty. For many, this average state of health has been accepted as the norm, and maintaining it is considered to be the best-case scenario.

The left side of the scale depicted in the Wellness Model represents a gradual decline from the neutral state of wellness through a series of signs and symptoms of degenerating health that can eventually lead to disability or even premature death. It is hoped that a person experiencing this slide into dysfunction will seek adequate care and return to the neutral point of wellness. The halting of physical and/or psychological breakdown and the

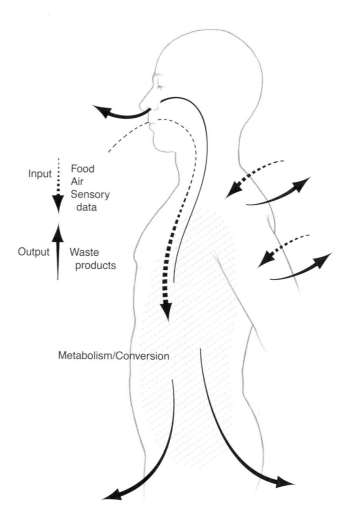

FIGURE 1-1 To maintain a state of health, the body must be able to freely take in and dispel energy.

rebuilding of health is called the Treatment Model. Most traditionally recognized physical and psychological therapies are based on this goal.

The right side of the scale depicted in the Wellness Model represents what Travis calls high-level wellness. This half of the continuum describes movement toward expanding states of greater well-being beyond the neutral stage of adequate functioning. These states of more complete fulfillment and happiness are motivated by increased awareness, pursuit of education, and personal growth. Achievement of these states is largely self-motivated as a person seeks out ways to explore opportu-

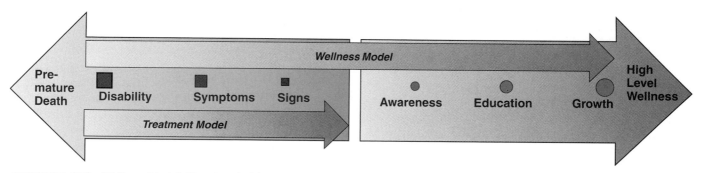

FIGURE 1-2 The Wellness Model. (Reprinted with permission from Travis JW, Ryan RS. Wellness workbook. Berkeley, CA: Ten Speed Press, 1981.)

nities for expansion of consciousness, creative expression, and productivity.

The Wellness Model describes a potential for personal excellence that we are all capable of achieving. Any method of treatment or intervention that leads a person back along the road to health can potentially provide the momentum to motivate that individual to seek the knowledge that will guide him or her to the highest level of wellness that person is capable of manifesting.

Integrated Deep Tissue System

The integrated deep tissue therapy method of bodywork encompasses the spectrum of the illness/wellness scale in that it can be used to provide assistance and education at almost any point along the continuum. This approach to massage therapy does not attempt to replace any form of medical treatment, whether physical or psychological. Massage therapists are not trained to diagnose, treat, or prescribe drugs for any kind of medical condition, nor are they qualified to provide psychological evaluations or counseling. Massage therapists are trained to work with the body's soft tissues to reduce tension and alleviate restrictions in the myofascial system and to increase fluid circulation within the body. Massage therapy education includes instruction on manual techniques applied to the body's myofascial tissues to improve their function as well as techniques for stretching and joint mobilization.

Massage therapists need to be familiar with the factors that lead to soft tissue dysfunction, including postural abnormalities and movement habits that can result in misuse, abuse, and injury to the body. They must also understand the role of the mind and emotions in creating heightened activity of the sympathetic nervous system that can lead to muscular tension and pain.

A person who practices integrated deep tissue therapy may be viewed primarily as an educator. Through manipulation and realignment of the body's soft tissues, the therapist teaches the client to experience the benefits of becoming more relaxed, balanced, and pain free. The client may then be motivated to gain the necessary information to make lifestyle improvements that will assist him or her in sustaining this higher state of well-being. These adjustments may include receiving regular massage therapy, instituting a fitness program, improving nutrition, and learning meditation or other forms of stress reduction.

Integrated deep tissue therapy incorporates viewpoints and methodologies from both Western and Eastern approaches to health. Many of the soft tissue techniques used here were developed within the context of the Western rehabilitative therapy model. A primary goal of these techniques is to improve muscle function through:

- Enhancement of oxygen and nutritive levels within muscle fibers
- Reduction of the effects of scar tissue and other adhering factors in the myofascia
- Decreased pain sensations by minimizing irritation to nerve endings caused by trapped waste products

The techniques of energy balance and enhancement are mostly drawn from Eastern bodywork modalities. The perspective on health provided by the Wellness Model and advocated by the integrated deep tissue therapy system is decidedly holistic, as are many traditional Asian healthcare practices. (For a good introduction to the holistic perspective offered by Chinese medicine, the reader is referred to Beinfield and Korngold.[3]) The holistic perspective views all aspects of a person—including the body, mind, lifestyle, and relationships—as important factors contributing to the overall state of health.

Origins

In embracing both the rehabilitative and holistic perspectives in healthcare, the integrated deep tissue therapy system follows in the tradition of many bodywork approaches that have been developed or promoted since the 1960s. A variety of sources have contributed to weave the tapestry that makes up this comprehensive style of body therapy. The techniques that have been incorporated are shown in Figure 1-3.

The overriding goal of integrated deep tissue therapy is to establish an internal environment whereby energy may be taken into the body, utilized, and dissipated back into the environment in a fluid, efficient manner. This is largely accomplished through assessing and removing restrictions in the myofascial system, which manifest as shortened or adhered areas within the muscles and fascia and result in limited function and, possibly, pain. As

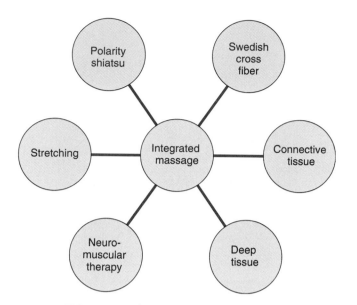

FIGURE 1-3 The Integrated Massage Wheel.

the physical body is restored to a condition of optimal performance capability, many signs and symptoms of malfunction often dissipate. A better self-image and a more positive outlook toward life in general may accompany this improvement in physical well-being.

One of the first people to develop a method of bodywork based on this concept of comprehensive, overall body assessment and realignment was Dr. Ida Rolf (Fig. 1-4). Her style of therapy is called structural integration, commonly known as Rolfing. Dr. Rolf was a biochemist who began to formulate the principles and techniques of structural integration during the 1940s. She developed a 10-session series of bodywork in which the fascial network is manipulated to realign the vertical axis of the body to the earth's gravitational field. Many of the newer styles of deep tissue therapy and myofascial work are at least partially derived from Dr. Rolf's pioneering concepts.

Neuromuscular therapy, or trigger point release work, rests on a foundation laid by Dr. Janet Travell (Fig. 1-5). Dr. Travell was a cardiologist who served two presidents as the White House physician. She did much research in the area of muscular involvement in pain causation and relief. Her two-volume work, *Myofascial Pain and Dysfunction, The Trigger Point Manual,*[4] coauthored with David Simmons, MD, serves as the seminal guide in this field.

A pioneering psychologist, Dr. Wilhelm Reich, developed many of the concepts of mind and body interaction that are incorporated in various styles of bodywork as well as several forms of somatic psychotherapy. Among other thought-provoking concepts, Dr. Reich proposed theories about how the shape and tone of the body are greatly influenced by the inner psychic structure. He also discovered that patterns of chronic tension based on restricted feelings become lodged in the neuromuscular system, contributing to conditions of neurosis. By confronting

FIGURE 1-4 Ida Rolf, PhD. (Reprinted with permission from the Rolf Institute.)

FIGURE 1-5 Janet Travell, MD. (Reprinted with permission from Virginia P. Street.)

these holding patterns in the soft tissues through physical manipulation, various exercises designed to amplify the tension, and conscious breathing, Dr. Reich found that the unconscious tension blocks could be released and the underlying feelings expressed.

Polarity therapy is a comprehensive, holistic healthcare practice that includes physical manipulations performed while the patient is on a massage table. It was developed by Dr. Randolph Stone (Fig. 1-6) and was based on his many years of studying traditional healing systems worldwide. The basic premise of polarity therapy is that health is built on freeing blockages in the underlying energetic pathways that provide organizational templates for the physical and psychological structures. Dr. Stone's writings and work have a broad interface with many styles of bodywork, including structural integration, acupressure, craniosacral therapy, myofascial release, and energetic forms of healing, like therapeutic touch.

The above list of pioneers whose works have illuminated the integrated deep tissue therapy system described in this manual is only a partial one. Many other talented individuals in the art of healing have also participated in the design and refinement of techniques that are incorporated in this fluidly adaptable synthesis of massage modalities. Their contributions are acknowledged and appreciated.

FIGURE 1-6 Dr. Randolph Stone. (Reprinted with permission from the American Polarity Therapy Association.)

Components of the Integrated Deep Tissue System

The techniques incorporated in the integrated deep tissue method are depicted on a wheel (see Fig. 1-3) rather than in a list. This is done to illustrate that they need not always be applied in a predetermined sequence; instead, they can be blended and mixed as required by the specific situation.

In each lesson of this text, the techniques are described in a prescribed order that is suggested as a general protocol for approaching the body. This sequence opens the body progressively, beginning with preparatory contact between the therapist and client, then warm-up of the tissues, and then work on the deeper layers. This basic structure allows much room for adaptability by moving through the techniques on the wheel according to the unique needs of the individual.

■ DEEP TISSUE THERAPY

The heart of the integrated deep tissue system is, naturally, deep tissue therapy. Many varying styles of deep tissue therapy have been developed over the years, but some characteristics are common to all of them. The primary function of deep tissue therapy is to reduce the level of stress imposed on the body by chronically shortened mus-

cles. This is accomplished by applying a combination of slow compressive and lengthening procedures to the involved musculature.

Results of Tense Musculature

The effects of chronically shortened, tense muscles are many. Circulation of blood and lymph is inhibited. Constricted muscles act as dams, blocking fluids from flowing freely throughout the body. It must be remembered that in an open system, energy exchange must be efficient for the system to function properly.

Muscles rely on a steady intake of oxygen and nutrients to provide the energy necessary for muscular contraction and relaxation to occur. The waste products of muscle metabolism are released into the venous blood supply to be transported out of the muscles and processed for removal from the body. If this cycle is disrupted, the muscles become toxic from lack of nutrition and build-up of waste products, and they can no longer perform their job effectively.

Toxicity within the muscle tissue irritates nerve endings, resulting in weakness and possible sensations of pain. This internal toxicity taxes the immune system and creates an environment in which disease can more easily take hold.

Role of Muscles

The primary function of muscles is to provide movement for the body. This is accomplished by paired groups of muscles alternately contracting and lengthening to move the bones to which they are attached. Muscles must be free to respond to stimuli from the nervous system, which sends the impulses that direct the muscles to contract.

The fine motor skills the body is capable of performing rely on this precise balancing act of muscular contraction and relaxation. Stated in a simplified manner, as one set of muscles contracts, it pulls a bone in a particular direction, causing the opposing muscles to lengthen and yield for the movement to occur. To move the bone in the opposite direction, the sequence of events is reversed, with the lengthened muscles receiving the stimulus from the nervous system to shorten. The currently contracted muscles then relax and lengthen to allow the bone to move.

Effects of Muscle Imbalance

Muscles that are chronically contracted disrupt the symmetry of balanced forces acting on the skeleton (Fig. 1-7).

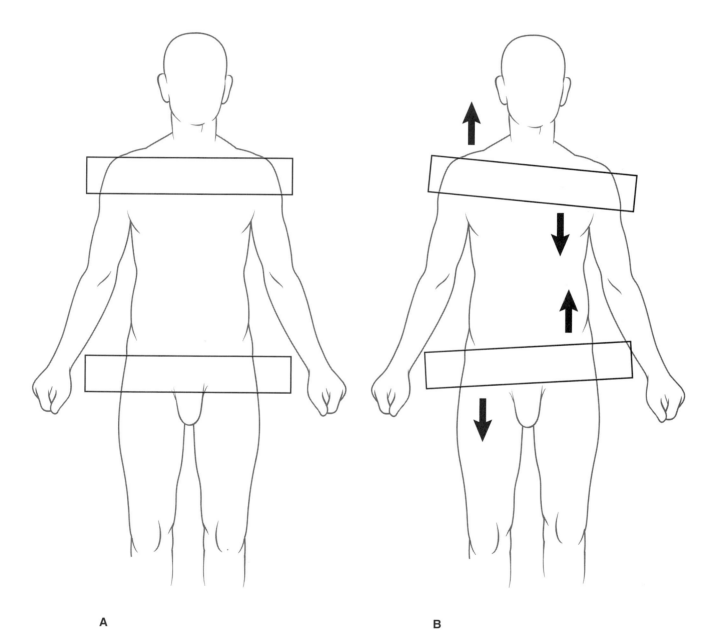

A

B

FIGURE 1-7 A. Normal muscle balance resulting in body symmetry. **B.** Uneven muscle relationships contribute to body assymetry.

They hold bones out of position, causing postural distortions that result in structural stress. Soft tissue integrity is compromised when the body is not in balance with the field of gravity. Fascial tissue builds up around points of stress to reinforce those areas from being pulled further out of alignment. Ligaments are also put under strain to brace misaligned joints.

Chronic uneven muscular pulls on the skeleton cause some muscles to remain contracted while their opposing muscles are stretched beyond their resting length and weakened. This results in lack of adaptability in movement, which makes the body more prone to injury. Muscle fibers that cannot lengthen are more likely to be torn during rapid, forceful movement. Injury is most likely to occur at the musculotendinous junction or where the tendon blends with the periosteum of the bone. Unless the factors creating these stresses on the soft tissues and skeleton are relieved, the body will continue to degenerate into states of greater dysfunction and pain.

Purpose of Deep Tissue Therapy

Deep tissue therapy is designed to return the body to a state of ease and balance by eliminating the uneven pulls on the skeleton caused by contracted muscles and constricted fascia. Muscular strain in the body may be assessed by watching how a person stands and moves. Manual testing of the degree of movement available at the joints also aids in determining which muscles are shortened or contracted. After recognizing the patterns of muscular distortion, the deep tissue therapist systematically releases the shortened muscles and stretches the constricted fascia to re-establish freedom of movement of the bones.

Application of Deep Tissue Therapy

Slow, compressive strokes applied along the length of a muscle recalibrate the nerve receptors that determine muscle length, allowing contracted muscles to relax. These receptors are called **muscle spindles** (Fig. 1-8), and they are located within the muscle belly parallel to the contractile, or extrafusal, fibers. Slow stretching of the muscle after the deep tissue strokes are applied also activates the **Golgi tendon organs**, which are the nerve receptors within the tendons that also help to determine the degree of tone in the muscle.

If a muscle is stretched quickly, causing the muscle spindles to lengthen rapidly, an impulse is sent through the nervous system directing the muscle to contract. This mechanism is known as the **stretch reflex.** It is a protective device that prevents muscles and tendons from being damaged by overstretching. If, however, a muscle is stretched slowly, causing the muscle spindles to lengthen slowly, the

FIGURE 1-8 A muscle spindle acts like a spring, being stretched when the extrafusal fibers around it are lengthened. (Modified from Bear MF, Connors BW, Parasido MA. Neuroscience: exploring the brain. 2nd ed. Philadelphia: Lippincott Williams & Wilkins, 2001, ch. 13.)

stretch reflex is overridden. In this case, a message is sent from the nervous system to allow the muscle to relax and lengthen further.

Deep tissue strokes are also performed along the borders of adjacent muscles to release fascial adhering and reduce build-up of scar tissue that may be preventing the muscles from moving independently. In deep tissue therapy, muscle groups are also freed in layers, from superficial to deep, to allow each muscle to perform its appropriate actions without restriction. Removing these glitches from the musculature frees obstructions that are binding the muscles and not allowing full movement capability.

Benefits of Deep Tissue Therapy

As the soft tissues of the body are realigned and balance is returned to the skeleton, much less strain is imposed on the nervous system. This results in better posture and freer movement, which greatly reduce the risk of injury. Coordination is also improved. Minimizing strain around joints reduces the incidence of osteoarthritis and the possibility of ligament tears as well, and reducing the amount of energy used in holding chronically contracted muscles increases the overall level of vitality and promotes clearer thinking. All the body's systems benefit from having more metabolic energy available to fuel them.

■ NEUROMUSCULAR THERAPY

Neuromuscular therapy is a specialized form of deep tissue work that treats a specific manifestation of muscular dysfunction known as trigger points. Trigger points are tiny areas of irritation that form within strained bands of muscle tissue. They refer sensations of pain, weakness, or numbness to surrounding or distant areas of muscle tissue.

Formation of Trigger Points

Trigger points are present in the majority of cases of chronic muscular pain. They are formed as a result of muscular strain, which in turn can be the result of some kind of trauma, including an accident, exposure to cold or infection, or overuse of a particular set of muscles. Areas of strain also form in misaligned areas of the body, where muscles have to work constantly to maintain distorted positions of the bones. Trigger points always manifest in areas of shortened musculature. It is common to locate trigger points in contracted muscles that are being treated by deep tissue therapy (Fig. 1-9).

The exact mechanism of trigger point activation is unknown. Dr. Travell postulated that the constant presence of waste products within a damaged group of muscle **fibrils**, apparently produced by unrelenting cellular metabolism in that section of the muscle, stimulates nerve endings in the area to send amplified input into the spinal cord.[5] This stimulus is then thrown back into the peripheral nervous system through weakened or **facilitated nerve pathways**. The impulses traveling along these nerve routes activate pain sensations in a specific portion of the muscles

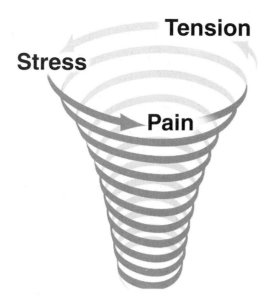

FIGURE 1-10 The stress-tension-pain cycle generates a self-perpetuating, downward spiral of dysfunction that often requires therapeutic intervention to be halted.

stimulated by those particular nerves. The areas affected by trigger points are called **referred pain zones.**

Trigger points are self-perpetuating. They accompany a phenomenon known as the **stress-tension-pain cycle** (Fig. 1-10). Stress can be generated by a number of factors, including physical trauma, as discussed above. Emotional trauma produces many of the same symptoms as physical stress, including muscular tension.

The body attempts to isolate areas of trauma through a process known as **muscle splinting.** This is a protective mechanism whereby muscles around the injured area contract to isolate the trauma and prevent movement that could lead to further damage. Scar tissue tends to build up in this area, as do taut bands of unyielding muscle fibers. The lack of circulation that occurs within these frozen bands of tissue, in addition to the cellular damage that results from the trauma, fosters the formation of trigger points.

The activation of trigger points produces discomfort and pain in the musculature. Sensations of pain in the body invariably raise a person's stress level. This leads to heightened tension, which fosters the conditions that increase pain, and thus the cycle is perpetuated.

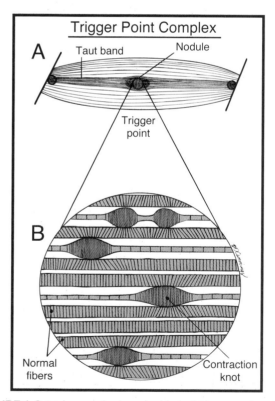

FIGURE 1-9 A trigger point is embedded within a taut band of muscle fibers. The contraction knots within the trigger point represent portions of a muscle fiber where the sarcomeres are fully contracted. (Reprinted with permission from Simons D, Travell J, Simons S. Myofascial pain and dysfunction: the trigger point manual. Vol. 1. Upper half of body. Philadelphia: Lippincott Williams & Wilkins, 1999:70.)

Treatment of Trigger Points

Neuromuscular therapy attempts to disrupt the stress-tension-pain cycle by locating trigger points and deactivating them. Manual pressure applied directly to the trigger point for 8 to 12 seconds disrupts the flow of nerve impulses activating the referred pain zone, thus diminishing the sensations of pain felt there.

Research conducted since Dr. Travell's findings were initially published has expanded our understanding about the physiology of trigger point activity.[6] It appears that muscular strain damage occurs at the neuromotor junction where **acetylcholine** is released, setting up a self-sustaining chain reaction that results in calcium flowing constantly within portions of muscle cells. This causes continual contraction of sets of **sarcomeres**, whereby **ATP** is used up and cannot be renewed. The presence of ATP is necessary to provide energy for all the cell's activities, including the return of calcium to its storage compartment, the sarcoplasmic reticulum, thus allowing the sarcomeres to resume a resting state.

Manual pressure on the trigger point provides the stimulus to pump ATP into the damaged cells and deactivate the positive-feedback loop between the acetylcholine and calcium. The flow of nerve impulses to the trigger point's referred pain zone thus ceases. Pressure on the trigger point may also instigate the release of **endorphins** and **enkephalin**, two of the body's natural pain fighters.

To prevent the trigger point from becoming reactivated, it is important to keep the muscle fibers around it lengthened. The therapist should stretch the affected muscle after treating it and instruct the client to continue to stretch that area on a regular basis.

The tissue breakdown that led to the formation of trigger points is not necessarily repaired by pressure point treatment. The goal of neuromuscular therapy is to reduce the active firing of trigger points to manage pain and stress levels in the body. This form of therapy works best when it is accompanied by other massage modalities that keep the muscles lengthened and relaxed, thus reducing the likelihood of future trigger point formation and activation.

■ SWEDISH MASSAGE

Swedish massage is classified as a circulatory style of massage. Its broad, sweeping strokes promote increased blood flow through muscle tissue, which facilitates metabolic efficiency. The Swedish style is also quite effective at inducing relaxation in the body by enhancing parasympathetic nervous system activity. It is often performed as a full-body massage, which helps to bring a sense of wholeness, continuity, and integration to the recipient.

Within the integrated deep tissue approach, Swedish techniques are used to warm up the tissues in preparation for deeper, more specific work. Swedish strokes are also incorporated to initiate the process of re-establishing the proper directions for the myofascial tissues to follow to eliminate stress-producing misalignment. The massage therapist can utilize these strokes almost like a sculptor, shaping and remolding the body into a better-organized configuration of muscle and bone.

Integrated deep tissue therapy is primarily a nonverbal form of communication with the body's nervous system and soft tissue components. It is designed to re-educate the **reflex arcs** to produce more effective movement patterns. The relaxing, pleasurable, lengthening sensations generated by Swedish massage strokes are the perfect vehicle for introducing sensations of ease and comfort.

■ CROSS FIBER

Cross fiber techniques are incorporated along with Swedish strokes to further relax the muscle groups and assist in the elimination of myofascial restrictions. The application of strokes perpendicular, rather than parallel, to the direction of muscle fibers is the distinguishing characteristic of all styles of cross fiber manipulation.

The cross fiber strokes used in the integrated deep tissue system are performed bilaterally. This means that they are applied across the muscle fibers in both directions, forward and backward, rather than in one direction only. The procedure consists of rolling bundles of muscle fibers over each other using either the fingers or the broad side of the thumb to release adhesions. Adhered muscle fibers diminish circulation of blood and lymph, and they inhibit the ability of the muscle to fully contract and lengthen.

■ CONNECTIVE TISSUE TECHNIQUES

Connective tissue manipulations are designed to stretch the fascial membranes that surround and penetrate the musculature. The fascial component of muscles is both strong and flexible and is responsible for providing support to all the body's structures. The degree of fascial mobility is an important factor in determining the shape of the body. As inhibiting factors in the fascia are released through slow stretching and low-force compressive movements, a renewed quality of expansiveness and freedom can be introduced to the body.

Many varieties of connective tissue release work have been formulated. The maneuvers presented here have been chosen for their effectiveness in spreading fascial membranes in conjunction with deep tissue therapy. Freeing the surrounding fascia is necessary to accommodate muscle lengthening that occurs from the release of contracted fibers brought about by the deep tissue strokes.

■ STRETCHING

Lengthening the soft tissues through stretching movements serves several important functions. The therapist stretches the recipient's muscles during a massage treatment for those muscles to better assimilate the neuromuscular changes that have occurred during the session, and the client stretching on his or her own after receiving a deep tissue therapy treatment is highly encouraged. Maintaining muscle length through stretching reduces the overall level of stress in the body and helps to eliminate many of the muscular imbalances that can result in pain and injury.

Massage is essentially a passive process for the recipient. During the session, the client's body is manipulated and moved, primarily by the therapist. For the changes brought about by deep tissue bodywork to become permanent, however, the client must activate the recalibrated reflex arcs achieved in the session through volitional movement based on the body's new alignment. Otherwise, the previous, aberrant muscle patterns will soon return, and progress toward greater body function will be halted.

■ ENERGY WORK

Techniques of energy balancing are based on the premise that the body is formed and nourished by patterns of energy currents that determine the state of health and vitality of the individual. When these energy pathways are flowing freely, all the body's systems are fortified, and continued growth and development are assured. Weakening or blockage of the energy currents eventually leads to breakdown within the body.

The two methods of energy balancing that are included in this course are polarity and shiatsu. Both are complete systems of bodywork and healthcare that require extensive specialized training to learn in their entirety. Practitioners of this integrated style of deep tissue therapy are not to be considered experts in either of these modalities unless they have acquired the education to meet the necessary requirements. A few techniques from both healing systems have been included here to enhance the effects of deep tissue therapy.

Polarity therapy likens the body's energy currents to the flow of magnetic forces, with positive and negative poles (Fig. 1-11). Balance between these two poles is mediated by a third, or neutral, pole. Blockage through any of these three poles weakens the natural flow of energy. This inhibition of energy flow manifests physically as myofascial restriction.[7] Most of the polarity procedures described in these lessons consist of contacts wherein the therapist places his or her two hands on the client's body at locations corresponding to this flow of energy to enhance the body's natural healing abilities.

Polarity procedures are applied at the beginning of the session to help induce relaxation and a state of readiness on the part of the client. The simple polarity holds described here are very effective at reducing sympathetic nervous system stimulation, allowing the client's body to assimilate the effects of the massage treatment more effectively. The sustained contact characteristic of the

FIGURE 1-11 Polarity energy currents.

opening polarity maneuvers, along with their innately nurturing quality, assists in building a bond of confidence and trust between the therapist and client.

Shiatsu is a Japanese style of bodywork that encourages the flow of the life energy, or **qi**, through a series of energy channels known as **meridians** (Fig. 1-12). It is administered through a combination of compressive strokes and stretching of the body along these pathways. The shiatsu procedures described in this course were chosen to bolster the effects of the accompanying deep tissue release work. By improving the flow of the vital life energies of the body, the release of soft tissue restrictions usually occurs more easily and is sustained for a longer period of time.

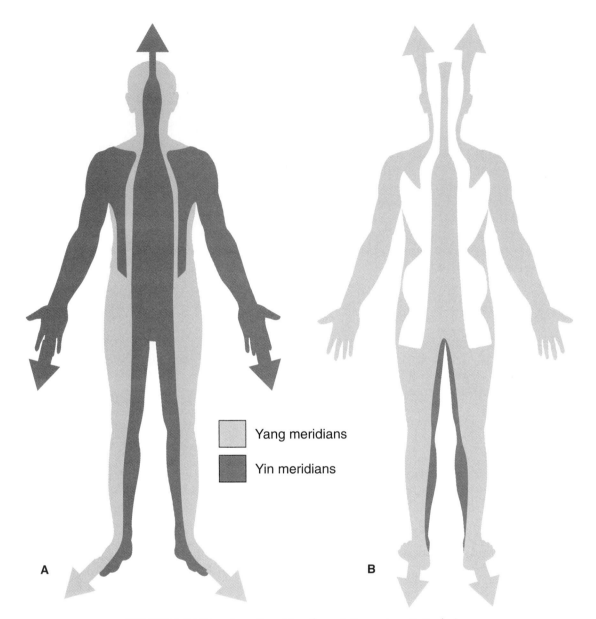

FIGURE 1-12 Direction of meridian flow. **A.** Front view. **B.** Back view.

Methods of bodywork exploring the combination of Eastern and Western modalities are becoming increasingly popular. The reader is referred to two books, *Informed Touch* by Finando and Finando[8] and *Acupuncture, Trigger Points and Musculoskeletal Pain* by Baldry,[9] for more information about this topic.

REFERENCES

1. Travis JW, Ryan RS. Wellness workbook. 3rd ed. Berkeley, CA: Ten Speed Press, 2004.
2. Travis JW, Ryan RS. Wellness workbook. 3rd ed. Berkeley, CA: Ten Speed Press, 2004: xxii.
3. Beinfield H, Korngold E. Between heaven and earth: a guide to Chinese medicine. New York, NY: Ballantine, 1992.
4. Travell JG, Simons DG. Myofascial pain and dysfunction: the trigger point manual. 2nd ed. Baltimore, MD: Lippincott Williams & Wilkins, 1999.
5. Travell JG, Simons DG. Myofascial pain and dysfunction: the trigger point manual. 2nd ed. Baltimore, MD: Lippincott Williams & Wilkins, 1999: 35.
6. Meyers T. Body Language N: an excursion through the alphabet in somatic terms. Massage Magazine September–October 2004, Issue 111: 134–140.
7. Stone R. The wireless anatomy of man and its function. In: Polarity therapy: the complete collected works. Sebastopol, CA: CRCS Publications, 1999: ZS1: charts 15 and 16.
8. Finando D, Finando L. Informed touch: a clinician's guide to the evaluation and treatment of myofascial disorders. Rochester, VT: Healing Arts Press, 1999.
9. Baldry PE. Acupuncture, trigger points and musculoskeletal pain. 2nd ed. London: Churchill Livingstone, 1993.

Learning the Work

The latter portion of this book consists of the integrated deep tissue therapy lessons. Each lesson contains information essential for learning and understanding this system of deep tissue therapy. This book is not to be considered a self-teaching guide. It is best used as a supplement to teaching by an experienced instructor who has mastered the system and can give the student the necessary guidance and feedback. While learning the work, the lessons should be read and practiced in the same order as they are presented in the book. The lessons have been organized to teach the student a logical, sequential approach to mastering the concepts of integrated deep tissue therapy.

The routines given in the lessons do not represent exact reproductions of specific bodywork sessions that would actually be performed on a client. Rather, they outline a general sequence of possible moves for an area of the body. Each routine describes techniques for releasing most of the muscles associated with that particular part of the body. Although the therapist needs to know all these techniques, he or she would not use every procedure described here on any one client.

The student will practice all the techniques in each lesson on a partner in class; this is done so that both students can learn the material effectively. There is no way to determine which techniques would be most beneficial for any individual without assessing that person according to his or her own particular needs.

Format of the Lessons

Each lesson is divided into two parts. The first portion presents information and assessment tools that provide the foundation for acquiring the skills of a deep tissue therapist. The second portion describes the techniques that are used in the integrated deep tissue system based on its six components.

The first part of each lesson is divided into the following sections.

■ GENERAL CONCEPTS

This section presents foundational information pertaining to the area of the body under discussion. It acquaints the student with the overall design of this body segment, and it describes the relationships between the muscles and bones.

■ MUSCULOSKELETAL ANATOMY AND FUNCTION

This portion of the lesson expands on the information mentioned in the General Concepts section. The material discussed here focuses on the anatomy and movement capabilities of the related muscles as they pertain to integrated deep tissue therapy.

■ CONDITIONS

These are common problems, diseases, indications, and contraindications that the deep tissue therapist may encounter. It is not an inclusive list; it is designed to point out highlights. The student is encouraged to do further research in this area as needed. (*Stedman's Medical*

Dictionary for the Health Professions and Nursing[1] is an excellent reference for medical conditions and terms.)

■ MIND/BODY CONNECTION

The holistic scope of the work is discussed in this section. Students are introduced to concepts involving the relationship between thoughts, beliefs, and emotions and the physical state.

■ POSTURAL EVALUATION

An outline for a full analysis of the body segments being studied is included in this section. Postural evaluation is one of the major assessment tools of the deep tissue therapist. It provides the necessary information to outline a plan of bodywork for an individual client. It also serves as a guide to assess changes in the client's body resulting from the application of integrated deep tissue therapy.

■ EXERCISES AND SELF-TREATMENT

Included in this section are exercises the client can do on his or her own that will stretch and strengthen the muscles that have been treated in the sessions. These exercises can be taught to clients so that they can be performed between massage sessions and will enhance the results of the deep tissue therapy.

■ QUICK REFERENCE BOXES/CHARTS

1. *Indications/Contraindications.* This box provides a brief synopsis of common reasons to perform massage treatments and conditions that could make receiving treatments inadvisable.
2. *Essential Anatomy.* This box lists the muscles, bones, and bony landmarks that will be referred to and/or worked on during the lesson.
3. *Conditions/Muscles Involved.* This chart outlines the most common muscles involved in certain postural deviations.
4. *Range of Motion.* Most of the possible movements for each major joint are listed, along with the muscles that perform those actions. Testing range of motion lets the therapist know if the client is restricted in normal movement and requires additional work on the muscles involved.

Lesson Sequence

The order of presentation for the integrated deep tissue lessons has been planned to maximize the learning process by giving the student a clear understanding about the organization of the body according to structure and function. The author is indebted to the pioneering work of Dr. Ida Rolf, who conceived a unique vision of the body's design and created a logical, effective plan to reorganize the soft tissues within the field of gravity.

Integrated deep tissue therapy is not considered to be a form of structural integration in the Rolfing tradition, in that it does not follow the progressive, 10-session series plan that is characteristic of that style of bodywork.[2] The overall layout of the lesson plans in this book does follow, in a very general way, the sequence of treatment that Rolf advocated. This sequence is suggested as an effective order in which to perform a series of deep tissue therapy sessions with a client over a period of time. It exemplifies the eighth guideline in *Principles of Conscious Bodywork* (see Chapter 3, page 24).

The sequence of the lessons is as follows.

■ THE TRUNK

- *Chest.* Opening the chest helps to establish better breathing habits. One of the first manifestations of inhibited feelings and bodily sensations is restricted breathing. Release of the breathing mechanism is crucial for the rest of the deep tissue work to be fully effective. The increased oxygen intake acquired by full, deep breathing is necessary to fuel the metabolic changes that are brought about by deep tissue therapy.
- *Spine and Back Muscles.* The spine supports the weight segments of the upper half of the body, and it must be aligned properly to perform this function properly. When the vertebrae are aligned, the nerves passing through the spinal column are unimpeded. Lengthening the spine helps to organize the soft tissues and bones of the trunk. Freeing the back muscles helps to further balance the chest area in the front of the trunk.

THE UPPER EXTREMITY

- *Scapula.* This is the root of the upper extremity. Many of the muscles that attach the arm to the body are anchored on the scapula. Freeing the scapula extends the range of motion of the arms and takes pressure off the rib cage.
- *Shoulder and Upper Arm.* Treatment proceeds progressively from the proximal portion of the arm to the distal portion. Release of the rotator cuff muscles and other shoulder muscles helps to reposition the arm and improve alignment of the upper body.
- *Forearm and Hand.* The muscles that control the hand are the smallest of the upper extremity. Re-establishing refined movement of the hand helps to strengthen its connection to the brain and contributes to the reduction of tension throughout the body.

THE LOWER LIMB

- *Foot, Leg, and Knee.* Reflexively, this body segment mirrors the hand and forearm. Massage work on both the feet and the hands helps to strengthen all the body's systems and contributes to an overall sense of well-being. The foot forms the foundation for vertical support of the entire body, and this area needs to be realigned to accommodate the shifts that have occurred by opening the upper body.

THE THIGH, ABDOMEN, AND PELVIS

Work on the thigh muscles accompanies release of the core muscles of the trunk. Many of the thigh muscles attach on the pelvis, and they greatly affect pelvic positioning and overall body alignment. The progression of the sequence on the lower extremity is upward, from the foot to the pelvis.

- *Posterior Thigh and Hip.* The posterior thigh muscles draw the base of the pelvis downward and flex the knees. They counterbalance the actions of the quadriceps muscles on the anterior thigh. The hip muscles control the movements of the femur and tend to accumulate tension.

The pelvis forms the body's center of gravity. Muscles that are attached to it tie the upper and lower portions of the body together. Increasing sensory awareness in the pelvic region facilitates well-coordinated, full-body movement.

The abdominal muscles provide support for the lower spine and assist in holding the viscera in place. The abdominal cavity is the seat of the **hara**, or vital life force. The body's ability to evolve to its full potential is greatly enhanced once the core has been freed.

- *Abdominal Muscles.* The abdominal muscles connect the chest to the pelvis and control the motions of the trunk. The rectus abdominus muscle assists the hamstrings of the posterior thigh in pulling the base of the pelvis anteriorly. The quadratus lumborum, which is the deepest abdominal muscle, forms the back wall of the abdominal cavity. It counterbalances the rectus abdominus by elevating the iliac crests and moving the base of the pelvis posteriorly.
- *Lateral Thigh, Adductors, and Intestines.* Balancing the lateral and medial thigh muscles helps to reduce lateral shifting of the pelvis and realigns the knee joint. The outer portion of the thigh is a reflex zone to the large intestine, so working on it during the same session with the intestinal region encourages better results.[3] The intestines are treated after the abdominal muscles have been relaxed.

  When the body is toxic as a result of sluggish elimination of intestinal waste, it adversely affects the ability of the muscles to metabolize the waste products that are squeezed out during deep tissue therapy. Proper function of the intestines aids in maintaining a more healthful internal environment in the body, which helps to sustain the chemical changes that are brought about by deep tissue therapy.
- *Anterior Thigh and Iliopsoas.* The abdominal muscles and thigh muscles should be released before work on the iliopsoas complex is attempted. Both the rectus femoris and psoas muscles tilt the iliac crests of the pelvis anteriorly, in opposition to the hamstrings and rectus abdominus, which tilt the iliac crests posteriorly. The psoas is the deepest core muscle. Its release can have profound effects on the entire body.

THE UPPER POLE—HEAD AND NECK

Work on the upper pole commences after balance of the pelvis has been achieved. The head and pelvis are the two weight segments that are positioned on either end of the spine, and they serve to counterbalance each other. The head and pelvis have a direct relationship to each other, both structurally and reflexively.

- *Neck and Head Extensors.* These muscles prevent the head from tipping forward. They are called into use often, and they tend to accumulate tension. It is difficult to maintain tension release in the rest of the body until the neck has been freed. It is recommended that some relaxation work on the neck area be done at the beginning of each massage session.
- *Neck and Head Flexors.* The front portion of the neck seldom gets addressed in standard massage sessions, but it is extremely important that it receive the same attention as the rest of the body. These muscles counterbalance the often-overused extensor muscles at the

back of the neck, and they are subject to damage from neck-related injuries.

- *Head, Face, and Jaw.* Release of the cranial, facial, and particularly, jaw muscles completes the balance of the upper pole and integrates the head to the neck. Relaxation of this area promotes increased parasympa-

thetic activity, reducing mental agitation and diminishing stress levels. The realignment of the head on the neck completes the process of total body re-education, allowing the client the opportunity to fully embrace the changes produced by the experience of integrated deep tissue bodywork.

Designing a Session

The lesson plans outline the full scope of the integrated deep tissue system, but they do not provide the step-by-step details of actual massage sessions. The plan for each bodywork treatment is constructed by the therapist with input from the client.

There are four parts to putting together an integrated massage session:

- The interview
- Client assessment
- The session
- Homework and follow-up

THE INTERVIEW

1. *Talk to the Client.* Before beginning to work on a client, a massage therapist needs to get to know the client somewhat. Find out why this person has come to receive bodywork. What are the expectations? Take a brief history of the client's previous experience with massage.
2. *Ask Questions.* Ask about previous injuries, surgeries, medical conditions, current medications, and so forth. Elicit as much information as possible about the client's state of health and any factors that will affect receiving massage.
3. *Talk About How the Client Is Feeling.* What is the client's emotional state? What factors are affecting it? Remember that people are not bringing just their bodies to the massage table—they are bringing their total selves. Factors affecting their well-being are important for the massage therapist to know.

   Feelings are a major component of how we experience ourselves through our bodies. The client's emotional state will play a part in the design of the sessions, and it may color the therapist's approach. For instance, if a person is expressing sadness, it may be determined that a nurturing style of touch would be more beneficial than a more forceful, penetrating approach.
4. *Establish Goals with the Client.* It is a good idea for the therapist to discuss what he or she would like to accomplish during the session, based on what the client has expressed. Then, the client has the opportunity to align with the goals, modify them, or add to them.

CLIENT ASSESSMENT

1. *Observe the Client.* The most important assessment tool the integrated deep tissue therapist uses is postural analysis. Through observing a client's posture and movement, it can be determined what the body's major tension patterns are and how to guide the client to more effective use of the body, reducing the likelihood of future problems and discomfort.

   Postural evaluation is used to monitor changes occurring during massage sessions. Take time to observe the client both before and after the session to assess the effects of the work. The body may respond differently than anticipated, and some modifications may need to be made.
2. *Use the Charts.* The range of motion and condition charts provided in the lessons should be used to assist in determining which muscles are contracted, based on the information gathered from the body reading. For example, if the client rolls his or her left shoulder forward, the therapist would check the range of motion chart for the shoulder joint and find which muscles medially rotate the shoulder. The client could also perform the same movements with his left and right arms to check if there is restriction in range of motion of both shoulder joints.
3. *Assess Other Factors.* Facial expressions, vocal tone, and gestures can all be indicators of a person's general state of being and can help in assessing the person's reaction to the bodywork, both while receiving it and afterward.

THE SESSION

There are two levels of organization within the integrated deep tissue therapy method presented in the lessons. The first level deals with the order of application for the six components of the integrated system within a massage session.

To open the body effectively, a suggested sequence of treatment is to:

1. *Open* the energy pathways to relax the body and prepare the soft tissues for the work that is to follow. The two techniques used to accomplish this are polarity and shiatsu.

2. *Warm up* the myofascia and enhance metabolic functioning by increasing blood flow through the body. Swedish and cross fiber techniques serve this purpose.

3. *Eliminate* restrictions within the fascial component of the soft tissues so that the muscles have room to lengthen. The connective tissue techniques are designed for this purpose.

4. *Relax* tension held in chronically shortened muscles. Deep tissue strokes achieve this result.

5. *Break up* cycles of pain generated by trigger point formation in the muscles. Neuromuscular therapy targets this phenomenon.

6. *Teach* the muscles and the mind to incorporate the newfound freedom that is created by the application of all these techniques. Stretching serves this purpose.

In a deep tissue session, this is a highly effective sequence to follow to achieve maximum results. After the initial sequence has been applied to an area, the techniques may be interwoven into the massage as dictated by the response of the client's tissues. This intermingling of the massage components gives a richer dynamic to the sessions, and it allows the therapist to tailor the approach to be maximally effective.

The second level of organization of the integrated deep tissue therapy method deals with the order in which the body is processed over a series of sessions. The recommended protocol is to process the body in the following sequence:

1. **The trunk**—chest and back
2. **The upper extremity**—shoulder, arm, and hand
3. **The lower limb**—foot, leg, and thigh
4. **The core**—abdomen and pelvis
5. **The upper pole**—neck and head

The above list refers to the order in which each body segment is emphasized over a progressive series of bodywork sessions. Following this sequence will assist in reorganizing the body effectively through reinforcing the counterbalancing relationships of the segments. The number of sessions required to bring satisfactory full-body integration varies. The therapist may choose to focus on any one segment for several sessions in a row—and may return to that area again in future sessions.

The deliberate omission of a detailed, nonflexible treatment plan is in recognition of the inherent organic nature of this style of bodywork. The therapist is encouraged to monitor the client's progress and work within his or her individual pattern of unfolding.

Although one specific body segment is emphasized in a single session, other areas of the body should also be addressed. The principle of working with counterbalancing relationships applies not only over a series of bodywork sessions but also within each individual session. This means that a degree of full-body balance and integration is sought with each treatment.

There are many ways that this can be accomplished. Some suggestions for achieving balance within each deep tissue session are:

- Follow the suggestions listed in the lessons under the category Accessory Work. They present useful ideas for creating complete bodywork sessions.
- Include some work on the neck and the feet in each session to more fully facilitate the experience of release and integration throughout the body.
- The suggested order in which to process the body over a series of treatments can also be applied within an individual session. In other words, in a 60- or 90-minute time span, the therapist may progress through the five segments of the body, selecting the appropriate type of work and amount of time to spend on each.

■ HOMEWORK AND FOLLOW-UP

After the massage session, the therapist may choose to show the client some exercises and self-care treatments he or she can do to further facilitate the release that took place in the session. The exercises described in the lessons were chosen specifically for this purpose. It is helpful to first demonstrate the exercise for clients and then watch them perform it, offering guidance on proper form and execution.

Always encourage clients to take the time to relax and reflect on their feelings and sensations after receiving bodywork. Strongly urge clients to allow time to rest after a deep tissue therapy session, because it takes time for all the changes brought about by massage to occur. A period of rest helps the body greatly during this period of assimilation. Suggesting that the client write about the experience in a personal journal can also enhance the effects of the massage by providing a means for the client to acknowledge consciously any internal differences that he or she feels as a result of the deep tissue work.

The therapist should let the client know that he or she is available if any questions or concerns arise in the days following the massage. The therapist may also want to call the client a few days after the session to check up on him or her and to allow discussion of the reactions to the work. Setting some mutually agreed-on, long-term goals for the time the client will receive therapy also is a useful endeavor.

REFERENCES

1. Stedman's medical dictionary for the health professions and nursing, illustrated 5th edition. Baltimore, MD: Lippincott Williams & Wilkins, 2005.
2. Rolf IP. Rolfing: the integration of human structures. New York, NY: Harper and Row, 1997.
3. Sills F. The polarity process: energy as a healing art. Berkeley, CA: North Atlantic Books, 2002: 122, Figure 6.16.

Guidelines for the Deep Tissue Therapist

Ethics

Massage therapy is becoming increasingly recognized by the medical community and by the population at large as a viable adjunct to standard stress reduction and rehabilitative programs. As allied healthcare practitioners, massage therapists need to maintain a strict code of professional standards. At times in the past, and even in the present, the intention of legitimate massage therapy has been called into question by certain lawmakers. Adherence to accepted rules of conduct and protocol will help to assure that massage therapists are afforded the proper respect this profession deserves.

Ethics are rules of behavior that define the parameters of effective interactions between people. All professions that deal with human relationships should have a formulated set of guidelines that clearly delineate the intentions and limitations of practice applying to that vocation. The intimate nature of touch therapies demands explicit descriptions of the type of service provided to assure protection for both the healthcare provider and the client.

The American Massage Therapy Association has created a code of ethics applicable to all massage professionals. It can be found in the Appendix. A few topics from the code are of special importance to beginning massage therapists, however, and are discussed below.

■ PROFESSIONALISM

A consummate professional projects an image of impeccable appearance and demeanor. Massage therapists should wear clothing that is neat, clean, and appropriate to their activities. Although some therapists prefer a medical-type look, for most of us a simple short-sleeved shirt and comfortable pants are adequate. Gym clothes or other exercise attire is generally not recommended.

Consistency is an extremely important quality to maintain. Timeliness is a vital aspect of this trait. The therapist should be fully prepared for each client a few minutes before the scheduled appointment time. The massage table should be fitted with clean sheets and set at an appropriate height, and any notes pertaining to the client should be readily available.

The time planned for a session should be closely adhered to, meaning that an appointment should begin and end on time. It is not a professional trait to give some clients extra time while perhaps short-changing others. A massage therapist must be reliable and accountable. Treating every client with the same consideration is imperative to maintaining a respected practice.

Fees for all services should be clearly stated and strictly followed. While it is certainly the option of each therapist to make individual payment arrangements in special situations, maintaining consistent pricing for all clients generally avoids disagreements and misunderstandings.

■ INTEGRITY

A massage therapist should always operate from a position of personal and professional integrity. Resolute professionalism fosters an environment of safety and trust that allows clients to be fully receptive to the benefits of massage therapy. Establishing clear boundaries greatly enhances the value of the therapeutic relationship and protects both client and therapist from inappropriate interactions.

Adherence to the following guidelines will help therapists to maintain proper boundaries in their practice:

- Always provide adequate draping for the client. Check with each client regarding the level of undress he or she is comfortable with, and maintain that level at all times.
- During a session, always respect a client's request to change the manner in which a technique is being applied or to stop work all together if the client so desires.
- Maintain a strictly professional relationship with clients. Do not date or socialize with clients.
- Do not discuss a client's sessions or private information with other people.
- Respect each other's time. Do not call clients at home unnecessarily. Do not encourage clients to call you at home or to spend excessive time at your office.

■ HONESTY

The primary role of the massage therapist is as an educator and facilitator for the body's natural healing processes. Massage therapy can be beneficial in treating many ailments and injuries, but it is not a cure-all. A clear understanding of the capabilities and limitations of massage therapy as a rehabilitative tool is integral to a healthy and productive relationship between the therapist and client. The therapist must be truthful with clients by expressing realistic outcomes of the therapy and the anticipated amount of time that will be required to achieve those goals.

Massage therapists also need to be diligent about staying within the scope of their education and ability when working with clients. When it becomes apparent that a client requires treatment that the therapist is not trained to perform, the therapist is obligated to recommend other sources for that treatment. Do not be afraid to refer clients to other qualified practitioners. Clients generally have much more respect for and loyalty to therapists who are honest about the limits of their skill.

■ EDUCATION

Massage therapy is a profession that affords the opportunity for continual learning and expansion. One could spend a lifetime studying and still not exhaust all the possibilities for growth in this field. It is the massage therapist's obligation to stay informed of advancements in the profession. This can be accomplished by reading massage periodicals and by participating in continuing education classes offered by massage training schools.

Many excellent resources on establishing ethical standards are available.[1,2] It is a good idea to discuss ethics questions with other professionals to learn more about the types of issues you may encounter. A massage therapist guides clients in establishing healthy behaviors not only by the massage techniques performed on the table but also by the example of their personal conduct.

Incorporating the Mind/Body Aspect of Integrated Deep Tissue Therapy

■ THE NATURE OF TENSION

One of massage therapy's primary values is its effectiveness at relieving tension in the body. Tension manifests physically as chronically contracted muscles, and it contributes to many problems, including pain, irritability, and diminished function. The manifestations of tension are often what prompt a person to seek massage therapy.

The mechanical techniques of massage therapy confront tension directly, through lengthening and relaxing contracted muscle fibers with a combination of pressure and movement. These results can be short-lived, however, because when the client is again confronted with stress-producing experiences, the tension and its ensuing problems often return. It may be necessary to explore the nature and sources of tension more fully with clients so that they are capable of neutralizing its effects when it invades the body.

Tension itself is a form of resistance. It is the body's attempt to defend itself against a perceived threat. Mild short-term tension, which accompanies low-level stress reactions, can be a useful response. The increased muscular tone and heightened activity of the sympathetic nervous system that accompany mild stress can actually improve a person's ability to respond to a threatening situation. For example, the tension we feel when driving in traffic, although not necessarily making us feel very good, does tend to improve our reflexes and mobilize our senses, letting us react to potentially dangerous events more quickly and effectively. Stress becomes a problem when it is overbearing and unyielding. Exposure to long-term stressful conditions produces chronic tension.

■ EMOTIONS AND TENSION

Psychological sources of stress can be as devastating as physical ones. Very often, people are unaware that the condition of their mind forges a direct link to their body. When worry, fear, anger, and other highly charged emotional states are unrelenting, they can have a devastating effect on the body through their tension-producing nature. As long as these emotional irritants are present, the body cannot maintain an environment of relaxation.

To complicate matters, areas of chronic physical tension lodged in the body may have been triggered by emotional stimuli that occurred years before. If a perceived threat is strong enough or has a sustained duration, or both, it can create an area of muscular tension that becomes locked in the body and is no longer responsive to a conscious directive by the mind to release. This type of unrelenting muscular tension was labeled armoring (Fig. 3-1) by psychologist Wilhem Reich.[3,4] Armoring refers to the protective nature of the muscle block. The block manifests to prevent the person from experiencing an unwanted or unacceptable feeling. There are many

FIGURE 3-1 The effects of armoring. Constricting bands of muscle tension reduce the capacity to feel and inhibit physiological functioning.

sources for these blocks, but the result is always the same—an area of deadened feeling caused by muscular restriction.

Deep tissue therapy offers an effective means to uncover places of frozen tension in the body. We all contain an invisible matrix of memories and emotions that hold our muscles in distorted positions. In some cases, these distortions may be necessary, because they allowed us to survive life experiences that would otherwise have been overwhelming to our fragile psyche. Much armoring occurs in childhood, before a person has acquired the necessary inner mechanisms that allow humans to effectively absorb or counter an intense emotional barrage.

As muscular tension softens during deep tissue therapy sessions, the underlying feelings sometimes resurface. In some instances, the client may choose to explore these feelings and their source. If this is the case, the therapist should recommend that the client talk to a qualified psychological counselor.

■ WORKING WITH EMOTIONAL RELEASE

Muscles that have become tense are painful. The lack of movement within the tense muscle belly prevents fresh blood, which is loaded with oxygen and nutrients, from reaching cells that are starving. Waste products that irritate nerve endings and dull the responsiveness of muscle fibers are trapped within the muscle, creating a swamp-like stagnation.

Over time, the uncomfortable feelings generated by the contracted muscles are repressed by the conscious mind, leaving only a vague blanket of numbness over the area. Any underlying feelings that may have triggered the initial tension are buried within deadened muscle tissue. The physical and emotional pain has not gone away. It is merely held suspended within steadily degenerating tissues, and it is still acting on the person at an unconscious level. Many people lack vitality or feel trapped in unproductive patterns of behavior because of the pervasive influence of these tension patterns.

As the muscle tissues are freed from their chronic gripping and the associated feelings surface, the client may experience a loosening of blocked emotions along with the muscular release. Depending on the source of the original inhibition, an emotional outpouring can manifest in a number of ways, including crying, laughing, a feeling of great relief, or even insight regarding the nature of the physical-emotional blockage. Muscular and emotional release are similar in many ways. Both represent a yielding of a restrictive pattern involving the mind, musculature, and nervous system.

Signs of Emotional Release

The signs of an impending emotional release are many and varied. Therapists need to be aware of them so that they will know how to act appropriately should an emotional outpouring take place.

- One of the first indications that inner feelings are surfacing is a change in the client's breathing pattern. He or she may begin to hold the breath, or he or she may take deeper or more rapid breaths.
- Blood flow to the skin may change. The client may become more flushed, or the skin may become more pale.
- The therapist may feel a change in the temperature level on the surface of the client's body.
- The degree of tension in the musculature, particularly in the jaw, chest, and abdomen, may suddenly increase.
- The client may begin to fidget or become unusually subdued.
- If the client's eyes are closed, the therapist can look for rapid movement under the eyelids.
- The client may suddenly open his or her eyes and begin to look around or stare off into space.
- The therapist should make note of changes in the level of communication offered by the client. A person who has been talkative and becomes uncharacteristically quiet, or one who was quiet and unexpectedly begins to converse, may be experiencing the surfacing of feelings.

There are many other signals of a possible emotional outpouring. Therapists should be attentive and note any changes in a client's demeanor that might indicate strong feelings are rising.

Handling Emotional Release

What is the proper course of action on the therapist's part if a client should experience an emotional release? First, the therapist needs to check with the client to make sure his or her needs are being met. Every massage office should be equipped with tissues, extra blankets, and water in case the client requires them. Beyond making sure that the client feels safe and comfortable, the therapist does not need to do anything except to be present and nonjudgmental.

It is not the therapist's responsibility to facilitate the client's feelings. The therapist should not try to push the client to express his or her feelings, nor should the therapist discourage an honest outpouring of emotion if it should spontaneously occur. It is important that the therapist stay calm and centered while the client is experiencing emotional release. Any attempt by the therapist to actively suppress emotional expression by the client can heighten the feelings of shame and embarrassment that many people experience when revealing withheld feelings.

The deep tissue therapist should deal with an emotional release in very much the same manner as he or she deals with a muscular release. The therapist should acknowledge the opening, give the client space to fully experience and absorb it, and be available to offer any assistance or support that may be required. It often is not necessary to verbally discuss the nature of the release or the reasons behind the emotions, unless the client wishes to do so. Most of the time, providing a compassionate and nurturing presence is all that the client requires from the therapist to process these feelings.

There is a component of fear accompanying much emotional release. Feelings are often suppressed because a person fears to express them, for whatever reason. That fear will resurface as the client lets go of the restricted emotions. With reassurance and support from the therapist, most clients feel a great relief once the feelings are expressed, as if a huge burden has been lifted off the person. If the client requires additional guidance in assimilating the feelings uncovered in the deep tissue session, the therapist may suggest that he or she seek the services of a professional counselor or psychologist.

Principles of Conscious Bodywork

The following principles provide guidelines for the most beneficial application of deep tissue therapy. They encapsulate many of the concepts discussed in this book, and they serve as important reminders to the deep tissue therapist in the endeavor to maintain the highest standard of excellence when performing integrated deep tissue therapy. The therapist should commit these principles to memory and strive to embody them in his or her deep tissue work.

1. **Respect the Client.** When a client chooses to receive bodywork, that person is entrusting his or her body to the therapist and also expressing vulnerability to the therapist. Your responsibility is to honor and care for that person to the best of your ability. Every opportunity given to you to work on someone in this manner should be viewed as a privilege. Honor your clients for their desire to grow and for allowing you to grow with them. Each individual is unique and precious. The gift that conscious bodywork offers is the reminder that we are all unfolding into our own perfection.

2. **Be Attentive.** The therapist needs to stay present and focused to be attuned to the process of opening that is

CASE STUDY 1 Emotional Release Work

 The subject is a 28-year-old man named Brian who works as a medical technician. He received a series of massage sessions several years ago and enjoyed them. He now wants to experience massage therapy again, because he is feeling out of touch with his body and thinks that receiving bodywork will help to bring him more physical awareness. Another reason he would like to achieve greater physical presence is that Brian has been experiencing problems with low self-esteem. He contends that a lack of assertiveness is causing problems at work and with his relationships. As a result, he feels weak and ineffective. As well as beginning massage therapy sessions, Brian has bought a health club membership and started a weight-training program to build himself up as part of his program to increase self-confidence.

Physically, there is a lack of symmetry between Brian's upper and lower body. His torso is rather well developed, with good muscular definition in the chest and arms. The abdominal region appears to be overly contracted. The lower ribs are drawn inward toward the midline, creating compression in the solar plexus region. This restriction is partially the result of tightness in the rectus abdominus.

Viewing Brian from the side, his back appears to be overly straight. Shortness in the abdominal wall has caused the pelvis to be drawn into a posterior tilt, causing a reduction in the lordotic curve. There is a band of tension wrapping around the midsection. The cervical curve is also reduced, and Brian's jaw is slightly retracted. The sternocleidomastoid muscles are clearly visible, with both tendons being prominent at the base of the anterior neck. His lower body lacks the definition of his upper body. His hips are broad, and the quadriceps muscles lack tone. His ankles are thick, and both feet are turned out. The piriformis and hamstring muscles appear to be contracted.

One of the initial goals in working with this client is to help him feel more supported by his legs and feet. He seems to control his body from the waist up, creating areas of tension in the torso and neck. When he walks, he throws each leg forward rather than swinging the thigh freely from the hip. Each step lands flat, on the entire plantar surface of the foot, rather than rolling smoothly from heel to toe to cushion the impact. In addition to receiving deep tissue therapy, Brian is encouraged to perform exercise activities in which he must use his legs and feet actively and with awareness. Tai chi classes and walking daily are recommended.

The plan for the first session was to begin the process of balancing the musculature of the legs. The initial contact was a polarity head hold followed by Swedish massage on the neck, with deep tissue strokes along the lamina groove in the cervical region. Next, the feet were addressed. Some time will be spent on the feet in each session to increase their mobility so that they become more active during walking actions. Freeing restrictions in the feet will also enhance Brian's feeling of being grounded and help build awareness through the lower body.

After the work on the feet was completed, focus was shifted to the tibialis anterior and peroneal muscles. These muscles were quite tense, contributing to a lack of fluidity throughout the feet. Next, the quadriceps muscles were massaged. This sequence was then repeated on the left leg.

As the quadriceps were reached on the left side, the client began to complain of an uneasy feeling in his abdomen, almost a feeling of light spasm. With Brian's permission, the therapist moved to the abdominal area to explore the feelings being generated there. The therapist lightly placed his right hand on Brian's abdomen while his left hand cradled the back of Brian's head. Brian was encouraged to breathe deeply into his abdomen, trying to push up the therapist's hand by expanding his abdomen as he inhaled and allowing the therapist's hand to sink toward his spine as he exhaled.

After a few rounds of deep breathing, Brian's breathing rhythm became choppy, especially on exhalation. He began to complain of tightness rising into his upper chest. The therapist asked him if he wished to continue to investigate these sensations. Brian responded that he would, so the therapist removed his left hand from behind Brian's head and placed it on the upper chest, just below the clavicles. Brian took a few breaths and began to clench his jaw. His neck and face were becoming flushed. The therapist asked if Brian was aware that he had begun to grit his teeth. Brian said no, he had not realized it and was only aware that it was a little difficult to take a deep breath, but he wanted to continue. The therapist asked him to open his mouth slightly and allow his lower jaw to drop. Brian did so, and at that point, he began to cry. The therapist removed his hand from Brian's chest, reached for a tissue, put the tissue in Brian's hand, and asked if Brian wanted to describe what he was experiencing. Brian said he wasn't sure what was happening but felt comfortable staying with the feelings. He closed his eyes and continued to breathe slowly and deeply. The therapist's right hand remained on his abdomen while the left hand lightly touched his shoulder in a reassuring manner. Soon, his body started shaking as waves of movement began to ripple through his trunk and legs. The crying became deeper.

After several minutes, the movement in his body calmed, and the crying subsided. Brian lay there for a while continuing to breathe rhythmically but more slowly. The therapist gradually removed his hands from Brian's abdomen and shoulder and asked him how he felt. Brian began to smile and said he could sense a buzzing, tingling sensation across his forehead and in his hands. He then related that his breathing felt much easier and that the tension in his abdomen was totally gone. He was very aware of the sensations in his body as he lay on the table. He said it felt as if a tight, heavy belt had been removed from around his waist, allowing him to sense his legs and feet much more fully. The therapist asked Brian if he would like to try to sit up on the table, and Brian answered that he would. The therapist helped lift him to a sitting position, with his legs hanging off the side of the table, and then brought him a glass of water, which Brian slowly sipped. When the therapist was sure that Brian was all right, he left the room to allow Brian to get dressed.

Upon entering the room again, the therapist encouraged Brian to walk around a little and relate what he was experiencing. Brian said his legs felt much freer and easy to move, and he could sense himself land lightly on each foot as he took a step. When he walked, he was also more aware of the movement of his arms coordinated with the swinging of his legs. He said he felt as if a huge amount of bottled-up tension had been released during this session. Brian is now looking forward to continuing to become better acquainted with his body through deep tissue therapy.

Topics for Discussion

1. How would you describe to a client the possibility that emotional release can occur as part of a deep tissue therapy session?
2. What are possible reasons why some therapists may never have clients who experience emotional release during a massage session?
3. Explain appropriate actions you should—and should not—take with a client who is experiencing emotional release.
4. Describe some potential situations in which it might be necessary to refer a client to a psychological counselor.
5. What would you say in a follow-up conversation or phone call to a client who has experienced an emotional release?

occurring within the session. Communication takes place continually between the therapist and client. This interchange happens in many ways. As much as possible, the therapist needs to be able to track the client's experience of the work through touch, observation, and communication. Through the hands, the therapist receives messages about the response of the client's tissues to the work being done. It is crucial that these messages be interpreted correctly for the therapist to make the appropriate choices about how to interact effectively with the client's body. The client will also be much more open to change if he or she feels that the therapist is attentive and responsive.

3. **Move Slowly**. Within a massage session, many different dynamics may be experienced in terms of pressure, speed, and flow. When working to change the state of the myofascial structures, the pace must be slow if it is to be effective. Connective tissue, deep tissue, neuromuscular, and stretching techniques are all performed at a slow rate. Time is required for the tissues to respond to the stimulus being applied. When deep

pressure is administered quickly, there is not adequate time to respond to the client's reaction to the force, so appropriate adjustments cannot be made. This is how injuries occur. If the therapist is moving slowly, however, there is enough time to ease up on pressure or to remove the hands from delicate tissues before damage results. A slow pace is also more conducive to the quality of self-awareness that fosters transformational growth by the client.

The massage experience establishes a relationship between the therapist and client whereby the client is often led into the same frame of mind as the therapist. Messages are received through the therapist's touch, quality of breathing, and inner attitude. A slow, fluid quality will transfer more of a feeling of integration and deep relaxation to the massage recipient. This encourages the state of healing that people seek from deep tissue massage.

4. **Never Force the Tissues**. There is an old saying that a blossom will open on its own when it is ready. Any attempt to pry the flower open from its bud will only ruin

the flower. The same is true with the body. An effective massage therapist learns how to interact with the soft tissues in such a way that they are encouraged to give up their holding patterns willingly. When the body is opening up freely, the therapist experiences a melting sensation under the fingers as they sink into the tissues, as if the hands were a boat being carried along by moving waters.

When resistance is encountered, the best tactic is to wait patiently for the internal conflict to be resolved before moving further. Pushing against resistant tissues sets up a tug-of-war situation between the therapist and recipient. In this kind of struggle, both the therapist and the recipient lose. The therapist may plow through the blockage with assertive force and may even succeed in creating an opening, but all the effort and pain produced during the attempt has probably lodged somewhere else in the client's body. Resistance in the muscles is a natural defense against invasion. It is the body's way of protecting itself against what it perceives as an intrusion, whether physical or emotional. Matching force with force is never very fruitful if the goal is to bring someone around to your point of view. Kindness, patience, and understanding are much more effective means to melt resistance.

5. **Work on "The Edge."** This guideline is closely related to the previous one. Working on "The Edge" describes an approach to soft tissue manipulation that creates the most productive environment for change to occur. Working in this realm means that the therapist has found the pace, pressure, and rhythm that provide the ideal stimulus for the client's tissues to release tension patterns and move into dynamic equilibrium. In other words, transformation is happening. When the qualities of pace, pressure, and rhythm are not in cadence with the client's tissues, the massage is not being very productive, and the results will be disappointing. Using the dynamic of pressure as an example, the client will not feel the muscles and fascia lengthening if the force of the stroke is too light and, consequently, will not feel tension melting in the tissues. If the pressure is too deep, however, the sensations of pain become overwhelming and block any other stimulus to the nervous system, inhibiting the positive benefits of the work. When the pressure is just right, the client's experience is that the body is becoming freer, and he or she is able to experience the pleasure of profound release.

6. **Move the Body Toward Greater Ease**. Massage should be an educational process. Through the medium of touch, the therapist is teaching the client what the body could feel like if it were in a better balance. When the mind and nervous system are presented with easy, pleasurable movement, they will tend to embrace and incorporate it, if given the opportunity. During any bodywork session, the therapist is monitoring the state of tension in the client's muscles and, through stroking and positioning of the body, is creating the greatest degree of comfort. Often, changing the position or angle of a body part on the table will relax the muscles around it and increase the effectiveness of any techniques applied to those muscles. Pads and bolsters can be used to change the alignment of the body on the table for more effective muscle release. Teaching the body proper positioning creates efficient pathways of movement for the muscles and fascia to follow as they start to move back to their natural positions.

7. **Elongate Shortened Tissues, and Strengthen Stretched Tissues**. Most deep tissue massage techniques are designed to bring balance to the body by lengthening shortened muscle fibers and the fascial sheaths that surround them. Muscles act in pairs. When a muscle contracts, its opposing muscle is stretched. If the muscle stays contracted, the antagonistic muscle will remain in an overly lengthened position, which usually has the effect of weakening it. Therefore, once the shortened muscles have been released, the stretched muscles should be strengthened with specifically targeted exercises.

Muscles need to be free to contract and lengthen at the slightest instigation for the body to maintain its ability to respond and adapt to stimulus. To bring harmony to muscular relationships, the massage therapist evaluates where tissues are shortened through observation and palpation and then elongates them through a combination of compression and stretching techniques. When the shortened muscles regain their proper length, the pull on the opposing muscles is reduced, and these muscles also return to a resting state. This allows the reflex arcs to once again do their jobs, and the body's full capacity for adjustment returns.

8. **Seek to Re-establish Balance**. As stated above, muscles operate in counterbalancing relationships. The body as a whole operates in the same way as well. When part of the body shifts in one direction, the rest of the body makes compensating adjustments to maintain some sort of functional integrity. Anyone who has tried to balance a stack of blocks knows that when one block is moved out of position, the whole stack has to be readjusted to prevent the blocks from falling into a pile. In organizing the body efficiently, the bodyworker is conscious of the body's counterbalancing nature and works accordingly. This means that massage sessions are structured so that the body's oppositional relationships are taken into account. When focusing on the top of the body, also do some work to align the bottom half of the body with it. Juxtapose work on the back of the body with work on the front. Integrate the right side of the body with the left side. Balance the deep, inner muscles with the more surface muscles, and so forth. Approaching the body in this manner within each session will give longer-lasting and much more profound results.

9. **Release Blockages so the Energy Can Flow.** An open body is analogous to a flowing river. The water in a river is constantly moving, finding its way along the path of the riverbed. The surface of the water may at times appear to be still, yet underneath, deep currents are always flowing. The river exhibits a quality of fluidity and ever-changing dynamics amidst a backdrop of timeless constancy. When the body is unified in harmonious balance, it exhibits the same ease of flow and adaptability as a rushing river. There is an ease of movement within an aura of tranquillity that appears to be almost liquid in nature. The tissues seem to ripple with a sense of aliveness.

   When the body is viewed with this image in mind, blocks to the flow of the life force become readily apparent. The breath may appear uneven or shallow, and muscles seem knotted in stiffness and immobility. The body structure is out of alignment. A feeling of strain emanates from it. The massage therapist develops an awareness of the areas of blockage, and he or she seeks to remove them in much the same way one would remove a log that is damming the flow of water in a stream.

10. **Approach the Body from the Perspective of Wholeness.** The words *heal* and *whole* are derived from the same root.[5] Therefore, *to heal* means *to make whole*. The ultimate goal of integrated bodywork is to help guide a person to a state of completeness, or wholeness. The body is the vehicle used for this healing to take place.

   In the process of learning various massage techniques, we break down the body into parts to be labeled and analyzed. The student learns how atoms make up molecules, which combine to create cells, which build all the physiologic systems. Muscles are delineated in the same manner. Bundles of muscle tissues are given special names and are described as performing specific actions. When massaging the body, the therapist may also compartmentalize his or her work by addressing individual systems with techniques designed to facilitate their specific functioning. However, a person is not just the sum of all these systems. We do not experience ourselves internally as a conglomeration of parts with strange Latin names. A human being is a locus of consciousness that transcends all the individual facets. It is this expansive quality that allows us to go beyond our limitations and fulfill our capabilities. Conscious bodywork offers the potential to tap into this experience of finding and expressing our unique qualities and individual natures.

REFERENCES

1. Benjamin B., Sohnen-Moe C. The ethics of touch. Tuscon, AZ: SMA, Inc., 2003.
2. McIntosh N. The educated heart: professional guidelines for massage therapists, bodyworkers and movement teachers. Memphis, TN: Decatur Bainbridge Press, 1999.
3. Lowen A. Bioenergetics. New York, NY: Penguin, 1993
4. Lowen A. The language of the body. New York, NY: MacMillan, 1971.
5. Neufeldt V, ed. Webster's new world dictionary of American english. 3rd college edition. New York, NY: Simon & Schuster. 1994:621.

The Lessons

Integrated Deep Tissue Therapy System Techniques

The integrated deep tissue therapy system, while incorporating many facets of stress-reducing relaxation styles of massage, embraces a broader vision of high-level wellness. It teaches a precise methodology for normalizing the muscular system, thereby reducing unbalanced pulls on the skeleton that lead to the loss of structural integrity and, eventually, physical breakdown. Circulation of fluids is improved, resulting in better metabolic functioning. Pain-producing elements within the myofascial tissues may be eliminated, diminishing excessive activity of the sympathetic nervous system, which is characteristic of high-stress states.

An important byproduct of a relaxed, stress-free body is a calm and powerful mind. Excessive firing of nerves brought about by the strain of holding muscles in distorted positions disturbs mental equilibrium and stimulates random mental chatter in the brain, which leads to unclear and unproductive thought patterns. As the body is brought into a state of dynamic equilibrium and poise through the deep tissue therapy techniques, the nervous system is able to return to its optimal, efficient state of low-level firing. This reduces the production of static within the central nervous system that creates disturbance in the mind.

Three Levels of Assessment Used in Deep Tissue Therapy

The systematic approach to processing the soft tissues presented here requires three levels of client assessment. Utilizing these assessment procedures with each client provides a plan of action and an ongoing means of evaluating progress. Modification of the plan may be made at any time to adapt to the client's rate of assimilation of the deep tissue therapy.

■ LEVEL ONE: DETERMINING PATTERNS OF MUSCULAR COMPENSATION

The first level of assessment that the deep tissue therapist must master is the ability to recognize the unique patterns of muscular compensation brought about by distortions in the myofascial system of each client. The characteristics of an individual's posture and movement are largely determined by the limitations imposed by restricted soft tissues. After the therapist has evaluated these patterns, he or she must determine which ones are most detrimental (i.e., causing pain, producing wear and tear on joints,

straining ligaments and muscle tissue, or leading to fascial build-up and bracing).

Deep tissue therapy sessions are built around minimizing these dysfunctional patterns of distortion. Because every person's muscular relationships are unique and ever-changing, no two deep tissue therapy sessions are exactly the same. Each treatment is designed to neutralize the counterproductive soft tissue patterns that are generating problems.

■ LEVEL TWO: CREATING A PLAN OF ACTION

The second level of assessment involves the ability to envision the body's progression to a balanced state over time by organizing a logical, effective plan of treatment. It takes time and patience to undo the effects of years of trauma and lack of education regarding proper movement. The therapist's job is to guide the client to the capability of pain-free, unrestricted movement through a combination of progressive deep tissue therapy treatments and supplemental stretching and strengthening exercises.

In Chapter 2, an effective protocol for efficiently reorganizing the body was introduced. To summarize, the spinal unit and upper extremity are approached first, followed by the lower extremity. Work on the lower extremity begins with the feet, because they form the structural foundation of the vertical body. The deep tissue therapy sessions then progress upward to the body's core, which consists of the abdominal cavity and pelvis. The pelvis, being the lower pole of the spinal column, is the body's movement and instinct control center.

After the core is freed up, work progresses to the upper pole of the spine—the neck and head region—which is the intellectual control center. Structural integrity between the two poles needs to be re-established for whole-body dynamic alignment to be realized fully. This sequence of learning and applying deep tissue therapy provides students with practical knowledge of how the natural counterbalancing relationships in the body manifest.

■ LEVEL THREE: CORRECTING MYOFASCIAL DISTORTIONS

The third level of assessment involves evaluating the state of the muscular system through observation and palpation. It takes place primarily while the therapist is working on the client's body. The deep tissue therapy techniques are designed to manipulate and stretch myofascial tissue. Just as an assortment of specialized tools are used by a mechanic to perform specific tasks, a variety of deep tissue strokes are incorporated by the therapist to address the full range of muscular qualities and conditions.

Part of the skill of mastering deep tissue therapy is acquiring the ability to recognize the manifestations of myofascial aberrations and the knowledge of proper application of the appropriate techniques to correct them. Remember that the primary goal of deep tissue therapy is to re-establish the proper balance of muscular forces around the skeleton. This is accomplished by lengthening chronically contracted muscles and treating other restrictive conditions, like scar tissue and trigger points, that are inhibiting the function of muscle fibers.

To release contracted muscles, slow compressive strokes are applied along their length, from origin to insertion, covering the tendons and muscle bellies. Shorter, focused strokes are then used to treat smaller sections of the muscle that may be aberrant. These strokes may be applied parallel to or across the muscle fibers, depending on the nature of the restriction. They are also used on the tendinous attachments to the bones to aid in minimizing scar tissue formation and to stimulate the Golgi tendon organs to send messages through the nervous system to direct the muscle to lengthen and relax.

Layers of Muscle Involvement

The muscular system is worked in layers, from superficial to deep. The deep tissue therapist must have a thorough knowledge of muscle anatomy to distinguish the various layers of muscles that are being affected. None of the layers should be neglected in a deep tissue treatment. Each has unique characteristics and tends to store different manifestations of tension (Fig. 4-1).

The superficial layer of muscle is the level that is most affected by the environment. It, along with the skin and adipose tissue, forms a barrier between the external world and the internal body. Invasions from the environment are often trapped in the superficial layer of muscle. These invasive elements include exposure to extreme temperatures and trauma resulting from accidents or falls. Tension tends to migrate from the surface of the body to the deeper levels. If the deeper layers of muscle are overemphasized in a deep tissue therapy treatment, the origin of many tension patterns in the surface muscles may be easily overlooked.

The deeper layers of muscle, which are often called on for maintaining postural positions, store stress patterns that result from trauma, faulty habits of movement, and psychological conditioning. The ropy, knotted fibers that are characteristic of tense muscles, along with trigger points, usually manifest at this level. Releasing these muscular conditions while reorganizing the superficial layer of muscle brings longer-lasting results. Imbalances between the layers of soft tissue distort the body with tension-producing compensations. By freeing all the soft tissue layers, the body becomes functionally integrated throughout.

Using the Lesson Material

Incorporating all three levels of assessment allows the therapist to perceive the continuum of myofascial influences acting on the client's body. In assessing a client and planning a course of action for treatment, the therapist moves from level 1 to level 3. The information presented here, in the lessons and the deep tissue routines, provides the necessary foundation to plan and execute a series of sessions effectively. Chapter 2 described how the lessons and routines are organized and provided an overview of the information they contain. The therapist's job is to adapt each routine to fit the specific requirements of the client based on the three levels of assessment.

FIGURE 4-1 Tension generally seeps through the body from the surface to the core. Tension patterns in the superficial layers are more spread out along the myofascial planes, whereas deeper tension congeals into ropy bands of fibers and knots.

TABLE 4–1	Timing a Deep Tissue Session	
Sequence	60-Minute Format	90-Minute Format
Opening	3 minutes	3 minutes
Warm-up	5 minutes	7 minutes
Connective tissue release	5 minutes	5 minutes
Deep tissue and neuromuscular therapy	38 minutes	65 minutes
Stretch	2 minutes	2 minutes
Accessory work	5 minutes	6 minutes
Closing	2 minutes	2 minutes

To determine the client's patterns of muscular tension and compensation, the therapist makes use of the postural evaluation outline along with the charts for range of motion and conditions. The sequence of the routines presented in this book provides an effective map for planning a course of treatment. It is a good idea to discuss with the client the approximate number of sessions that will be required to bring his or her body to a state of better functioning so that a level of commitment to deep tissue therapy is agreed to at the beginning. Most people experience a significant improvement in their state of health and well-being within 5 to 10 sessions.

A deep tissue therapy session is generally scheduled in a 60- or 90-minute format, depending on the preference of the therapist and the needs of the client. The session is structured as follows:

- Opening: polarity and shiatsu
- Warm-up: Swedish and cross fiber techniques
- Connective tissue release
- Deep tissue and neuromuscular therapy
- Stretch
- Accessory work
- Closing: foot reflexology move or polarity

Table 4-1 provides an approximation of the amount of time spent on each section.

This timeline is very flexible. It is only meant as a general guideline to help the therapist use the session time efficiently. The large block of time given to deep tissue and neuromuscular therapy allows the therapist to intersperse techniques from the other sections as needed. In addition to the time given to work on the massage table, the therapist must factor in the time spent with the client both before and after the session, which could add up to an additional 30 minutes to the appointment time.

Each routine contains instructions for deep tissue release on all the muscles in that particular body region. It is not necessary to perform deep tissue therapy on all the muscles listed in a routine. Contracted muscles are chosen for focus based on the therapist's observation of the client's unique patterns of distortion. The client's history of traumas and reported areas of pain are also taken into account when deciding which muscles should be targeted for deep tissue release and neuromuscular therapy treatment.

The illustrations accompanying the descriptions of the strokes demonstrate the full technique performed on a willing recipient. In this way, the student can see the completed stroke. Therapists must also take into account the client's level of comfort in receiving massage. For some clients, draping may need to be adjusted so that less of the body is exposed, and some strokes may need to be stopped before the therapist reaches the muscle attachment, particularly in the pelvic region. The therapist and client should discuss these issues before the massage so that the client can be assured his or her boundaries will be respected.

Postural and Movement Muscles

Understanding the characteristics of skeletal muscles helps the therapist to anticipate the types of problems that are likely to be encountered in specific muscles. Skeletal muscle serves two important functions: movement and support. The skeletal muscles move the human structure through space. They exhibit an extraordinary dynamic range, capable of producing large bursts of motion that propel the body against the force of gravity or controlling tiny, subtle movements that allow the fingertips to trace the contours of a single strand of hair. The skeletal muscles also support the position of the bones in relation to each other against the force of gravity to maintain postural integrity.

To carry out these functions, two distinct types of skeletal muscle have evolved. The muscles that are mostly responsible for movement are called **phasic**, whereas the support, or postural, muscles are known as **tonic**. As the roles of the muscles become defined, their biochemical properties diverge. A muscle's role as phasic or tonic is not strictly determined at birth; it can change depending on the types of movement activities in which a person engages.[1] For instance, a long-distance runner will not have exactly the same distribution of movement and postural muscles as a computer operator has, because they use their muscles in vastly different ways.

CHARACTERISTICS OF POSTURAL MUSCLES

- Postural, or tonic, muscles support the body against the force of gravity. They are referred to as the workhorse muscles, because they have to be able to perform for long periods, sustaining a semicontracted state (Table 4-2).
- These muscles are made up of a large percentage of slow-twitch red fibers, which have a plentiful blood supply, so they do not produce a large amount of fatiguing waste products.
- These muscles maintain a high level of endurance, because their fibers do not contract in unison but, rather, segmentally. The motor units in the fibers fire irregularly, like blinking holiday lights. As one section of the muscle contracts, other portions of it relax. (Think of long-distance runners passing the baton to each other at intervals to distribute the workload among several athletes.) Because the fibers contract in relay fashion, these muscles do not tire easily and, therefore, can offer long-term support to the body. Not enough fibers contract at one time to produce movement of the bones, but they are able to maintain a continuously toned state that braces the structure against the force of gravity.
- Tonic muscles are slow to respond to a reflex stimulus. They cannot contract and relax quickly, like phasic muscles can.
- The movement capabilities of these muscles are limited, as is their ability to sustain heavy loads.

- These muscles tend to cramp easily if called on to move quickly or exhibit great strength.
- When a person's posture is distorted, the postural muscles have to work very hard to brace misaligned joints and tend to become hypertonic.
- This permanent, highly contracted state of muscles fosters the formation of trigger points.
- The body also produces additional connective tissue in these muscles to bolster their bracing capability. The overabundance of connective tissue confines the muscle in its contracted state, preventing it from being able to lengthen. Thus, the body becomes congealed into a distorted shape. Because of the unyielding nature of built-up connective tissue, the person cannot willfully move the body into the proper position. Slow, focused stretching exercises must be performed by this person on a regular basis to release bonding within the fascial tissues. In addition, the person must receive connective tissue release work to release the muscles from their confinement and return the body to its natural, lengthened state.

CHARACTERISTICS OF MOVEMENT MUSCLES

- The movement, or phasic, muscles are responsible for moving the body through space.
- These muscles are made up predominantly of fast-twitch red fibers, which contract and release rapidly in response to stimulus. The movement muscles are linked to the body's many reflex arcs. They can move the body quickly to adapt to unanticipated events, like stepping off an unseen curb.
- The fast-twitch fibers have a relatively low blood supply available to them, causing these fibers to fatigue quickly and produce large amounts of lactic acid that are not flushed out of the muscles quickly. Although the movement muscles have more short-term strength than the postural muscles, they tire much faster and need more recovery time.

TABLE 4–2	Major Postural Muscles
Adductor longus	Pectoralis major
Adductor magnus	Piriformis
Erector spinae muscles	Quadratus lumborum
Gastrocnemius	Rectus femoris
Hamstrings	Soleus
Iliopsoas	Sternocleidomastoid
Levator scapulae	Upper trapezius

- In a person with muscular imbalance, movement muscles tend to weaken in response to postural muscles shortening. Because the deep tissue compressive manipulations are designed to lengthen contracted muscles, the postural muscles are often the focus of deep tissue sessions. As postural muscles are released, allowing the musculoskeletal relationships to become more integrated, the movement muscles naturally become stronger. If particular movement muscles remain weak even after treatment, additional strengthening exercises may be recommended to improve their function.
- Because the phasic muscles often have to make quick

adjustments, their fibers are prone to microtearing. This tearing often occurs at the musculotendinous junction. The constant pull of the muscles against the attached bones can lead to inflammation of the tendon, known as tendinitis.
- Like the postural muscles, movement muscles can also become hypertonic. Repetitive use of certain muscle groups for a specific activity, such as hammering nails, can lead to chronic contraction of those muscles. The quick changes in length that are sometimes required of movement muscles to stabilize the body's equilibrium can lead to spasms and permanently contracted states.

Palpation

Palpation is the art of sensing or feeling changes in the tissues. It is incorporated with the massage strokes to generate an instantaneous feedback loop. In other words, to gauge the effect of a stroke, a massage therapist is sensitive to the reaction of the client's tissues, as perceived through the therapist's hands, while various techniques are performed. If necessary, the therapist can make adjustments to the stroke in terms of pace, pressure, or intention to yield the desired outcome, which is the resolution of aberrations in the myofascia.

The hands are extremely sensitive instruments for performing massage—particularly the fingertips, because they contain a high percentage of nerve receptors. These nerve receptors are capable of perceiving temperature differences, textural qualities and variations, degrees of hardness or softness, moisture, degrees of depth, and minute movements. The ability to register all these characteristics allows the therapist to tune into the client's tissues at a very subtle level.

Skill in palpation is developed through practice. Over time, the brain develops the capacity to absorb more and more input from the nerve receptors, increasing the capacity of the therapist to distinguish and assimilate all the signals coming through the hands. Although the fingers and palms contain a higher number of nerve receptors compared with other parts of the body used to perform massage strokes, palpatory proficiency can also be acquired with the elbow, knuckles, and forearm through regular, concentrated practice. Chaitow et al.[2] provide a large selection of palpatory exercises.

Accurate palpatory assessment requires the ability to visualize clearly the soft tissues that are being targeted. Therefore, a thorough knowledge of anatomy is necessary to train the hands to move through the layers of the body both accurately and safely. The therapist must be able to palpate the condition of the skin and the underlying layers of adipose and fascia. Sensing the qualities of the skin can yield much information about the underlying tissues.

An abnormally warm area on the skin may indicate inflammation in the soft tissues beneath it, and skin that feels tight and cannot slide easily over the underlying tissues may indicate binding in the superficial fascial membranes.

To palpate the muscles accurately, the therapist needs to be familiar with their shape, the directions of their fibers, and their points of attachment on the bones (Fig. 4-2). The therapist must also be able to distinguish the differences

FIGURE 4-2 Examples of common shapes and organizational patterns of skeletal muscles. (Reprinted with permission from Premkumar K. The massage connection: anatomy and physiology. 2nd edition. Baltimore, MD: Lippincott Williams & Wilkins, 2004: 187.)

between normal and abnormal muscle tissue. A normal muscle that is free of tension and restrictions has a springy, resilient quality. It yields to pressure, and it maintains even tone. Healthy muscles have a translucent quality when palpated, meaning that other tissues can easily be felt through them. They do not feel painful to the touch, even when deep pressure is applied.

Abnormal muscle tissue embodies the effects of strain and imbalance. Unhealthy muscles can be weak and flaccid, or they can be dense and tough. Their fibers are more pronounced than those of healthy muscles. They may feel stringy or ropy and crunch when rolled across. Highly contracted muscles feel thick and hard. They are not resilient when pressed; rather, they are resistive. Muscles that are under tension, being held in a stretched position, can feel like taut cable wires. Unhealthy muscle tissue usually feels painful to the touch, but it can also feel numb or deadened, particularly if the abnormal condition is long-standing. With experience, the various states of muscle health can be palpated accurately, and appropriate techniques can be applied to counteract the effects of strain and improper usage.

Knowledge of the shape and function of the skeleton is equally as important as the ability to visualize muscles when palpating the body. All muscles are anchored to bones, which the muscles pull on to move them. Much of the damage done to muscles through trauma and stress occurs at their attachments to the bones. Tracing the contours of the bones is an extremely important aspect of deep tissue therapy. Repairing damage at the tendinoperiosteal junction helps to reduce much of the pain experienced as a result of pulled muscles.

Guidelines for Performing the Modalities

■ ENERGY WORK

Polarity and shiatsu moves are used at the beginning of each deep tissue therapy session to prepare the client for the massage work that is to follow. The initial contact between client and therapist establishes the quality of their interaction. It allows the client time to relax and become accustomed to the therapist's touch. The therapist uses this time to establish rapport with the client and build an environment of trust and safety.

The goal of energetic styles of bodywork is to allow the body to open up so that energy can flow more effectively. Whether one wishes to think of energy as life force or merely as conscious awareness of the body's internal activities, the opening moves establish a bond between the therapist and client that enhances the level of receptivity in both parties.

Polarity

The polarity contacts introduce each deep tissue session. Polarity techniques are described at the beginning of each routine for the part of the body being emphasized in that lesson. The polarity touch is very soft and is usually administered with full, open hands. The therapist should place the hands on the client's body slowly and lightly. The therapist's palms and fingers touch the surface of the body with only enough pressure to make contact with the client's skin. The therapist's hands should have the quality of hovering on the surface of the client's body. A useful image is to imagine placing your hand on a leaf floating on the surface of a pond. Use only enough pressure to feel the leaf against your palm without submerging it in the water.

Dr. Randolph Stone, the developer of polarity therapy, used terminology from magnetism when describing the direction of energy flow through the body. The direction of outwardly flowing energy was described as the positive pole. The inwardly flowing direction was called the negative pole. Described in bodily terms, the upper portion of the body is the positive pole, whereas the lower portion is the negative pole. The right side and front of the body are considered positive, and the left side and back are considered negative. To enhance the flow of energy between the therapist and client, opposite poles should be connected whenever possible, just like connecting batteries in an electronic device (Fig. 4-3). In other words, the therapist's right hand (positive pole) makes contact with the negative pole of the client's body, while the therapist's left hand (negative pole) makes contact with the client's positive pole. Directions for appropriate placement of the therapist's hands are given in the description of each polarity move in the lessons.

After the therapist establishes contact with the client's body, the polarity move is generally held for 1 to 2 minutes. During this time, the therapist sits or stands upright in a relaxed, receptive stance, and his or her pattern of breathing should be even and calm. There should be no strain on the body or distractions in the mind so that the therapist may be fully sensitive to the sensations in his or her hands. Feelings of warmth or mild vibration in the therapist's palms and fingers while contacting the client's body are common sensations, as is heightened attunement to the rhythms of the client's various pulses. The

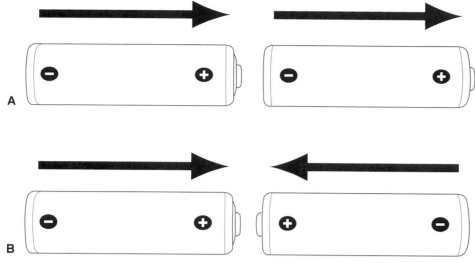

FIGURE 4-3 A. Aligning a negative pole to a positive pole allows a continuous flow of current. **B.** Aligning two like poles to each other blocks current flow.

therapist may also become aware of subtle shifts and movements in the client's body. These movements emanate from the fascial layers of the body. Clients often report becoming deeply relaxed and more in tune with the feelings in their body as a result of the focused contact.

No analysis of the sensations is necessary for treatment to be effective. The therapist's focus is on being receptive to all the input that is being received from the client's body to become more in tune with the client. Receptivity and compassion are the qualities the therapist should cultivate while administering polarity therapy. To release the polarity hold, the therapist very slowly removes his or her hands from the client's body while maintaining focus on the client's comfort and welfare. It is helpful to time the release of the hands to the client's inhalation, as if the client is gently pushing the therapist's hands off the surface of the body as it expands to take in a breath.

Shiatsu

The shiatsu moves are performed after the polarity hold is released. A few easy-to-perform techniques have been chosen from the vast repertoire of shiatsu procedures. As explained in Chapter 1, the goal of shiatsu is to enhance the flow of qi, or life force, through a complex series of channels, or meridians, that run through the body. This is accomplished by applying a series of compressive moves that trace the course of the channels. Whereas some shiatsu techniques move very specifically along the path of a meridian, the techniques chosen for this course are more general, usually covering several channels at a time.

Many of the shiatsu moves incorporated in the lessons involve compression moves done with the hands along the

length of a limb, moving proximal to distal. To begin the sequence, the therapist faces the client's body and holds the limb with both hands. The thumbs are placed on the lateral side of the limb, the palms cover the center of the limb, and the fingers wrap around the medial side. A combination of compression, squeezing, and slight medial rolling of the limb is used in coordination with both therapist and client exhalations. The stroke begins by pressing the thumbs into the lateral side of the limb. The stroke is continued by pressing down on the top of the limb with the palms. As the thumbs maintain contact, the therapist adds a squeezing action with the fingers to embrace the limb fully with the hands. The stroke is completed by rolling the limb slightly medial while maintaining the pressure on it with the hands.

Effective shiatsu incorporates the therapist's whole body, not just the hands. The weight and motion of the body into the stroke, not the contraction of arm or hand muscles, supply the necessary compressive force. The correct body motion for the move described above begins with the stance (Fig. 4-4). The therapist's feet are placed a little wider than hip-distance apart and separated from each other lengthwise by the distance of a comfortable walking stride. Both knees are slightly flexed, with awareness focused on the pelvis as the initiator of movement. At the beginning of the stroke, about 70% of the body's weight is on the back foot. As the stroke continues, the weight is shifted forward, timed with the pace of the stroke and with exhalation. At the completion of the stroke, about 70% of the therapist's weight is on the front foot. The spine stays long, and the shoulders, arms, and hands remain relaxed throughout the entire stroke. The therapist slides the hands a little further down the limb, shifts his or her weight back to the back foot, and begins the compression sequence again. The therapist continues in this manner to the wrist or ankle.

FIGURE 4-4 Proper body position for the application of shiatsu strokes.

■ SWEDISH MASSAGE

The Swedish strokes are introduced immediately following the polarity and shiatsu maneuvers. Although Swedish massage is only mentioned in the routines after the energy techniques, it may be incorporated throughout the session at the therapist's discretion. The strokes should be applied with a sense of fluidity and continuity to promote a quality of integration throughout the soft tissues. More than any other technique, Swedish massage generates a sense of unity in the body, and its use enhances the benefits of every other modality.

Swedish massage contains a huge repertoire of strokes. The three basic Swedish techniques—effleurage, pétrissage, and friction—are utilized in the integrated deep tissue therapy system to warm up the tissues, enhance fluid circulation, and create a unifying bridge between the other modalities used in this therapeutic approach.

Effleurage strokes are smooth, gliding strokes that are executed over the surface of the skin. One or both hands may be used, depending on the particular pattern of the stroke. Effleurage is used to warm up the tissues, soothe the nervous system, and relax tense muscles. Various degrees of pressure may be applied depending on the purpose of the stroke and the preference of the client. Lubricant is utilized to prevent friction or the therapist's hands sticking to the client's skin. Although the palmar surfaces of the hands are the most commonly employed tools,

other parts of the hand or arm may be used as well, including the knuckles, thumbs, and forearms.

Basic effleurage patterns should move from bone to bone whenever possible to stroke the entire length of the muscles. Effleurage strokes are used to delineate muscular arrangements to the client's nervous system, promoting relaxation-inducing sensations of length. An effleurage stroke that is stopped before it reaches a muscle's bony attachment tends to generate feelings of shortness and tightness that are counterproductive to the goal of massage.

The following are descriptions of effleurage-style strokes used in this course that may not be familiar to all readers:

- *Shingles* is an effleurage variation in which one hand replaces the other by gliding under it every 2 or 3 inches throughout the length of the stroke (Fig. 4-5). It creates a pattern reminiscent of overlapping roof shingles.
- *Swimming* is a forearm variation of effleurage that is commonly performed on the back or thighs. The therapist places both forearms parallel to each other on the midback or midthigh (Fig. 4-6). The therapist simultaneously shifts his or her weight forward and slides and rolls the forearms apart, allowing them to glide over the skin until they are shoulder-width apart. At that point, the therapist draws the arms back together, without losing contact with the skin, to begin the stroke again. The motion is somewhat similar to the arm movement used by swimmers in the breaststroke.
- *Thumb gliding* is an effleurage stroke incorporating the full lengths of the thumbs. The thumbs alternately glide over the skin in an overlapping pattern similar to the path of windshield wipers (Fig. 4-7). This stroke is commonly used on smaller body parts, such as the palm of the hand, the plantar surface of the foot, and around the knee.
- *Draining* is a two-handed effleurage stroke that is performed on either the arm or the leg, moving from the distal to the proximal end. Both hands are wrapped around the extremity at either the ankle or the wrist, with the fingers embracing the sides of the extremity while the thumbs cross each other over the midsection (Fig. 4-8). The webbing between the thumb and index fingers of both hands makes full contact with the central, rounded contour of the limb. Light pressure is maintained as the hands glide up the limb toward the proximal end. Upon reaching the proximal end, the hands separate and slide down the medial and lateral sides of the limb to begin the stroke again. Contact with the skin is never broken.

Swedish pétrissage strokes are used to further relax muscles and pump fluids through them with grasping, squeezing motions of the hands. One- or two-handed variations are commonly employed. Knuckle kneading is

FIGURE 4-5 Shingles stroke.

FIGURE 4-7 Thumb gliding stroke.

a form of pétrissage that uses the knuckle side of an extended-finger fist position. The knuckles are rolled back and forth over a small section of the body at a comfortable pace and pressure.

Friction strokes are used to relax contracted muscle fibers and realign scar tissue. The therapist presses into the client's tissues, pinning the skin directly under the fingers or palm to the underlying muscle and fascia. The skin and muscle are then moved as one unit to separate

adhered muscle fibers. The pressure is firm so that the skin does not glide independently over the muscle tissue, which can cause irritation. Friction strokes are performed in circular motions or in back-and-forth, cross fiber patterns.

FIGURE 4-6 Swimming stroke.

FIGURE 4-8 Draining stroke (shown on the forearm).

■ CROSS FIBER

Cross fiber techniques form a bridge between circulatory styles of massage therapy and deep tissue therapy. They are utilized to release adhesions in bundles of muscle fibers, which reduce fluid flow through the muscle and hold it in a contracted state. The two primary strokes incorporated in the integrated deep tissue system are fingertip raking and a rolling technique using the full length of the thumb. These techniques are based on strokes developed by Therese Pfrimmer,[3] one of the originators of cross fiber style therapy. Both strokes require a generous application of lubricant to provide a smooth, back-and-forth, gliding motion across the muscle fibers.

Fingertip raking is executed with a hand position formed from a cupped palm and curved fingers that are spread slightly apart. The fingertip pads roll across the muscle at a 90° angle to the direction the fibers are running in a continuous, back-and-forward motion that progresses along the full length of the muscle between its two attachments (Fig. 4-9).

The rolling stroke uses the broad side of the thumb all the way from its tip to the thenar eminence on the palm. To execute the stroke, the entire palmar surface of the hand is placed on the body with the thumb straight and comfortably extended from the hand in its natural position, an approximately 60° angle (Fig. 4-10). The length of the thumb lies parallel to the direction the muscle fibers are running. As the hand glides back and forth across the muscle, the thumb rolls over the muscle fibers. This causes the bundles of fibers to slide against each other,

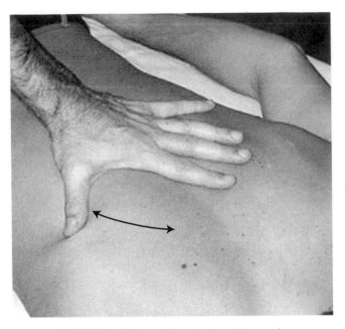

FIGURE 4-10 Cross fiber thumb rolling stroke.

spreading them and releasing fascial restrictions that may be keeping them bunched together. A helpful image in performing the stroke properly is a rolling pin being rolled back and forth across a ball of dough, flattening it out.

Both cross fiber strokes are performed at a moderate pace. The therapist should be able to cover the entire length of an average-sized muscle in five or six back-and-forth strokes. Because they roll across muscle fibers, cross fiber strokes allow the therapist to feel the condition of the fibers more effectively than strokes that run parallel to the fibers. Stringy or ropy fibers are signs of adhesion and should be focused on for several consecutive strokes.

Cross fiber strokes should not be performed over the same section of muscle for more than five or six passes in a row, or they can lead to irritation of the skin. If the fibers still feel dry and stringy after several passes, the therapist should move on, perhaps returning to that section of fibers later to recheck it.

■ CONNECTIVE TISSUE

The goal of working on the body's fascia is twofold—to make the ground substance more fluid, and to release the collagen bonds that are causing muscles to adhere. The techniques that are used to spread fascial membranes often incorporate slow stretching and pulling actions.

Steady, sustained stretching of fascial membranes helps to free restricting links that form within the collagen mesh. The key to successful fascial release is the ability to

FIGURE 4-9 Cross fiber fingertip raking stroke.

FIGURE 4-11 Fascial lift and roll technique.

sense the limit of the tissue's ability to stretch and then hold the stretch until a yielding or lengthening sensation is felt. The tissues should never be forced with more pressure or stretch than they can comfortably accommodate.

Connective Tissue Strokes

1. *Fascial Lift and Roll Technique.* This is a skin and muscle rolling technique designed to release adhered areas in the superficial fascia. Both hands are used. The thumbs are placed end to end on one side of the tissue to be rolled, and the fingers are positioned on the other side. The tissues are lifted and pressed toward the fingers with the thumbs. They are then rolled between the fingers and thumbs (Fig. 4-11). If the skin can be lifted easily off the underlying tissues, it may be rolled independently. Otherwise, the skin, adipose, superficial fascia, and muscle tissue may all be lifted and rolled. Always move slowly and deliberately. Adhered areas may feel quite painful. Begin the rolling action on a section of tissue that is relatively easy to lift, and gradually move toward the more resistive areas. Never force the tissues.

2. *Myofascial Spreading.* This stroke may be executed using fingers, knuckles, or the base of the palms. A very small amount of lubricant may be used. The therapist's hands should be able to pull the client's skin without slipping over it. Press into the midline of the section of tissue to be released until slight resistance is felt. Allow the hands to draw apart evenly until the client's tissue will not stretch any further. Hold at that point until the resistance yields and your hands can slide further apart (Fig. 4-12). This stroke is designed to release binding in the fascial membranes.

3. *Myofascial Mobilization.* The fingers, knuckles, palm, or forearm may be used for this stroke. The myofascial tissues are rolled against the underlying muscles and bones with a back and forth or a circular movement (Fig. 4-13). This technique is used to free myofascial tissue that is adhering to itself. It re-establishes the ability of tissues to slide freely over each other.

David Rini

FIGURE 4-12 Myofascial spread.

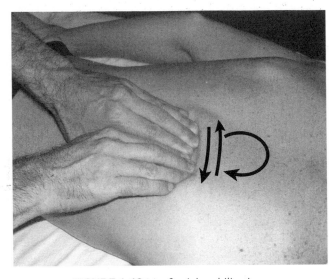

FIGURE 4-13 Myofascial mobilization.

■ DEEP TISSUE

The term *deep tissue therapy* has many connotations. It may be interpreted as the application of deep pressure to muscles or as therapy to the deeper-lying muscle groups in the body. Perhaps the most encompassing description of deep tissue therapy is that it is therapy that has a *deep* impact on the client. At its core, deep tissue therapy is transformative in nature. It has the capability to transform the dysfunctional characteristics of the body's soft tissues to minimize pain and stress as well as to enhance function on many levels. To accomplish these goals, deeper pressure on the tissues may be required at times. However, the pressure of strokes should never feel uncomfortably painful or at all intrusive to the client.

Pain is subjective. There is no constant, measurable amount of pressure to which every person will have the same response. The experience of touch as painful or pleasurable depends on many factors, including the degree of tension in the tissues, possible injurious conditions in the muscles, and the person's interpretation of the quality and intent of the touch. To be able to relax and willingly accept deeper gradations of pressure, the client must be assured that the therapist is mindful of the effects of his or her touch on the client's body. The therapist must be capable of making the necessary adjustments to prevent his or her touch from becoming painful, harmful, or intrusive. The organic, ever-changing nature of the interaction between the therapist and client during a deep tissue session requires constant vigilance to ensure that the therapy remains productive.

Application of Deep Tissue Therapy Strokes

After the warm-up phase of the session is completed, the deep tissue strokes are implemented. The lessons provide descriptions of the application of the strokes to specific muscles. They do not give details about the pace, depth, or number of repetitions of each stroke, because as stated above, those factors are variable, depending on the receptivity of the client's tissues and the client's attitude toward the work. Palpatory assessment and on-going verbal communication with the client are necessary to determine the precise quality of the deep tissue techniques. The approach to deep tissue therapy will be different with every individual, and even the same client will require varying degrees of pressure on different muscle groups, depending on their condition.

The overall goal of the deep tissue strokes is to relax contracted muscles. This is accomplished by the application of slow, compressive force into the muscles, accompanied by gradual movement of the stroke along the length of the muscle. This compressive force slowly lengthens the fibers in the muscle belly, similar to sustained stretching of a muscle.

Deep tissue strokes that are designed to lengthen shortened muscles are performed parallel to the muscle fibers. In this book, they are referred to as elongation strokes. They must be performed very slowly; otherwise, the stroke will activate the stretch reflex, causing the muscle to contract even more and defeating the purpose of the deep tissue therapy.

When an elongation stroke is being performed at the appropriate pace, the tissues feel as if they are yielding, or melting, under the therapist's touch. If resistance is encountered while stroking along the muscle, the therapist should stop at that point and hold the stroke steady until the resistance melts. The therapist may need to lessen the degree of pressure being used to achieve the requisite softening of the muscle tissue before continuing the stroke.

Muscle Layers

Muscles are released in progression from the surface to the deeper layers. The therapist must be thoroughly familiar with the musculature and able to picture the muscles' shapes and positions in relation to each other so that he or she knows when a particular muscle is being reached. Deeper muscles cannot be palpated directly. Their fibers are felt *through* the layers of muscle above them. If the surface muscles are contracted and tense, their fibers are not pliable enough for the therapist to feel through them to the deeper layers. Therefore, the surface layers must be released before the deeper layers are accessible.

As the therapist applies pressure, he or she sinks into the tissues only to the level of mild to moderate resistance. The feeling of resistance is a result of the muscle's contracting to defend itself against potentially harmful pressure. Deep tissue strokes may be applied with more force than connective tissue strokes, but never to the point at which the client has to tighten the muscles against the pressure. As soon as the soft tissues contract to defend themselves, tension is reintroduced into the body, and deep tissue therapy starts to become counterproductive.

Client Response

The client will sometimes experience sensations of pain during the work. Unhealthy conditions in muscle tissue are usually painful when touched. These include trigger points, scar tissue, bands of taut fibers, and spasms. When these conditions are encountered, the therapist should explain to the client the cause of the painful reaction. An element of fear associated with painful sensations, and educating the client about the nature of the painful response often calms the feelings of apprehension, lessening the subjective sensation of pain. The therapist always works with the client's input to ensure that the threshold of uncomfortable pain sensations is not crossed.

Signs of muscle relaxation are varied. As a muscle releases, it feels like it is able to spread more easily and has a softer tone when pressure is applied to it. Contracted fibers may fibrillate, or visibly jump, as they are relaxing. Sometimes, a pulsation runs through the entire length of the muscle. Stringy, taut fibers become less pronounced as fluid circulation is enhanced.

Knots, or lumps, within a muscle belly are indications of deeply contracted fibers with accumulated waste products caused by fatigue, overuse, or trauma. These areas are usually painful to the touch, and they respond well to static compression maintained within the client's tolerance level for up to 30 seconds. Tiny lumps within the fibers that feel like crystals, or grains of sand, may be the result of waste product build-up or indications of scar tissue formation. They can also be found in tendinous fibers near the tendon's insertion on the bone. These small knots are usually tender when pressed, and they respond well to small, precise cross fiber strokes directly over them.

Evaluation of the Work

During the deep tissue session, the therapist should periodically pause to assess the progress of the work. These pauses also allow the client to relax and assimilate the experience more fully. Softly palpating the muscles worked with the palms of the hands enables the therapist to assess the degree of relaxation that has been produced. The therapist may choose to ask the client for feedback about his or her feelings or reactions in response to the work done thus far. To enhance the assimilation process, a polarity contact may be administered to an area of the body after deep tissue therapy is completed.

Assessment of change may include range of motion stretches that use the muscles just released to evaluate the degree of lengthening and relaxation that has occurred. Additional effleurage strokes performed from the muscles' origins to their insertions reinforce the nervous system's reprogramming of the muscles' resting lengths.

■ DEEP TISSUE STROKES

On Muscle Bellies

1. *Elongating/Lengthening.* This stroke is a slow, gliding, compressive movement that is performed parallel to the muscle fibers, from origin to insertion (Fig. 4-14). The fingers, knuckles, base of the palm, thumbs, elbow, or forearm may be used. It is the primary technique used to return a contracted muscle to its resting length.
2. *Spreading.* These techniques are used to palpate aberrations in small sections of muscle fibers. They are in-

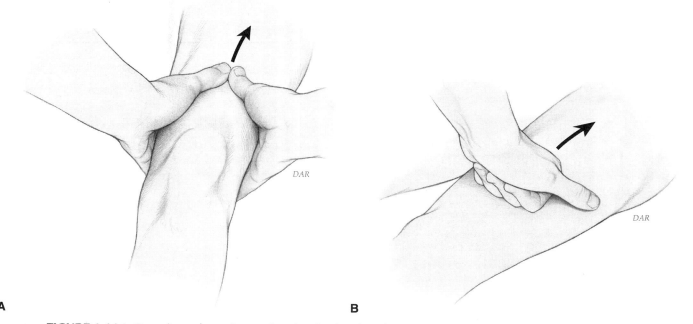

A   B

FIGURE 4-14 A. Deep tissue elongation stroke using the thumb pads. **B.** Deep tissue elongation stroke using the knuckles.

FIGURE 4-15 Hand position for spreading techniques.

FIGURE 4-16 Fanning stroke.

corporated within taut bands of fibers to locate trigger points precisely (Fig. 4-15).

The fingers, thumbs, knuckles, or elbow may be used. Although the thumb pads are the most sensitive part of the body used for delivering deep tissue strokes, it is best to perfect the use of these other body parts to save wear and tear on the thumbs.

- *Up-and-Down.* Move parallel to the muscle fibers, covering 1-inch sections at a time.
- *Side-to-Side.* Move perpendicular to the muscle fibers using back-and-forth motions in 1-inch segments.
- *Combination.* Perform up-and-down and side-to-side strokes on the same section of muscle, creating a 1-inch square.

- *Fanning.* The hands spread apart from each other in an arc pattern 3 to 4 inches wide (Fig. 4-16). This stroke stretches fascial membranes.
3. *Static Compression.* Lean directly into the muscle tissue at a 90° angle to the surface of the body (Fig. 4-17). Thumbs, fingers, knuckles, or elbows may be used. This stroke is used on extremely contracted sections of muscle fibers. It is also used to treat trigger points and acupressure points.
4. *Sifting.* This is a cross fiber style stroke. Grasp a section of muscle tissue between your fingers and thumb, and then roll the fibers to release adhering factors and locate trigger points within taut bands of tissue (Fig. 4-18).

FIGURE 4-17 Static compression using the thumb.

FIGURE 4-18 Sifting technique.

FIGURE 4-19 Hand position for treating a tendon.

Tendons

The following deep tissue procedures are used to treat tendons:

1. Stroke on the tendon toward the insertion point on the bone.
2. Do short, cross fiber strokes across the tendon.
3. Hold static compression where the tendon attaches to the bone.

The thumbs, elbow, fingers, or knuckles may be used (Fig. 4-19).

Separating Muscles

Stroke along the borders of muscles to separate them from each other. Use elongation strokes with the thumb, elbow, or knuckles (Fig. 4-20).

■ NEUROMUSCULAR THERAPY

The purpose of neuromuscular therapy is to seek out and treat any trigger points, which may be causing pain or muscular weakness. A description of trigger points and their formation was provided in the introduction to neuromuscular therapy in Chapter 1.

David Rini

FIGURE 4-20 Deep tissue elongation stroke between muscle bellies.

Finding Trigger Points

Trigger points are located in one of two ways. First, they may be encountered while performing deep tissue strokes on a muscle. A trigger point is always found within a taut band of muscle fibers that are tender to the touch. An indication that a band of fibers houses a single trigger point, or a group of trigger points, is that the fibers will twitch and elicit a pain response when the therapist's finger strums across them. Once the taut band of fibers is located, the therapist carefully seeks out the point within the fibers that delivers the most pronounced pain sensation when compressed.

If active, the trigger point will also produce painful feelings within a particular, remote site, known as a referred pain zone. A trigger point found in a specific location will always refer sensations to the same distant site. Travell and others have spent much time mapping the referral patterns of trigger points; these maps are available in many books and in chart form (trigger point charts are available at medical bookstores and massage supply stores). The predictability of trigger point referral patterns provides the key to the second method of locating trigger points.

During the interview that takes place before the deep tissue session, the client may describe areas of soft tissue that commonly cause pain and discomfort. This pain may be active or most pronounced after certain physical activities or when the person's stress level is high. The client is probably describing referred pain sites that are activated by trigger points. The therapist should try to pinpoint the exact location and dimension of the pain zone. A practical way to accomplish this is by the therapist tracing the perimeter of the pain zone on the client's body, with permission, while the client describes it. The therapist can also draw the area of pain on a piece of paper containing a blank figure of the human body. Once the location and size of the referred pain pattern are known, the associated trigger point can be found with the use of a trigger point chart.

Deactivating Trigger Points

The procedure for treating trigger points is simple. Once the location of the trigger point is pinpointed, the therapist presses on it directly, using the thumb, finger, or elbow (Fig. 4-21). The degree of pressure applied should elicit a mild pain response at the site of the trigger point and at the referral zone. After explaining this to the client, the therapist may incorporate a simple pressure-determining scale graded from 1 to 3 (1 signifying too little pressure, 2 signifying appropriate pressure, and 3 signifying too much pressure). By using this scale with the client, the therapist can always gauge his or her pressure perfectly to the client's reaction. This scale can also be used when performing deep tissue strokes to determine the proper amount of pressure.

Trigger points are always painful when pressed, but they are not usually noticeable otherwise. The pain pro-

FIGURE 4-21 Hand position for neuromuscular therapy trigger point release.

duced by a trigger point is registered at the referral site, not at the location of the trigger point itself. Treatment performed solely at the referral site may offer temporary relief or comfort. It will not relieve the pain permanently, however, because the source of the irritation (the trigger point) has not been deactivated.

Trigger points are treated with static compression for approximately 8 to 12 seconds. That is usually enough time to interrupt the pain messages being delivered by a trigger point to its corresponding referral zone. During the holding period, the client should experience a significant drop in the level of pain sensation. The therapist needs to monitor the client's experience of the pain pattern to measure the effectiveness of the treatment. Again, a simple verbal device can be used to gain information about the level of pain sensation. Every few seconds, as the therapist continues to press, the client is asked if the degree of pain is more, the same, or less. If the treatment is successful, the client should report a continual lessening of the pain.

Immediately after deactivating the trigger point, the therapist should stretch the affected muscle to attain its natural resting length. Trigger points manifest within contracted bands of fibers. The more regularly a muscle is stretched, the less likely it is to harbor trigger points. The client should be taught exercises to perform between treatments to stretch the affected muscles.

Charting Trigger Points

Mapping and treating trigger points can become rather complex, especially if the trigger points have been active for a long time and the client has several areas of chronic pain. Stacks of trigger points can develop in muscles that overlay each other. In these clients, each trigger point in the stack needs to be treated in succession, from the surface muscles to the deeper layers. Several trigger points can also be clustered around each other within the same muscle, and they may have the same or different referral zones connected to them. Referral pain zones themselves can even develop trigger points, known as satellite trigger points.

Satellite trigger points develop their own patterns of pain referral that extend into other areas of the body. If left untreated, trigger point activity can gradually spread throughout the body. The therapist must carefully map each pain zone and track down the trigger point, or trigger points, that are causing it to fire. Maintaining a body map for each client that charts each pain zone and the associated trigger points is very helpful in dealing with cases of chronic pain.

Evaluation of Treatment

The length of time that pain relief from trigger point treatment lasts is variable. Among other factors, it depends on the activities and lifestyle of the client. Job-related, repetitive movements that are aggravating trigger points may have to be relearned or curtailed. Stress management techniques should be incorporated to reduce excessive stimulation within the nervous system. Regular exercise, including slow, sustained stretching, should be practiced on a regular basis. If the necessary steps are taken, relief from trigger point pain may last anywhere from several days to forever.

At the client's next deep tissue therapy session, the therapist should ask about the duration of pain reduction in the referral zones. If necessary, trigger points can be retreated. If no pain relief is reported, the therapist should suggest a consultation with a physician to examine possible causes of the pain other than musculoskeletal dysfunction.

Body Mechanics

Of all the essential skills necessary to become a competent deep tissue therapist, one of the most important is learning to use proper body mechanics. Correct body alignment and movement support efficient execution of the strokes, minimizing wear and tear on the therapist both physically and mentally. Straining to perform the techniques not only is detrimental to the therapist's body, it interferes with the qualities of relaxation and openness that the therapist strives to transmit to the client through the strokes.

Almost all massage strokes require the transmission of weight from the therapist's body, moving from the feet and legs to the spine, then passing from the shoulder girdle through the arms and hands to the recipient. Leaning into the client's body is the means by which pressure for the strokes is generated. The study of body mechanics is largely based on learning how to transfer weight through the body structure without creating strain in the muscles.

Problems that occur because of a misaligned skeleton are compounded while performing massage. In addition to contending with the force of gravity, the therapist's body structure must distribute many extra pounds of pressure generated by the compressive movements of the strokes. When the body is not properly positioned, strain around unstable joints can become tremendous, leading to tissue breakdown and, eventually, disability.

The basic principles of alignment that apply when standing upright are also utilized in performing massage. The best way to understand correct alignment is to become familiar with the proper position of the skeleton to minimize structural stress. When correct placement of the bones is sensed or visualized, the nervous system di-

rects the muscles to perform the necessary actions to maintain that position.

The complex, precise coordinating actions the muscles must perform to move the body are carried out almost entirely at an unconscious level. Any attempt to consciously control the muscles severely inhibits the nervous system's job of orchestrating smooth muscle function. Using this principle in mastering massage techniques requires learning the correct position of the body for delivering each stroke and developing the kinesthetic awareness to sense when the body is deviating from this position.

The major principles of good body mechanics have been divided into five questions the therapist can easily memorize and recall when performing massage to quickly assess if he or she is using the body properly.

▪ THE FIVE-QUESTION CHECKLIST

1. Are the centers of my joints aligned?
   - My thumb is comfortably extended, not flexed or hyperextended.
   - My spine is straight from the sacrum to the atlas.
   - When my knee is flexed, it lines up over the second toe of the foot.
   - When my leg is straight, the knee is not hyperextended.
   - The tips of my elbows are pointed outward, not rolled inward.
   - My scapulae are relaxed and dropped, and the humerus is resting comfortably in the shoulder joint.
   - My wrists are in a neutral position.

2. Is my body facing the direction of my stroke?
   - My shoulders and hips line up in the same direction.
   - My hands line up with my center of gravity (a point at the midline of the body, 2 inches below the navel).
   - My legs and feet are moving in the same direction as my upper body.
   - My legs are approximating a parallel position, with my feet at least hip-width apart (imagine standing on skis).
3. Am I moving with my whole body?
   - At the beginning of the stroke, most of my weight is on my back foot.
   - My weight shifts forward as I apply pressure and/or as the stroke travels forward.
   - The force needed to perform the stroke flows upward, from my feet to my hands.
   - The more relaxed I am, the more easily the force can flow through my body.
   - Body movement is fluid and continuous; I am never *locked* in a position.

4. Am I lengthening as I apply pressure?
   - For every action, there is a reaction:
     - As I reach my back foot into the floor, my body lengthens upward.
     - As I reach forward, I lengthen backward.
   - My joints feel properly aligned and not compressed.
   - My body expands and softens as I apply pressure.
   - My shoulders are relaxed, my shoulder girdle wide, and my spine long.
   - My muscles feel loose and long, not contracted and tense.
5. Am I breathing from my center?
   - The rhythm for each stroke comes from my breathing pattern.
   - I allow myself to relax and fall forward as I exhale into the stroke.
   - My lower body and upper body come into balance at my pelvis.
   - I breathe all tension out of my body as I work.
   - I yield rather than force.

Therapist Self-Care

Massage therapy is a demanding profession. It requires intense mental concentration and regular physical conditioning. As with any care-giving job, there is always the danger of burnout if the therapist does not provide adequate self-care. People who are constantly giving to others often neglect to take the necessary time to replenish themselves. A few simple practices, if done on a regular basis, will assure that the therapist remains healthy and able to sustain a full-time massage practice:

1. *Exercise Daily.* Daily exercise is a requisite for taking care of the body adequately. Practicing proper body mechanics minimizes stress to the therapist's body, but it is not enough to counteract the compressive forces generated by performing massage therapy. The therapist's muscles and joints need to be lengthened and stretched regularly.

   Tai chi and yoga are both excellent practices that maintain a person's flexibility and strength while reducing the build-up of stress. These systems also encourage deep breathing, which is extremely important for rejuvenating the body and the mind. The self-awareness and mental control that tai chi and yoga foster help the massage therapist to increase his or her capacity to empathize with and stay focused on the client throughout the entire deep tissue therapy process.

2. *Take Time for Daily Reflection.* Daily reflection helps the therapist to remain centered, enthusiastic, and committed while caring for others. There are many different ways to clear the internal clutter that accumulates from intense work involving constant interaction with other people. Activities like walking, gardening, reading, and meditating all have the capacity to provide an outlet for the therapist to unwind and relieve potentially toxic mental and emotional build-up.

3. *Eat Vitalized Food and Drink Water.* Massage therapy is intensive work. It involves constant physical activity, moment-to-moment decision making, and unwavering vitality. In short, being a massage therapist calls on all of one's resources. The body must have adequate reserves of energy through intake of nutritious food and clean water to sustain the level of activity required for this work. Maintaining a well-balanced diet is one of the cornerstones of healthy living.

4. *Receive Bodywork Yourself.* Along with the activities mentioned above, the experience of receiving regular massage therapy keeps the body operating at peak performance levels. It also reminds the therapist what the experience of being a massage recipient is like—and what a profound impact he or she is having on clients by sharing deep tissue therapy skills.

REFERENCES

1. Chaitow L. Muscle energy techniques. 2nd edition. New York, NY: Churchill Livingstone, 2001: 38–39.
2. Chaitow L, Freyman V, Chambers G. Palpation and assessment skills. 2nd edition. New York, NY: Churchill Livingstone, 2003.
3. Pfrimmer T. Muscles: your invisible bonds. Blyth, ON, Canada: Blyth Printing, 1983.

Connective Tissue

Role of Fascia

The connective tissues provide shape, support, strength, and continuity to all the structures contained within the human form. In a sense, it is the connective tissues that hold the body together. They include the bones, cartilage, ligaments, tendons, and fascia. Taken as a whole, the connective tissues are the most pervasive class of tissue in the body.

Fascia is a sheet-like membrane that wraps and interweaves all the muscles in the body (Fig. 5-1). (For an informative description of the composition and role of fascia, see Chapter 3 in *Job's Body: A Handbook for Bodywork*.[1]) It can be thought of as a multilayered net that encases and connects all the soft tissue structures, from just below the skin all the way down to the bones. Within the muscles, it binds the muscle fibers together (Fig. 5-2). Fascia even forms the walls of the individual muscle cells, and muscle is often referred to as myofascial tissue in acknowledgment of the inextricable relationship of muscle fibers and fascia.

To release constricted muscles fully, the distinct qualities and functions of muscle fibers and fascia must be considered. Muscle fibers actively shorten, or contract, to move the bones; they are passively lengthened by the shortening of other muscle fibers. Deep tissue massage techniques are designed to release chronically shortened muscle fibers through manual compression and slow stretching. However, a muscle cannot regain its resting length, even when contracted fibers are relaxed, if the surrounding fascial membranes are binding it. The constricted fascial casing will prevent the muscle fibers from expanding and, thus, maintain the restricted condition of the muscle. Techniques that address the unique characteristics of fascia must be applied to fully lengthen myofascial tissue.

Fascia is composed of three primary constituents: a fluid material called ground substance, and two proteins (**collagen** and **elastin**). Each of these contributes a specialized property that gives fascia its diverse characteristics of fluidity, strength, and elasticity. Ground substance is the primary component of fascia. Chemically, it is classified as a **mucopolysaccharide,** and it is the same liquid that forms the interstitial fluid bathing every cell of the body.

This ground substance is a gel, which means it has the capability of moving between a more fluid and a more solid state. The degree of viscosity of the ground substance is largely dependent on three factors: temperature, movement, and hydration. When the body is in motion, heat is generated, which tends to promote a more fluid state in the ground substance. Greater fluidity within the fascia promotes freer muscle tissue. Exercise helps the body to remain supple, partly as a result of this effect. Lack of movement causes the ground substance to thicken, which tends to inhibit muscular freedom. Because of this phenomenon, the body feels stiffer when a person has been sitting or lying still for long periods. The elements of pressure and stretching used in fascial release techniques replicate natural muscle movements and help to return the ground substance to a fluid state.

Within the ground substance lie mesh-like layers of collagen, a protein that is composed of long, ropy strands. Depending on the form of connective tissue, collagen can be configured in different patterns, but its basic role is to provide strength and support. Adjacent molecular chains of collagen readily link together because of the strong bonding capability of hydrogen, one of collagen's primary components. This creates an extremely durable webbing

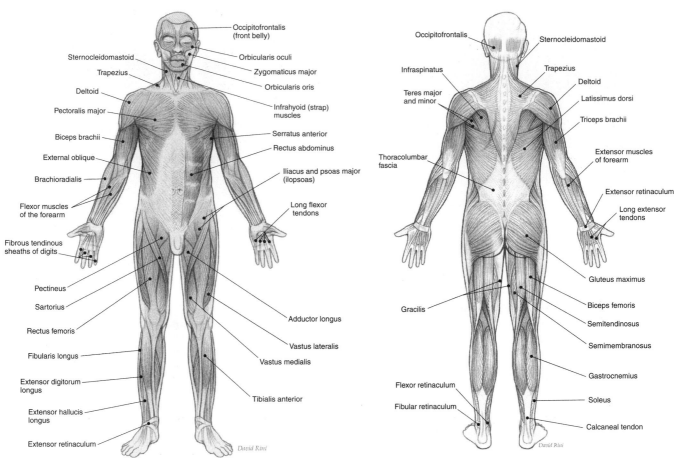

FIGURE 5-1 A. Anterior superficial muscles. **B.** Posterior superficial muscles.

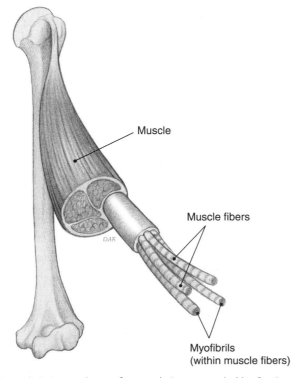

FIGURE 5-2 Every layer of a muscle is surrounded by fascia, from the surface down to the cellular level.

that can resist stretching even better than steel wire can.[2] Ligaments and tendons contain a high concentration of collagen, making them very effective in holding the skeleton and muscles together.

Distributed within the collagen mesh of fascial membranes is another protein, elastin, which has much greater flexibility than collagen. Elastin gives fascia more stretchiness compared with other forms of connective tissue, allowing it to change shape as muscles contract and expand. Fascia can be envisioned like the surface membrane of a jelly-filled balloon, having the ability to stretch and mold in response to internal changes but also having strong resistive force to contain and give shape to its largely fluid contents.

In addition to giving fascia strength, collagen's affinity to bond causes fascial membranes to stick together like plastic wrap. This can lead to muscular and postural problems. Under conditions of compression, which are aggravated by gravity's downward pull on the body, adjacent muscles tend to adhere to each other, causing them to lose their differentiation. As muscles meld together, the body's movement capability is diminished, and the structure begins to pull toward the ground.

CASE STUDY 2 Connective Tissue Release

The client is a 36-year-old woman named Margaret, who works in sales. She views her job as fairly high stress. She is constantly dealing with people, either in person or on the telephone. Although she exercises regularly, doing stretching and aerobics at least three times a week, she feels unable to relax fully. At times, it is difficult to take a deep breath, because her chest cavity feels muscularly tight and constricted. Her blood pressure is borderline high. Her goal in seeking massage therapy is to be able to relax and reduce the feelings of muscular tension that build up on a daily basis.

On observation, her muscles appear to be well toned. She was athletic in high school, having been on the swimming team, and her body still has an athletic quality. The musculature in her upper trunk and shoulders appears constricted. Her shoulders are medially rotated, with a slight degree of kyphosis in the upper back, and her sternum is depressed, causing her chest to appear somewhat sunken. Her head projects forward, causing the T1 vertebra to be prominent. There is a build-up of connective tissue around the upper thoracic vertebrae. Her pelvis is posteriorly rotated, and she stands with her knees slightly flexed. This postural stance points to short hamstring muscles. Overall, she appears vertically compressed when standing, as if she were carrying a heavy load on her shoulders.

The plan for the initial session was to help relieve the feelings of muscular constriction caused by built-up stress and to open the chest and shoulder region so that she can experience fuller breathing. Future sessions will deal with lengthening the spinal column and bringing the head and pelvis into a better relationship with each other.

Soon after the session began, it became apparent that the client was unable to accept deep, direct pressure to the muscles. The muscles were held tightly, in a seemingly protective mode. When moderate pressure was applied, the client reported feeling uncomfortable pain, and her upper body retreated further into its medially rotated stance. The therapist decided that a connective tissue approach was the preferred treatment for this client. The fascial compartments needed to be stretched so that her muscles could lengthen and relax. The client was uncomfortable with firm pressure and did not like sustained pressure to specific areas of soft tissue, even when the contact was light.

Myofascial mobilization and spreading techniques were applied to the pectoralis major, pectoralis minor, and serratus anterior to help expand the chest region and widen space across the shoulder girdle. The fanning stroke was also used in the upper thoracic region to help lift the sternum. Long Swedish strokes, combined with connective tissue spreading, were used on the rest of the body to promote feelings of length and relaxation. Overhead stretching of the arms was used at the end of the session to stretch the chest.

The client reported feeling much lighter at the end of the session. Her breathing felt much fuller without forcing it. Her comment was, "I feel like a burden has been lifted off of me."

Topics for Discussion

1. What are some indications that a connective tissue approach should be the primary course of treatment for a particular client?
2. Explain the reasons for performing connective tissue strokes slowly.
3. What kind of self-care treatment would be most beneficial for a client receiving connective tissue massage?
4. How would you explain to a client why connective tissue strokes feel different from other massage techniques that he or she may have received?
5. Why is connective tissue therapy a useful addition to any other form of massage treatment?

The continuity of the fascial membranes throughout the body provides a medium to absorb and distribute evenly the impact arising from falls and from everyday movements such as walking or jumping, much like the role of shock absorbers in a car. Fascial planes thicken in areas of the body that are under stress as a result of postural misalignment, poor movement mechanics, or injury; this thickening occurs to provide additional bracing.

These denser layers create a break in the flow of forces through the structure, resulting in areas of weakness at the points of discontinuity. The weakened tissues are vulnerable to breakdown, causing degeneration and injury. Realigning the lines of force that flow through the fascia adds immeasurably to the body's overall state of health and vitality by minimizing wear and tear on the muscles and skeleton.

Working with Fascia

The goal of working on the body's fascia is twofold: to make the ground substance more fluid, and to release collagen bonds that are causing muscles to adhere. The techniques used to mobilize fascia often incorporate slow stretching and pulling actions. Steady, sustained stretching of fascial membranes helps to free the restricting links that form within the collagen mesh.[3] The key to successful fascial release is the ability to sense the limit of the tissue's ability to stretch and then hold the stretch until a sensation of yielding or lengthening is felt. The tissues should never be forced with more pressure or stretch than they can accommodate comfortably.

Because contractile muscle fibers and fascial membranes are so intricately intertwined, it is physically impossible to touch one without affecting the other. The therapist's intention while manipulating tissues is the key to distinguishing which component of the myofascial unit is being emphasized. Helpful images for sensing tissue release when working on fascia can include visions of an ice cube slowly melting on a sidewalk or butter melting in a frying pan.

As the therapist's hands are placed on the body, pressure is applied only to the point at which resistance is first felt in the muscle tissue. This might be registered as a slight recoil or a feeling of the tissue thickening. The therapist then waits for a softening of the resistance, which allows his or her hands to continue to glide through the tissue until further resistance is encountered. This slow, methodical sensing of the tissue's reaction to the therapist's manipulation assures that the state of the fascia is being affected.

Connective Tissue Routine

The description of the connective tissue procedures does not include the specific muscles being worked on, because the goal of these strokes is to stretch the fascial membranes that wrap all of the muscles. The therapist's focus while performing these strokes is on sensing the softening and stretching of the tissues in response to the slow movements of the hands. The following chapters focus on lengthening and repatterning specific muscles.

◼ NECK

Position

- The client is lying supine on the table.
- The therapist is sitting at the head of the table.

1. *Longitudinal Neck Release.* Place the fingers of both hands under the occipital ridge. Allow the fingers to sink into the tissues until a slight resistance is felt.

   Move the tissues of the neck with short up and down strokes but without sliding over the skin (Fig. 5-3). Move the fingers down a couple of inches to the next section of the neck, about an inch below the first section, and repeat the up and down stroke. Continue with this pattern to the base of the neck.

   Return to the occiput, and place the fingers farther away from the midline than on the first pass. Repeat the sequence down the neck.

2. *Lateral Neck Release.* Place the fingers lengthwise, from underneath, on either side of the spinous processes of the neck. Let the fingers sink into the tissues. Slowly spread them laterally, away from the

David Rini

FIGURE 5-3 Longitudinal neck release.

spine (Fig. 5-4). Slide farther down the neck, and re-peat. Continue, spreading in horizontal strips, to the base of the neck.

3. *Horizontal Neck Release.* Turn the client's head slightly to the side. Using your fingers, sink in along the ante-rior border of the sternocleidomastoid muscle. Slowly

glide the fingers in a posterior direction as far as you can reach (Fig. 5-5). Repeat, in horizontal strips, throughout the length of the neck.

4. *Laterally Flex the Client's Neck.* Place your fingers into the front portion of the trapezius muscle on the flexed side, slightly behind the clavicle. Gradually sink in un-

FIGURE 5-4 Lateral neck release.

FIGURE 5-5 Horizontal neck release, with the working hand moving posteriorly.

FIGURE 5-6 Lifting and rolling the superficial fascia of the upper chest.

til mild resistance is felt, and perform the short up and down movements with your fingers.

Repeat moves 1 through 4 on the other side.

■ CHEST

Position

- The client is lying supine.
- The therapist is standing at the side of the table.

1. *Fasial Lift and Roll Technique.* Grasp the skin of the upper chest lightly between your thumb and fingers. Slowly, roll it superiorly toward the clavicle (Fig. 5-6). Cover as much of the chest as you can. When working with female clients, avoid the breast tissue.

2. *Fanning Strokes on the Upper Chest.* Place the fingers of both hands on the sternum. Sink into the tissues, and spread slowly outward from the midline with a fanning stroke (Fig. 5-7). Repeat the stroke several times, moving in a superior direction toward the clavicles.

FIGURE 5-7 Fanning stroke on the chest.

FIGURE 5-8 Myofascial mobilization of the tissues over the ribs.

3. *Myofascial Mobilization of the Tissues Over the Ribs.* Beginning at the lower portion of the rib cage, place your fingers on the lowest ribs, and slide the tissues up and down over the rib (Fig. 5-8). Feel for areas where the tissue either does not move or feels like it is sticking to the rib. Work to free all the tissue. Progress up the rib cage, working over each rib until you reach the clavicle. Repeat on the other side of the chest.

4. *Compress and Spread the Chest Tissues.* Holding the wrist, abduct the client's arm 90°, and flex it at the elbow. Move the arm into various stretched positions while you compress and spread the stretched myofascial tissues of the chest with the heel of your other hand (Fig. 5-9).

ABDOMEN

Position

- The client is lying supine, with a bolster under the knees.
- The therapist is standing at the side of the table and is facing the client's abdomen.

1. *Fascial Lift and Roll Technique.* Reach across the client's body, and grasp the skin at the waistline between your thumb and fingers. Roll the skin, moving slowly toward the midline (Fig. 5-10). When you encounter tightness or resistance, slowly lift the skin away from the underlying muscle, and hold until a softening is felt. Cover the entire side of the abdomen thoroughly, working in horizontal strips from the side of the trunk to the midline. Walk around to the other side of the table, and repeat the procedure on the other half of the client's abdomen.

2. *Myofascial Stretch of the Abdomen.* Place the right palm on the abdomen, over the navel area. Place your left palm on top of your right hand. Begin to make a slow,

David Rini

FIGURE 5-9 Compressing and spreading the myofascial tissues of the chest.

FIGURE 5-10 Lifting and rolling the abdominal tissue.

clockwise, spiraling motion, moving the skin over the underlying tissues (Fig. 5-11). Do not glide over the skin. Gradually increase the size of the spiral, stretching the skin and fascia to their maximm degree.

3. *Abdominal Stretch of the Abdomen.* With the client's knees flexed, have him or her stretch both arms overhead and reach fully. Encourage the client to take a deep breath, lifting the chest and pulling the abdomen in while continuing to stretch the arms overhead until a stretch is felt in the abdominal muscles (Fig. 5-12). A useful image to aid this stretch is to tell the client to imagine the navel touching the front of the spine as he or she reaches.

FIGURE 5-11 Myofascial stretching of the abdomen using the palms of the hands.

FIGURE 5-12 Abdominal stretch.

■ ARM

Position

- The client is lying supine.
- The therapist is standing at the side of the table, next to the client's hand.

1. *Myofascial Spreading of the Palm.* The client's palm is facing away from the therapist. Using both hands, curve your fingers under the client's hand, pressing your fingertips into the palm. Slowly slide your hands apart, stretching the tissues of the palm (Fig. 5-13). Perform this move very slowly, and pause to allow the fascia to stretch.

FIGURE 5-13 Spreading the fascia of the palm.

FIGURE 5-14 Lifting and rolling the forearm tissues.

2. *Fascial Lift and Roll Technique.* The client's arm is resting on the table. Place your hands in the skin rolling position, parallel to the muscle fibers, above the client's wrist. Roll and lift the tissues of the forearm, in horizontal strips, from wrist to elbow (Fig. 5-14).

3. *Myofascial Spreading of the Forearm.* Flex the client's arm at the elbow. Place your hands around the forearm at the wrist, with your fingers sinking into the midline of the palmar side of the forearm using the same hand position as described in move 1. Slowly spread the fingers away from the midline, stretching the tissues (Fig. 5-15). Continue, in horizontal strips, to the elbow. Repeat the move on the other side of the forearm.

FIGURE 5-15 Myofascial spreading of the forearm.

FIGURE 5-16 Myofascial spreading of the upper arm.

4. *Myofascial Spreading of the Upper Arm.* The client's arm is lying on the table. Begin the stroke just above the elbow. Using the heels of your hands or the broad side of your thumbs, spread the tissues evenly from the midline out to the edges of the upper arm (Fig. 5-16).

■ BACK

Position

- The client is lying prone.
- The therapist is standing at the head of the table.

1. *Myofascial Mobilization of the Back.* With your fingertips or palms, sink into the tissues enough to be able to move the skin without sliding over it. Using a short up and down and side to side motion, move the skin over the underlying tissues (Fig. 5-17). Work in small sections, and cover the entire back. This procedure can also be performed with a rolled-up towel to move the skin.
2. *Myofascial Spreading of the Back.* Standing at the side of the table, sink into the tissues with your fingers or knuckles. Glide through the tissues with a spreading motion, moving as the fascia softens and pausing at resistance. Begin the stroke at the spine, and move outward in horizontal motions across the back (Fig. 5-18). If using the fingers, work on the opposite side of the client's back from the side of the table where you are standing, and stroke from the spine away from yourself. When using the knuckles, work on the same side of the back, and stroke from the spine toward yourself.
3. *Myofascial Release of the Tissues Over the Bones.* Using a circular friction motion, roll the myofascial tissue over the bones. In the upper back, roll the tissues over the ribs and scapulae. In the lower back, roll against the 12th rib, the lumbar spine, and the iliac crest.
4. *Back Stretch.* Have the client lift up onto his or her hands and knees while under the sheet and then sit back on the heels, resting the chest on the thighs and the forehead on the table in front of the knees to stretch the muscles of the back (Fig. 5-19).

DAR

FIGURE 5-17 Myofascial mobilization of the back.

DAR

FIGURE 5-18 Myofascial spreading of the back.

■ FOOT

Position

- The client is lying supine.
- The therapist is standing at the side of the table next to the client's foot and is facing away from the client's head.

1. *Myofascial Spreading of the Plantar Surface of the Foot.* Stand at the side of the table, and face the dorsal side of the client's foot. Curve the fingers of both hands around the underside of the foot. Sink your fingers into the sole of the foot until mild resistance is felt. Slowly spread your fingers from the midline to the outer edges of the foot (Fig. 5-20).

David Rini

FIGURE 5-19 Back stretch from a kneeling position.

FIGURE 5-22 Position for foot stretch (a).

FIGURE 5-20 Myofascial spreading of the plantar surface of the foot.

2. *Myofascial Mobilization on the Dorsal Side of the Foot.* Standing at the base of the table, place your fingers on the dorsal surface of the foot. Slide the tissues up and down and side to side in small sections (Fig. 5-21). Cover the entire surface of the foot.

3. *Fascial Stretching of the Foot*
   a. Grasp the client's toes with one hand while holding the metatarsal portion of the foot with the other hand. Flex the toes forward and back to stretch the foot (Fig. 5-22).
   b. Hold both sides of the client's foot with your hands. Shift the bones of the foot back and forth by alternately moving one hand toward you and the other hand away from you in a continuous motion (Fig. 5-23).

FIGURE 5-21 Myofascial mobilization on the dorsal side of the foot.

FIGURE 5-23 Position for foot stretch (b).

FIGURE 5-24 Myofascial spreading of the leg.

FIGURE 5-25 Myofascial mobilization of the leg.

■ LEG

Position

- The client is lying supine.
- The therapist is standing at the side of the table next to the client's ankle.

1. *Myofascial Spreading of the Leg.* Place the hands around the tibia, with the heels of the hand meeting at the midline of the leg. Slowly spread the hands apart, with pressure against the base of the palms (Fig. 5-24). Begin the sequence at the ankle. Moving in horizontal strips, work your way up the leg to the knee.

FIGURE 5-26 Lifting and rolling the myofascial tissue of the anterior thigh.

David Rini

FIGURE 5-27 Myofascial mobilization of the anterior thigh.

2. *Myofascial Mobilization of the Leg.* Using the fingers or knuckles, roll across the lateral leg muscles until they slide freely over the bone (Fig. 5-25). Begin at the ankle, and work in horizontal strips up to the knee.
3. *Fascial Stretches for the Leg.* With one hand on the ankle and the other hand on the metatarsal, alternately flex and extend the client's foot. Place one palm on the dorsal surface of the foot and the other palm on the plantar surface of the foot. Invert the foot, and then hold, allowing the myofascial tissues to stretch. Evert the foot, and hold.

■ ANTERIOR THIGH

Position

- The client is lying supine.
- The therapist is standing at the side of the table next to the client's knee.

1. *Fascial Lift and Roll Technique.* Place your hands in the skin rolling position on the thigh, parallel to the muscle fibers. Lift and roll the tissues of the thigh (Fig. 5-26). Move from the knee to the hip, and work in horizontal strips, covering the entire thigh.
2. *Myofascial Spreading of the Thigh.* Place the hands around the thigh, with the heels of the hand meeting at the midline. Applying pressure with the base of the palm, slowly slide the hands apart, spreading the

tissues of the thigh. Begin the stroke at the knee. Repeat the spreading action in horizontal strips to the hip.
3. *Myofascial Mobilization of the Thigh.* Using the fingers of both hands, roll the muscles of the thigh over the bone until they slide freely (Fig. 5-27).

■ MEDIAL THIGH

Position

- The client is positioned supine, with the leg to be worked on bent at the knee and turned out, or in side posture, with the top leg flexed 90° and the bottom leg straight. The underneath leg is the one to be massaged.
- The therapist is standing at the side of the table next to the client's knee.

1. *Myofascial Spreading of the Medial Thigh.* Place the sides of the thumbs next to each other on the midline of the medial thigh. Slowly spread the thumbs apart, stretching the myofascia (Fig. 5-28). Begin the stroke at the knee. Working in horizontal strips, continue to the groin.
2. *Myofascial Mobilization of the Medial Thigh.* Using your finger pads, roll the muscles against the bones, helping them to slide freely.

FIGURE 5-28 Myofascial spreading of the medial thigh.

■ LATERAL THIGH

Position

- The client is placed in side posture. The upper leg is flexed, with a bolster under the knee. This is the leg that will be massaged.
- The therapist is standing on the front side of the table and is facing the thigh of the client's top leg.

1. *Fascial Lift and Roll Technique.* Place the hands in the skin rolling position along the lateral thigh, parallel to the muscle fibers. Lift and roll the muscles (Fig. 5-29). Start at the knee, and continue, in horizontal strips, to the hip.
2. *Myofascial Spreading of the Lateral Thigh.* Place the heels of the hands against the midline of the lateral thigh. Slowly spread the hands apart (Fig. 5-30). Begin the first stroke at the knee. Repeat, in horizontal strips, to the hip.

    Variation—Spread each half of the thigh individually. Place the hands parallel along the midline of the thigh. Using the fingertips, spread from the midline outward. Work in horizontal strips, and continue to the hip. Repeat on the other side.
3. *Myofascial Mobilization of the Hip.* Standing behind the client, place the forearm across the hip area. Slowly roll the muscles in a back and forward motion (Fig. 5-31). Place the forearm farther back into the gluteal area, and repeat.

■ CALF

Position

- The client is lying in a prone position.
- The therapist is standing at the side of the table next to the client's calf.

1. *Fascial Lift and Roll Technique.* Lift and roll the skin and muscles of the calf, the gastrocnemius and the soleus, moving in horizontal strips (Fig. 5-32).

DAR

FIGURE 5-29 Lifting and rolling the tissues of the lateral thigh.

FIGURE 5-30 Myofascial spreading of the lateral thigh.

FIGURE 5-32 Lifting and rolling the calf tissues.

FIGURE 5-31 Myofascial mobilization of the hip.

FIGURE 5-33 Myofascial spreading of the calf.

2. *Myofascial Spreading of the Calf.* Placing the heels of the hands on the midline of the calf, spread laterally.

    Variation—Use the fingertips to spread each side of the calf separately, from the midline laterally (Fig. 5-33).
3. *Myofascial Mobilization of the Calf.* Using your fingers, roll the muscles against the underlying muscles and bones. Work to release any areas that feel adhered.
4. *Flex the Knee, Bringing the Leg Perpendicular to the Table.* Dorsiflex the foot, and hold the stretch.

■ POSTERIOR THIGH

Position

- The client is lying prone.
- The therapist is standing at the side of the table next to the client's thigh.

1. *Fascial Lift and Roll Technique.* Lift and roll the skin and muscles, working parallel to the fibers. Begin the stroke slightly above the knee joint. Move in horizontal strips to the hip.
2. *Myofascial Spreading of the Posterior Thigh.* Use either the heels of the hands or the knuckles. Place your hands on the midline of the thigh, just above the knee. Slowly and evenly spread the hands apart. Move in horizontal strips, from the knee to the hip.

    Variation—Stand at the side of the table, and face the client's thigh. Place the fingertips of both hands on the midline of the thigh. Allow the fingers to sink into the tissues until mild resistance is felt. As the tissues soften, let the fingers slowly slide in a medial direction. Walk around to the other side of the table, and repeat the stroke on the posterior thigh in the opposite direction.
3. *Myofascial Mobilization of the Posterior Thigh.* Using the fingers, roll the muscles of the thigh over each other and against the femur. Work to free the individual muscles from adhering.

FIGURE 5-34 Lifting and rolling the gluteal tissues.

■ POSTERIOR HIP

Position

- The client is lying prone.
- The therapist is standing at the side of the table next to the client's pelvis.

1. *Fascial Lift and Roll Technique.* Lift and roll the gluteal muscles in a superior direction (Fig. 5-34).
2. *Myofascial Spreading of the Posterior Thigh.* Using your knuckles or the heels of the hands, spread the tissues from the sacrum to the trochanter (Fig. 5-35).

FIGURE 5-35 Myofascial spreading of the gluteal area.

David Rini

FIGURE 5-36 Myofascial mobilization of the gluteal tissues.

3. *Myofascial Mobilization of the Posterior Thigh.* Using your fingers, roll the muscles to re-establish individual action (Fig. 5-36).

REFERENCES

1. Juhan D. Connective tissue. In: Job's body: a handbook for bodywork. 3rd edition. Barrytown, NY: Station Hill Press, 2003.

2. Juhan D. Connective tissue. In: Job's body: a handbook for bodywork. 3rd edition. Barrytown, NY: Station Hill Press, 2003: 72.

3. Juhan D. Connective tissue. In: Job's body: a handbook for bodywork. 3rd edition. Barrytown, NY: Station Hill Press, 2003: 88.

The Fundamentals—Breath and Support

The Chest

■ GENERAL CONCEPTS

The deep tissue series begins with the chest. Because the overall goal of deep tissue therapy is to bring a person's body to a condition of better balance and function, the logical place to begin is with the breathing mechanism. It is primarily through the breath that the body receives and metabolizes the energy that is necessary to carry on its vital processes. The first breath we take marks our entry into this world, and the last breath signals our departure. How we manage all the breaths in between has much to do with determining the quality of the lives we lead.

The movement of the breath in and out establishes a primary rhythm, or flow, through the body. It represents our ability to take in and assimilate as well as to give out and let go. The smooth flow of breath is also crucial to the bodywork process. During a deep tissue session, the recipient is called on to absorb pressure, process change, and release stored tension. If the breath is inhibited, this sequence of events is blocked, and consequently, the person cannot obtain the full effects of the deep tissue work.

Tension in the muscles of the chest inhibits the movement of the lungs and constricts the capillaries, diminishing the amount of oxygen that is taken into the body. Decreased oxygen affects metabolism all the way to the cellular level. With less oxygen available, the body's connective tissues become less pliable, restricting muscular action. Over time, a person becomes encased in muscular tension that severely limits full interaction with the surrounding environment and diminishes the capacity to feel. Through observation and palpation, the deep tissue therapist evaluates the patterns of myofascial constriction that are limiting full breathing capacity and then focuses on reducing or eliminating them.

The effects of open, full breathing are many. The amount of stress and tension stored in the body is reduced while levels of endurance are often substantially increased. The body's ability to eliminate toxins is greatly improved. As much as 70% of the body's toxins are released through the breath. When breathing capacity is reduced, other organs of elimination, such as the skin and the kidneys, have to overwork to flush toxins out of the system. This can leave the body in a weakened state and more vulnerable to disease. Full breathing helps to keep the blood pressure normalized. A structure in the brain, called the medulla, oversees the size and tone of the arteries. The medulla responds to the condition of the blood circulating through it. If the carbon dioxide level is high, for instance, the blood pressure becomes elevated as well. Full, rhythmic breathing also plays an important role in managing states of anxiety and panic, which can influence positively conditions like depression and asthma.

■ MUSCULOSKELETAL ANATOMY AND FUNCTION

The chest, or thoracic cage, is one of the three major weight segments supported by the spine. It consists of 12 pairs of ribs, the 12 thoracic vertebrae, the costal cartilage, and the sternum (Essential Anatomy Box 6-1 and Fig. 6-1). The thoracic portion of the spine is its least moveable segment, providing a stable attachment for the ribs in the back of the body. The ribs join the sternum on the anterior side by means of the costal cartilage. The cylindrical, cage-like design of the chest forms a protective housing for the heart and lungs. Refer to Figure 6-1C for an illustration of the bones of the thorax.

BOX 6-1 ESSENTIAL ANATOMY The Chest Routine

MUSCLES
Pectoralis major
Subclavius
Intercostals
Diaphragm
Serratus posterior superior
Serratus posterior inferior

BONES AND LANDMARKS
Ribs
Sternum
Manubrium
Xiphoid process
Sulcus intertubercularis
Locations of vertebrae T1–T3, T11–L2
Clavicle

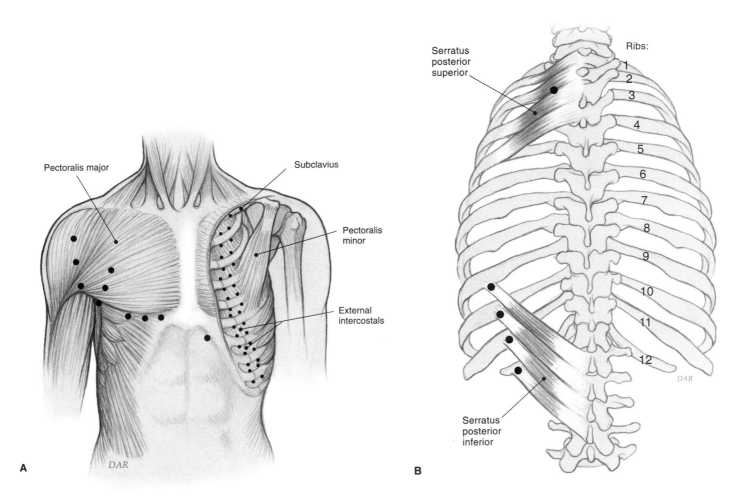

FIGURE 6-1 A. Muscles of the chest with areas of possible trigger point formation indicated. **B.** Posterior breathing muscles with areas of possible trigger point formation indicated.

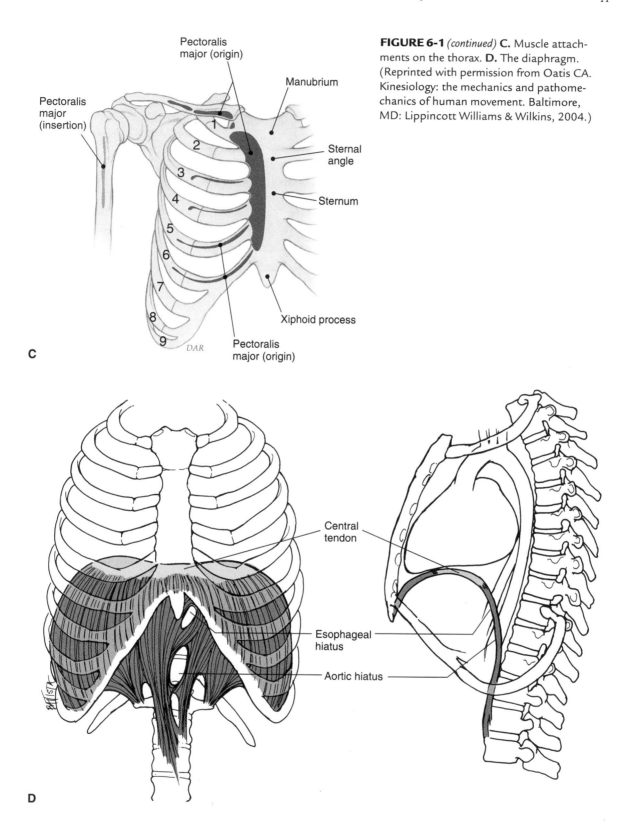

C

Pectoralis major (origin)

Pectoralis major (insertion)

Manubrium

1
2
3
4
5
6
7
8
9

DAR

Sternal angle

Sternum

Xiphoid process

Pectoralis major (origin)

FIGURE 6-1 *(continued)* **C.** Muscle attachments on the thorax. **D.** The diaphragm. (Reprinted with permission from Oatis CA. Kinesiology: the mechanics and pathomechanics of human movement. Baltimore, MD: Lippincott Williams & Wilkins, 2004.)

D

Central tendon

Esophageal hiatus

Aortic hiatus

BATISTA

The **pectoralis major** muscle is made up of three overlapping sections that fan across the anterior chest cavity. All three sections attach on the lateral side of the upper humerus, on the lateral side of the bicipital groove. The upper section originates on the medial half of the clavicle and is the most superficial of the three sections. The middle section attaches along the sternum. The lower section, which is also the deepest, attaches to the costal cartilages. The broad, fan-like arrangement of the pectoralis major fibers allows it to act on the arm from numerous angles. This design also distributes force coming from the arm over the entire anterior rib cage, minimizing impact stress to the thorax.

All three sections of pectoralis major contribute to horizontal flexion and internal rotation of the arm. In these actions, it is opposed by the latissimus dorsi, which extends and laterally rotates the arm. Both muscles work together to adduct the arm and lift the thorax toward the arm in pull-ups. Chronically contracted pectoralis major muscles are characterized posturally by a collapsed chest, with the arms drawn forward and rolled inward when hanging at the sides of the body. The **subclavius** muscle lies deep to the clavicular section of the pectoralis major. It attaches on the first rib and to a groove on the underside of the clavicle. It fixes the clavicle to the chest wall and depresses it.

Breathing is a vital and complex activity that involves not only all the bones and muscles of the chest area but also accessory muscles in the abdomen, shoulder girdle, and neck. The respiratory muscles function continuously throughout life. These muscles must be free to carry out the coordinated actions necessary to achieve full breathing.

Although 46 muscles are involved in the breathing process, the primary breathing muscle is the **diaphragm.** This dome-shaped muscle is connected to the lower ribs, sternum, and lumbar spine in a rim around the body. The bases of the lungs attach to the upper surface of the diaphragm. The diaphragm forms the floor of the chest cavity and the roof of the abdominal cavity. The movement of the diaphragm creates a bellows action in the chest and lungs that allows air to be drawn in and forced out of the body.

The diaphragm has two main portions (Fig. 6-1*D*). The central tendon, which is noncontractile tissue, forms the central roof of the dome and blends with the pericardium. Being firm, the central tendon helps the diaphragm to maintain its shape.

Surrounding the central tendon are muscular fibers that are arranged in a radial design like spokes on a wheel. This muscular portion of the diaphragm consists of two sections, the crural part and the costal part. The crural portion forms a muscular extension of the diaphragm that runs in two sections down the anterior surface of the lumbar spine, attaching on the vertebral bodies and disks of L1–L3 and on the aponeurotic arcuate ligament. The crura form a connection for the breathing apparatus between the upper and lower spine.

As the diaphragm contracts during the inspiration phase of breathing, the fibers are drawn downward toward the crura (Fig. 6-2). The dome flattens, causing the lungs

Left lung

External intercostal muscles

During inspiration the diaphragm presses the abdominal organs downward and forward.

Action of rib cage in inspiration

Left lung

Internal intercostal muscles

During expiration the diaphragm rises and recoils to the resting position.

Action of rib cage in expiration

FIGURE 6-2 Mechanics of normal breathing. (Reprinted with permission from Weber J, Kelley J. Health assessment in nursing. 2nd edition. Philadelphia, PA: Lippincott Williams & Wilkins, 2003.)

to be stretched downward, increasing their surface area and diminishing the internal air pressure in the lungs. Air from outside the body rushes in to fill the vacuum, thus equalizing the internal and external pressure. As the diaphragm descends, the amount of space in the abdominal cavity is decreased, thereby increasing internal abdominal pressure and causing the abdominal wall to distend, making room for the squeezed abdominal contents.

During inspiration, the **external intercostal** muscles contract, elevating the ribs and causing the lower portion of the rib cage to lift and extend laterally. The intercostal muscles attach to adjacent ribs all the way around the circumference of the rib cage. They are extensions of the abdominal oblique muscles into the chest cavity. The fibers of the external intercostals angle obliquely downward and inward. The fibers of the internal intercostals angle obliquely upward and outward.

The **serratus posterior superior** also contributes to inspiration. It lies deep to the rhomboids in the upper back. Serratus posterior superior connects the C7–T3 vertebrae and ribs 2–5 at a 45° downward angle. When the serratus posterior superior contracts, it lifts the upper ribs, thus expanding the chest. This muscle can be strained when a person engages in too much forceful, high chest breathing without incorporating the abdominal muscles.

On exhalation, the abdominal muscles contract, pushing the abdominal contents inward and upward, thus causing the diaphragm to be lifted back to its dome-shaped position. This diminishes the size of the lungs and decreases the internal air pressure, causing the air to rush out of the lungs to re-establish air pressure equalization. The **internal intercostals** contract, causing the ribs to move downward and inward and assisting in diminishing the size of the lungs. Refer to Figure 6-2 for a visual representation of the breathing process.

The **serratus posterior inferior** muscle attaches to the T11 and T12 and the L1 and L2 vertebrae. Its fibers angle upward at about a 45° angle, mirroring the serratus posterior superior, to attach to ribs 8–12. It stabilizes the lower ribs, and it assists in expiration. Serratus posterior inferior can be strained during lifting, twisting, and reaching actions, such as stretching to grasp an item located on a high shelf. Figure 6-1, *A* and *B*, illustrates the muscles of the chest.

As mentioned previously, many other muscles are involved in the breathing process, assisting in the essential movements and stabilizing muscles and bones. Full, unrestricted breathing is actually a full-body phenomenon. The breath is experienced as a pressure wave moving throughout the entire body. Watching a small baby breathe demonstrates this effect beautifully. The deep tissue massage therapist should be aware of how the client's body is moving as he or she breathes and where the breath is inhibited. The reintegration of full-body breathing is a primary goal of deep tissue massage.

■ CONDITIONS

1. *Asthma* is a respiratory disorder that is characterized by periodic bouts of difficulty in breathing accompanied by coughing and a build-up of mucus secretion. Attacks are precipitated by an inflammation of the bronchial tubes triggered by factors such as allergens, strenuous exertion, or emotional factors. Massage is beneficial if performed between attacks, when the bronchial tubes are not inflamed. It can help to expel excess mucus, release tension in the chest muscles, and reduce stresses that may contribute to attacks.

2. *Emphysema* is a condition affecting the lungs. The alveoli or air sacs are overexpanded to the point at which the walls begin to break down, making breathing difficult. Cigarette smoking is a major contributing factor. Breathing exercises and massage can be helpful if the condition is not too advanced.

3. *Acute bronchitis* is an inflammation of the tubes leading from the trachea to the lungs in the upper respiratory tract. It is short in duration but severe. It is accompanied by coughing and heavy mucus production along with a low-grade fever and constriction behind the sternum. Because it is an inflammatory condition, deep massage is contraindicated until the inflammation begins to subside and the patient starts to expel built-up mucus.

4. *Pleurisy* is an inflammation of the pleurae, the membranes covering the lungs. It is accompanied by difficulty in breathing and sharp pain under the ribs and extending into the abdomen. Massage is contraindicated.

5. *Cracked ribs* are best left alone. They usually heal easily, but taping is sometimes required.

6. *Weak respiratory tract caused by pollution.* The toxic substances floating around in the air from industry, aerosols, cigarette smoke, and many other sources are irritants to the lungs. These substances can generate the respiratory conditions listed above as well as many others. Good diet, breathing exercises, stretching of the chest muscles, and regular massage greatly benefit the respiratory tract.

Please refer to Indications/Contraindications Box 6-2 for an additional list of indications and contraindications for the chest region.

■ POSTURAL EVALUATION

1. Describe the general shape of the chest.
   - Do the right and left halves match?
   - Are the upper and lower portions symmetric?
2. Check the position of the sternum.
   - Is it lifted?
   - Is it depressed?

BOX 6-2 INDICATIONS/CONTRAINDICATIONS
Conditions Affecting Chest Massage

INDICATIONS
Shallow breathing
Tightness in the chest
Chronic cough
Pain in the chest
Difficult or painful breathing
Heaviness around the heart

CONTRAINDICATIONS
Inflammatory conditions of chest tissues
Broken ribs
Tuberculosis
Recent surgery
High fever
Severe illness

The chest region has two primary functions: It serves as a container, and it serves as a pump. The heart is housed and protected by the chest. We identify the heart with feeling, primarily with our capacity to experience and radiate love. Love is considered to be a warm emotion. It is often associated with fire. We feel the fires of passion burning or the warm glow of a smoldering ember in our chest when we are in love. When the chest is open, our feeling expands outward to others and is returned to nourish our heart center.

A chest that is tight, closed, and shut off squeezes the heart and reduces its capacity to produce warm, loving emotions. The fire has died, and we are left with the experience of cold-heartedness, a lack of warmth. As chronic tightness in the muscles of the chest cavity is released, one often feels an energizing of the heartfelt emotions. Tears may accompany the reconnection to the capacity for joy, sadness, affection, and intimacy.

The chest also serves as a pump for the oxygen and blood that flow through the body. The heart is situated between the lungs. Therefore, each breath we take massages the heart and helps to increase circulation. The outward, expansive movement of the body that accompanies inspiration represents our capacity to give outwardly of ourselves, to share. The inward, contractive movement of expiration denotes our ability to receive, to surrender, to take in.

Balance of the mind/body system is reflected in a full, integrated breathing rhythm that allows us to shift easily between these two phases. The rib cage and abdomen are mobile, with the ability to change shape and size easily.

3. Observe the position of the ribs.
   - Do the ribs hang from the manubrium?
   - Where do the ribs appear to be squeezed together?
   - Where are the spaces between the ribs expanded?

FIGURE 6-3 Stretching the pectoral muscles in a door frame.

TABLE 6–1	Body Reading for the Chest	
Conditions		**Muscles That May Be Shortened**
Overexpanded chest—the sternum is lifted, ribs are expanded, shoulders drawn back		Scalenes External intercostals Rhomboids
Hollow chest—the sternum is depressed, upper ribs are compressed, shoulders are pulled forward		Pectoralis major Pectoralis minor Subclavius Internal intercostals Anterior deltoid Diaphragm Rectus abdominus

4. Observe the breathing pattern.
   - Which phase of breath (inhalation or exhalation) is favored, if any?
   - Which portions of the chest appear to move easily with the breath?
   - Which portions of the chest appear to be rigid and not moving with the breath?
5. Look at the region of the diaphragm, at the level of the lower ribs.
   - Are the lower ribs spread apart and pulled up?
   - Do the lower ribs appear to be relaxed and hanging downward?
   - Are the lower ribs squeezed or drawn together?

Refer to Table 6-1 for a description of common distortions of the chest and possible muscles involved.

EXERCISES AND SELF-TREATMENT

1. *Stretch for the Pectoralis Major Muscles.* Stand in a doorway with your arms spread apart and your hands or forearms resting against the sides of the door frame (Fig. 6-3). Shifting your weight forward from your pelvis, allow the back to arch slightly and the chest to lift and stretch. Breathe deeply. Positioning the arms higher or lower along the sides of the door frame will alter the muscle fibers being stretched.
2. *Stretch for the Chest and Abdomen.* Lie on your back across a bed with your midthoracic spine on the side edge of the mattress so that your upper body can hang down toward the floor, with the arms extended. Take deep breaths. Alternative surfaces are an exercise ball (Fig. 6-4), the arm of a large couch, or several blankets rolled up tightly into the shape of a cylinder at least 18 inches in diameter and fastened with belts or rope.
3. *Release for the Contracted Diaphragm and Serratus Posterior Muscles.* Lie on your back on the floor. Place two tennis balls on either side of the low back, at the level of the 12th rib. Slowly allow your weight to sink into the balls as you relax, and breathe fully.

CHEST ROUTINE

Objectives

- To restore the chest cavity to its full volume
- To release inhibiting factors in the breathing muscles
- To integrate effective breathing patterns
- To realign the shoulders and ribs

Energy

POSITION

- The client is lying supine on the table, with a bolster under the knees.
- The therapist is standing at the side of the table next to the client's chest.

POLARITY

The left palm is placed over the manubrium, and the right palm slides under the back and is positioned between the shoulder blades. Envisioning the smooth, pump-like motion of the lungs, the therapist's hands move in accordance with the rising and sinking of the client's thorax with each breath. The position is held for at least 1 minute, allowing the client time to relax and focus on the breath.

SHIATSU

Moving to the head of the table, the therapist presses the finger pads into the intercostal spaces on both sides of the upper chest simultaneously to stimulate points on the lung, stomach, and kidney channels (Fig. 6-5). The fingers move to different spaces, covering the upper chest area thoroughly. Each set of fingertip compressions is held for the length of the client's exhalation and is released as the client inhales.

FIGURE 6-4 Stretching the chest and abdominal muscles.

Swedish/Cross Fiber

1. *Shingles Stroke on the Pectoralis Major Muscles.* The therapist stands on the side of the table at the client's shoulder level. One hand is placed on the opposite side of the upper chest from the side on which the therapist is standing, with the heel of the hand against the sternum and the fingers facing the client's shoulder. Perform short, alternate strokes with the palms across the chest to the client's shoulder. Repeat several times.
2. *Pétrissage Strokes on the Pectoralis Major Muscles.* Each side of the chest may be worked individually, or both sides may be worked simultaneously.
3. *Fingertip Raking Across the Upper Chest Muscles.* Slide the fingers in both directions perpendicular to the di-

rection of the pectoralis major muscle. Avoid the breast tissue when working on a woman.

Connective Tissue

Perform the fanning stroke on the upper portion of the chest. Begin with the sides of the thumbs touching each other. The tips of the fingers of both hands may be used as an alternative to the thumbs. Slowly spread them apart, stretching the tissues. Keep the strokes small, spreading the thumbs or fingers 2 or 3 inches apart with each stroke.

Start at the midline of the chest over the sternum, just above the level of the breasts. The fanning strokes move upward toward the clavicles. Repeat the stroke a number of times, covering the entire upper segment of the chest.

FIGURE 6-5 Fingertip compressions in the intercostal spaces.

CASE STUDY 3 The Chest

The client is a 10-year-old boy named Joey, who has asthma. His mother wants him to receive deep tissue therapy to help alleviate the condition and possibly boost his self-esteem. He has been picked on in school because of his small stature and because he cannot participate fully in sports activities.

Postural evaluation of Joey reveals that his chest area is severely constricted. There are noticeable hollow areas under the clavicles and along the borders of the anterior deltoids, indicating that the pectoralis minor muscles are extremely contracted. The central sternal region of the chest is lifted, but in a strained manner as a result of the boy's conscious attempt to make himself appear bigger. This position of the chest may also partly be a consequence of struggling to breathe during asthma attacks.

The focus of the session was to relieve tension in the chest and ease restrictions in the breathing muscles. The boy, being rather shy, was afraid to be left alone; therefore, his mother sat in on the session. Based on observation and the information gathered about his asthmatic condition, the areas chosen to focus on included the pectoralis major and minor, subclavius, scalenes, intercostals, and diaphragm. A connective tissue approach to these muscles was mandated because of the child's age and his sensitivity to touch in the chest area.

Joey responded well to the front to back polarity contact on his sternum and upper back. He visibly relaxed, and his breath deepened. Swedish massage strokes were used to warm up the muscles thoroughly before the deep tissue/connective tissue strokes were applied. The deep tissue protocol was followed, but with full attention given to sensing a melting of the tissues before applying any further pressure or moving through the muscle fibers.

The chest muscles were released in layers, from superficial to deep. Many trigger points were encountered in the intercostal muscles. As a trigger point was pressed, Joey was encouraged to breathe deeply and imagine the point melting. He enjoyed participating in the process and felt a sense of accomplishment when the uncomfortable feelings generated by the trigger points dissolved. The diaphragm was contacted and massaged very carefully. (It is not advised to work that area intensively on children because much of their muscular tension is emotionally rooted and deep, aggressive work on the diaphragm confronts that tension too strongly.[1] See Kogan[2] for Reich's caution to therapists about approaching the diaphragm aggressively.)

The session was concluded with long, Swedish strokes along the erector spinae and with fingertip raking into the intercostal spaces between the ribs in the back to balance the release work performed on the front of the chest cavity. After the session, Joey's mood was much lighter. He was thrilled to be able to take fuller breaths without struggling, and he commented to his mother how much broader his chest and shoulders felt. He was extremely proud of himself. Joey was shown the door frame stretches for the chest muscles, and it was suggested that he practice them every day to maintain the newfound length in his pectoralis major and minor muscles.

Topics for Discussion

1. Give at least three reasons for beginning a series of deep tissue sessions with chest work.
2. Describe several possible manifestations of chest constriction along with the muscles involved.
3. What precautions should be taken when performing deep tissue therapy on the diaphragm muscle?
4. How might restricted breathing patterns be revealed by observing a client's thorax?
5. Where are the most likely areas for trigger points to form in the thoracic region, and why?

The intention is to free the fascia of the upper thorax, creating a sense of lift in the chest.

Deep Tissue/Neuromuscular Therapy

SEQUENCE

1. Pectoralis major (attachments and belly)
2. Subclavius
3. Intercostal muscles (from supine and side position) 💿
4. Diaphragm 💿
5. Back muscles (serratus posterior superior and inferior)

It is likely that the chest muscles will be restricted in many areas, because the breathing mechanism is compromised in the majority of the adult population as a result of stress and the lack of encouragement of full expression of feeling and sensation. The release of trigger points not only assists in opening up the breathing but also is instrumental in rebalancing the shoulder girdle and freeing the ribs.

1. Pectoralis Major (Attachments and Belly)

Origin: Clavicular—medial half of the clavicle. **Sternal**—sternum to the seventh rib, cartilages of upper six ribs.

Insertion: Lateral lip of the bicipital groove of the humerus.

Action: Adduction of shoulder. Medial rotation of shoulder. **Clavicular**—shoulder flexion, medial rotation of shoulder, horizontal adduction of humerus. **Sternal**—adduction of humerus diagonally downward, anterior shoulder stabilizer.

Pectoralis Major (Origin)

Strokes

- Elongation stroke on the sternum, just lateral to the midline, from the xiphoid process to the manubrium, using the fingers or the thumb (Fig. 6-6).
- Elongation stroke along the inferior border of the medial half of the clavicle, using the fingers or the thumb. Move medial to lateral. Feel for small knots and stringy fibers. If they are tender or refer pain, work on them with cross fiber strokes and direct compression.
- Insertion of the pectoralis major. Perform the side to side stroke and static compression with the fingers on the lateral lip of the bicipital groove of the humerus (Fig. 6-7). To locate it, take the client's arm to an abducted position. Slide your fingers along the border of the pectoralis major and the anterior deltoid to reach the point of attachment on the humerus. It is superior to the deltoid tuberosity on the lateral lip of the bicipital groove. Check for trigger points. If any are found, hold them for 8 to 12 seconds while checking with the client about the level of pain reduction.

Pectoralis Major (Belly)

There are three sections to the pectoralis major muscle. They are named after their sites of origin: clavicular, sternal, and costal. Trigger points in the upper or clavicular portion may be found along the lateral border, underneath the edge of the anterior deltoid

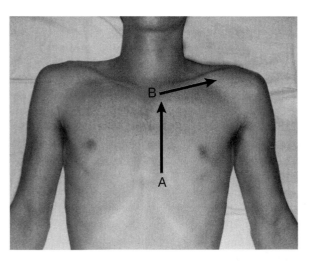

FIGURE 6-6 Directions of elongation strokes on the sternal and clavicular attachments of the pectoralis major.

FIGURE 6-7 Contacting the insertion of the pectoralis major on the lateral lip of the bicipital groove of the humerus.

muscle. They refer pain throughout the anterior deltoid and into the area of the pectoralis major near the trigger point.

Trigger points in the sternal section tend to accumulate in the medial and lateral portions between ribs 3, 4, and 5, near the insertion points of pectoralis minor. Check along the inferior border of the costal section of the muscle for trigger points. The pain pattern is into the front of the chest and down the arm.

Trigger points in the lower section of the muscle tend to form along the lateral border. They refer pain into the breast and nipple.

Heavy lifting, prolonged holding of the arms in an abducted position, and emotional stress may all contribute to the formation of trigger points in this muscle.

Strokes

- The client's arm is still in the abducted position. Using your knuckles, perform the elongation stroke from the sternum to the insertion on the humerus in several strips (Fig. 6-8). Begin the first strip just inferior to the clavicle. Begin the last strip across the muscle at the xiphoid process.
- With a female client, the knuckle stroke should only be done on the upper chest, superior to the breast tissue. At the level of the breast, stroke outward, using the fingers or thumb, from the sternum to the medial border of the breast.

2. Subclavius (Fig. 6-9)

Origin: Upper border of the first rib.

Insertion: Groove on the inferior surface of the clavicle.

Action: Depresses and moves the clavicle forward. Stabilizes the clavicle during shoulder movements.

FIGURE 6-8 Elongation stroke on the clavicular, sternal, and costal sections of the pectoralis major.

A commonly occurring trigger point is found on the medial side of the muscle, near the manubrium. Its referral zone is along the inferior border of the clavicle and down the arm into the thumb side of the hand.

Strokes
- Stand at the side of the table, and face the inferior border of the client's clavicle. The client's arm is flexed at

90°. Hold it slightly inferior to the elbow. Drawing the clavicle slightly away from the chest wall for easier access to the subclavius muscle, traction the arm toward the ceiling.
- Using the pads of the index and middle fingers or the pad of the thumb, stroke under the inferior border of the clavicle from the medial to the lateral end.

3. Intercostal Muscles

Origin: External—from the lower border of each of the upper 11 ribs. **Internal**—from the cartilages to the angles of the upper 11 ribs.
Insertion: External—superior border of the rib below the origin. **Internal**—superior border of the rib below the origin.
Action: External—elevation of ribs during inspiration. **Internal**—depression of ribs during exhalation.

Intercostals (Supine Position)

Trigger points are likely to be found in concentration along the borders of the ribs where the intercostal muscles attach. Contracted muscles related to inhibited breathing are the probable cause of their formation.

Strokes
- Begin at the base of the rib cage, in the rib space between the 10th and 9th ribs. Place your fingers between the two ribs. Allow the fingers to sink into the tissues until resistance is met (Fig. 6-10).
- Perform a short side to side stroke, feeling for deviations in the tissues (i.e., stringy fibers, tiny knots). Hold with static compression on tender points until pain diminishes. The thumbs may be used instead of the fingers if more pressure is required.

FIGURE 6-9 Accessing the subclavius.

FIGURE 6-10 Releasing the intercostals (supine position).

- Continue with this procedure, working between each pair of ribs, to the clavicle. Be thorough.

Intercostals (Side Posture)

Position

- The client is put in side posture, with the knees flexed and a pillow placed between them. The top arm is positioned in front of the client, allowing access to the side of the chest. A pillow may be placed under the side of the head for comfort.
- The therapist stands behind the client.

Strokes

- Perform fanning strokes with the fingers or heels of the hand in a superior direction on the side of the chest, from the base of the rib cage to the axilla, to soften the superficial fascia and prepare the tissues for deeper work.
- Find the space between ribs 10 and 9 (Fig. 6-11). Sink the fingers into the tissues until resistance is met, and begin short side to side strokes, working the intercostals in sections. Continue, working in each rib space, to the top of the axilla to reach the spaces between the upper ribs.

4. Diaphragm

Origin: Sternal part—inner surface of the xiphoid process. **Costal part**—inner surfaces of the cartilages of ribs 7–12. **Lumbar part**—L1–L3 vertebrae.

Insertion: Central tendon.

Action: Increases volume of the thoracic cavity on inspiration by drawing the central tendon down.

> **An active trigger point along the diaphragm attachment on the underside of the costal cartilage may be found approximately 1 inch lateral to the xiphoid process.**

DAR

FIGURE 6-11 Releasing the intercostals from side posture.

FIGURE 6-12 The diaphragm release.

Position

- The client is placed back in a supine position with a bolster under the knees.
- The therapist is standing at the side of the table facing the client's rib cage.

Strokes

- With the palm supinated, slide your fingers under the border of the costal cartilage of ribs 7–10, just lateral to the xiphoid process. The finger pads must stay in contact with the underside of the costal cartilage to avoid pressing into the underlying organs. Take time to let the fingers sink into the tissues (Fig. 6-12).

> **Avoid pressing directly on the xyphoid process, because it is not well supported.**

- Do short, side to side motions with your fingers, feeling for tightness and trigger point activity. Move laterally along the border. Place the palm of your nonworking hand over the lower ribs to give additional support to the upward pressure of your working hand.
- Work with the client's breath. On the exhalation, sink into the tissues with your fingers until resistance is felt. On the inhalation, allow the client's abdomen to push your fingers out from under the ribs.

5. Back Muscles

Position

- The client is lying supine.
- The therapist is standing or sitting at the side of the table.

Serratus Posterior Superior

Origin: Spinous processes of the C7 and the T1–T3 vertebrae. Ligamentum nuchae.

Insertion: Upper borders of ribs 2–5, just lateral to their angles.

Action: Elevates upper ribs. Possible assistance in inspiration.

This muscle may house a trigger point just medial to the superior angle of the scapula. It is a common cause of shoulder pain. The pain is felt deep, under the upper portion of the scapula. It can also extend over the posterior deltoid and down the triceps.

Strokes
- Slide your hands under the client's back at the level of the upper thoracic spine (T1–T3). Beginning at the spinous processes, perform short back and forth motions with your finger pads moving toward the vertebral border of the scapula.
- Hold static compression over sensitive points as the client breathes deeply.
- As an alternative move, use the knuckles instead of the fingers.

Serratus Posterior Inferior
Origin: Spinous processes of T11–T12 and L1–L2 vertebrae.
Insertion: Inferior borders of ribs 9–12, lateral to their angles.
Action: Depresses lower ribs and moves them dorsally. Possible assistance in expiration.

 To locate trigger points, examine the serratus posterior inferior's attachments along the inferior borders of ribs 9–12. The pain pattern is throughout the muscle itself and over the lower ribs.

Strokes
- Slide your hands under the client's back at the level of the lower thoracic and upper lumbar vertebrae (T11–T12 and L1–L2). (If the client is too large or heavy to slide your hands under his or her trunk effectively, you may position the client in side posture to release the serratus posterior superior and inferior muscles.) Beginning at the spinous processes, perform short back and forth motions with your finger pads in a diagonally upward direction, toward the muscle's insertion on the inferior borders of ribs 9–12 (Fig. 6-13).

⚠ When performing the strokes on ribs 11 and 12, be careful to contact only the inferior edge of the ribs. Do not press down on the body of the ribs, because they have little support underneath them.

- Hold with static compression over sensitive points as the client breathes deeply.
- As an alternative procedure, use the knuckles instead of the fingers.

STRETCH

1. The therapist stands at the head of the table. The client extends his or her arms overhead toward the therapist. Take hold of the client's arms slightly superior to the elbow joints. Pull the arms toward you and slightly

David Rini

FIGURE 6-13 Hand position for accessing the serratus posterior inferior along ribs 9–12.

downward while the client takes full breaths, focusing on expanding the chest (Fig. 6-14).
2. The client turns onto his or her side, with the knees flexed. The client's straightened superior arm reaches behind him. The therapist stands behind the client's

FIGURE 6-14 Thoracic stretch with the client supine.

David Rini

FIGURE 6-15 Pectoralis major stretch in side posture.

shoulder. Hold the extended arm, and slowly increase the stretch while your fist is placed against the client's scapula to prevent the client from rolling backward too far (Fig. 6-15). This position stretches the pectoralis major muscle.

ACCESSORY WORK

1. Perform an elongation stroke on the erector spinae and paraspinal muscles. Using the forearm, begin the stroke between the scapula and spinous processes on one side of the back. The forearm is parallel to the spine until you clear the inferior angle of the scapula. Then, it is rotated perpendicular to the spine to make contact with a broader section of the back. Continue the stroke to the iliac crest of the pelvis (Fig. 6-16). Repeat on the other side of the back.
2. Press points along the inferior border of the 12th rib, which is near the attachment of the diaphragm muscle (Fig. 6-17). Both sides may be palpated simultaneously. Begin with the thumbs on either side of T12, and move them apart laterally.

3. Concentrate on diaphragm reflex points on the foot (Fig. 6-18). Press points along the diaphragm line on the plantar surface of the foot, moving medial to lateral. The line is located slightly inferior to the metatarsal bones, and it runs all the way across

FIGURE 6-16 Elongation stroke for the erector spinae muscles.

FIGURE 6-17 Pressure points for diaphragm release.

FIGURE 6-18 Reflex zone for the diaphragm.

the surface of the foot. It is easy to distinguish, because the color of the skin is darker above the diaphragm line and lighter below it.

CLOSING

Sitting at the foot of the table, lightly hold the heels of the client's feet in your hands for 30 to 60 seconds. Remove your hands slowly.

The Back and Spine

■ GENERAL CONCEPTS

The spine acts as the primary support structure for the entire body. Proper alignment of the spine is essential so that it can carry the weights that are connected to it (the head, rib cage, and pelvis) without producing stress in the muscles of the trunk. A poised, balanced spine results in the effortless elongation of the trunk that is associated with correct posture. The muscles attached to the spine must be free of restrictions to achieve the equalization of forces along the spinal column that is necessary for a balanced relationship between its components. This is the next goal in the deep tissue series.

The spine is constructed so that many muscles and ligaments attach to it in a lattice-like pattern, allowing a great deal of mobility and flexibility. The spinal column is capable of forward and side flexion, extension, and rotation. One reason for this tremendous movement versatility is to protect the spinal cord. The spinal column's high degree of flexibility reduces the risk of spinal cord and nerve injuries.

■ MUSCULOSKELETAL ANATOMY AND FUNCTION

Spinal Column

The spinal column consists of 33 bones. There are 7 cervical vertebrae, 12 thoracic vertebrae, 5 lumbar vertebrae, and at birth, 5 modified sacral vertebrae and 4 small vertebral remnants forming the coccyx. The bones of both the sacrum and the coccyx fuse later in life, leaving 24 functional vertebrae in the adult. There are also 23 intervertebral disks sandwiched between the vertebral bones (Essential Anatomy Box 6-3 and Fig. 6-19).

Most vertebrae are composed of two parts, a round body and a posterior segment, called the vertebral arch. The vertebral arch is a complex structure. It includes the spinous and transverse processes, which provide attachment sites for many muscles and ligaments. The opening between the vertebral body and arch is called the vertebral foramen. Lined up within the spinal column, the foramen form a tunnel, called the vertebral canal, within which the

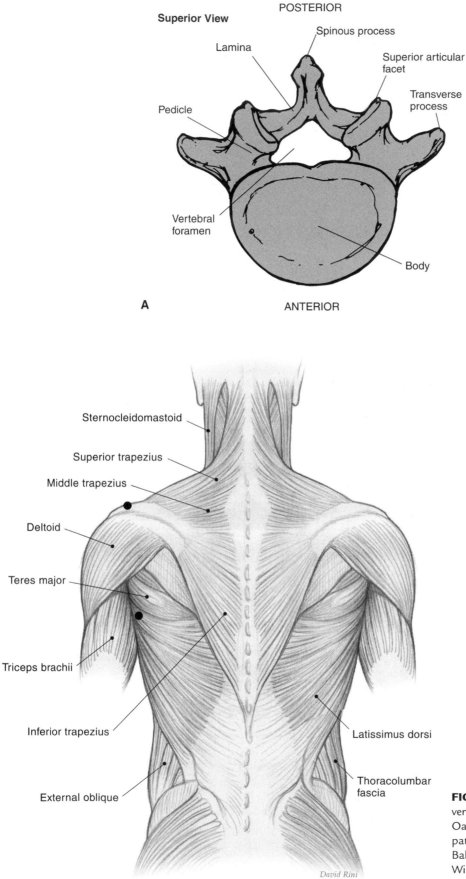

Superior View

POSTERIOR

Lamina

Spinous process

Superior articular facet

Transverse process

Pedicle

Vertebral foramen

Body

A

ANTERIOR

Sternocleidomastoid

Superior trapezius

Middle trapezius

Deltoid

Teres major

Triceps brachii

Inferior trapezius

External oblique

Latissimus dorsi

Thoracolumbar fascia

David Rini

B

FIGURE 6-19 A. Superior view of lumbar vertebra. (Reprinted with permission from Oatis CA. Kinesiology: the mechanics and pathomechanics of human movement. Baltimore, MD: Lippincott Williams & Wilkins, 2004.) **B.** Muscles of the back—superficial layer with areas of possible trigger point formation.

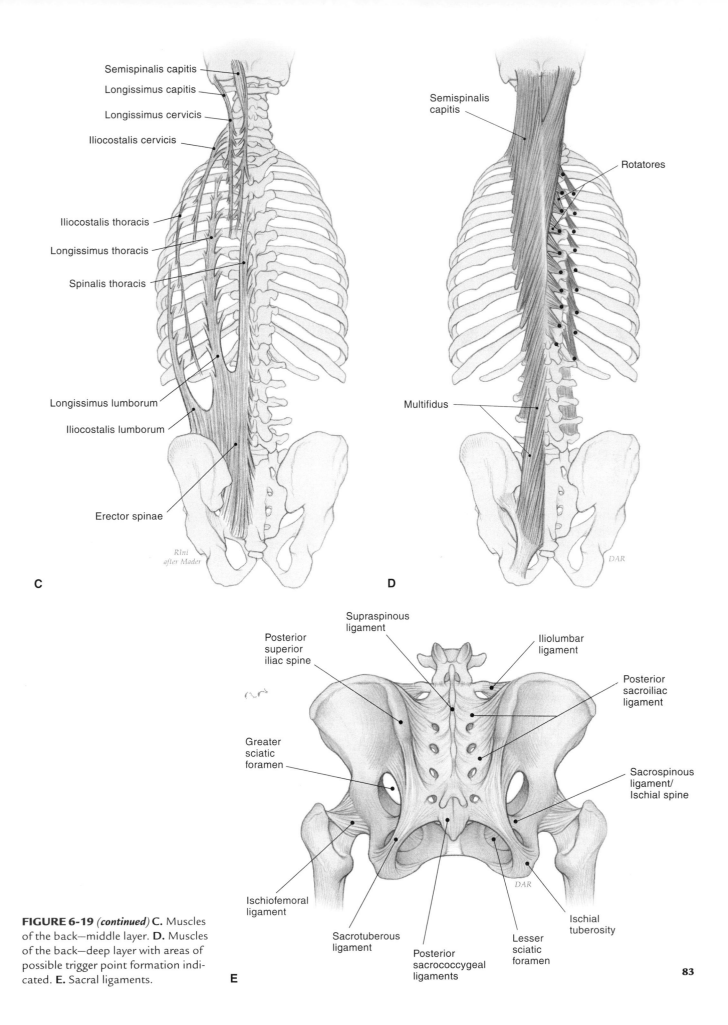

Semispinalis capitis
Longissimus capitis
Longissimus cervicis
Iliocostalis cervicis

Iliocostalis thoracis
Longissimus thoracis
Spinalis thoracis

Longissimus lumborum
Iliocostalis lumborum

Erector spinae

Rlni after Mader

C

Semispinalis capitis

Rotatores

Multifidus

DAR

D

Supraspinous ligament
Posterior superior iliac spine
Iliolumbar ligament
Posterior sacroiliac ligament
Greater sciatic foramen
Sacrospinous ligament/ Ischial spine
Ischiofemoral ligament
Sacrotuberous ligament
Posterior sacrococcygeal ligaments
Lesser sciatic foramen
Ischial tuberosity

DAR

E

FIGURE 6-19 *(continued)* **C.** Muscles of the back—middle layer. **D.** Muscles of the back—deep layer with areas of possible trigger point formation indicated. **E.** Sacral ligaments.

BOX 6-3 ESSENTIAL ANATOMY

The Back/Spinal Column Routine

MUSCLES
Trapezius
Latissimus dorsi
Erector spinae
Rhomboid minor
Rhomboid major
Intercostals
Quadratus lumborum
Sacral ligaments

BONES AND LANDMARKS
Vertebral column
Spinous processes
Transverse processes
Lamina groove
Scapula
Ribs
Iliac crest
Sacrum
Coccyx

---

spinal cord is located. Please refer to Figure 6-19A for an illustration of a vertebra.

The vertebral bodies are separated by collagenous disks. The two components of the disk are a central, compressed fluid core, called the nucleus pulposus, and a fibrous covering, called the annulus fibrosus. The disks act as cushions, helping to transfer weight evenly between the vertebrae and preventing adjacent bones from rubbing against each other. The disks in the lumbar and cervical segments of the spine are thicker in relation to the height of the vertebrae, allowing greater movement between the individual vertebrae, but the disks in the thoracic segment are smaller, decreasing the amount of possible motion. When adjacent vertebrae are properly aligned, compression on the intervertebral disk is distributed evenly, allowing a smooth downward transfer of weight.

Vertebrae that are chronically displaced put uneven pressure on the intervertebral disk that is sandwiched between them, causing it to bulge and, possibly, to slip out of position. This can produce pain if the disk presses against a nerve. It also diminishes the ability of the disk to maintain space between the vertebral bodies, another major source of spinal pain.

One of the spinal column's primary functions is to provide an anchor of support and stability for the cranium, thorax, and pelvis. These body segments are displaced along the spinal column in the sense that none falls directly through the body's central line of gravity. Therefore, to support them effectively, the spinal column is composed of a series of four opposing curves that offset the uneven size and placement of these three weights (Fig. 6-20).

There are two concave curves, the cervical and the lumbar, and two convex curves, the thoracic and the sacral. This is an ingenious design, creating continuity of weight transfer throughout the spinal column. The

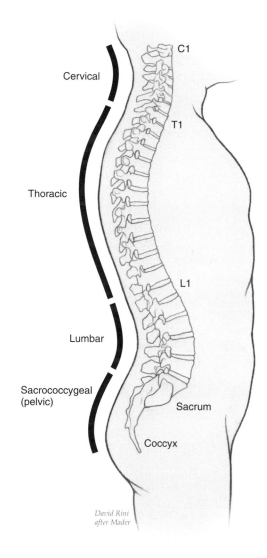

FIGURE 6-20 The four counterbalancing spinal curves.

vertebrae where the curves change (C7–T1, T12–L1, and L5–S1) bear the greatest weight load and must remain aligned for the spine to act as an integrated, stress-free unit.

Mechanically speaking, all the bony weights of the trunk should be placed as close to the central axis of the body and as close to each other as possible to minimize stress on the weight-bearing spine. This is an important factor in determining correct posture and movement. For this balance to occur, the soft tissues of the back must be able to contract and lengthen freely to accommodate all the shifts of weight and movements that are necessary to maintain this dynamic equilibrium.

Although the spine is referred to as a column, this is not a completely accurate description. A column transfers weight vertically through its central axis by internal compression of its structural components. It does not rely on outside forces to distribute weight. The spine does not function this way. Because of its curved design, it is not aligned with the body's central axis and, therefore, cannot maintain balance on its own. It must rely on the aid of the attached muscles, which constantly transfer and redistribute forces to maintain equilibrium of the trunk.

The concept of tensegrity provides a more precise description of the relationship between the bones and muscles of the back.[3] In a tensegrity structure, weight is transferred through the tension members, or the stretching components of the structure, rather than through the compression members. The compression members act as spacers and points of attachment for the tension components to maintain the necessary shape and distribution of force in the structure. An example of this design in architecture is the geodesic dome.

In the back, the bones serve as the compression members. The spine, ribs, cranium, and pelvis act as spacers, maintaining the proper lengths for the muscles that are attached to them, which serve as the tension members. Thus, the bones are suspended in a web of soft tissue support. When the muscles become chronically shortened and dysfunctional, they are unable to distribute weight effectively, and the spine begins to act more like a compression-style column, setting the stage for breakdown and injury.

Chronic compression of the spine is the cause of many back difficulties. The ligaments, which are the reinforcing supports for the spine, and the intervertebral disks take over the job of transferring weight, which should be done by the muscles. The ligaments may become inflamed and even tear, because they have to reinforce and carry weight beyond the maximum load they were designed to support. The disks become chronically compressed, losing their springiness and ability to cushion the vertebrae.

Spinal Muscles

The muscles that move the spine consist of two groups, the superficial and the deep paraspinal muscles. The superficial group is called the **erector spinae** (Fig. 6-19C). It is made up of three muscles, the **iliocostalis**, **longissimus**, and **spinalis**. Depending on their location along the spine, these muscles are subdivided into segments called the **cervicis**, **thoracis**, and **lumborum**. They span the entire length of the back with iliocostalis lumborum, extending all the way down to the sacrum.

The longissimus and iliocostalis muscles are the strongest of the group as well as the most likely to be injured and to develop trigger points. The spinalis is a smaller and weaker muscle. It is the most medially placed, attaching to the spinous processes of the L2–T2 vertebrae. Collectively, the erector spinae muscles extend the vertebral column. The iliocostalis and longissimus are also responsible for lateral flexion of the spinal column.

The deep paraspinal muscles, also known as the transversospinalis muscles, connect the transverse processes of the vertebrae to the spinous processes in a layered, upwardly angled pattern. From the most superficial to the deepest-lying, they are the **semispinalis**, **multifidi**, and **rotatores** (Fig. 6-19D). The semispinalis span five to six vertebrae. The multifidi span three vertebrae, and the rotatores connect adjacent vertebrae. All three muscles extend, laterally flex, and rotate the vertebrae. They also serve to elongate the spinal column. These muscles are active most of the time, because they are responsible for maintaining the alignment of the spinal column as the body shifts its position.

A primary purpose of deep tissue therapy on the back is to relieve compression and other stresses along the spine by re-establishing effective muscle function. Massage work, along with exercise and proper spinal mechanics, can help to relieve the majority of back problems.

■ SOURCES OF BACK PROBLEMS

The underlying cause of most back pain is instability of the spinal joints.[4] The disks and ligaments alone provide minimal support for the amount of force exerted on the vertebral joints in everyday movements. Adjacent spinal vertebrae are constantly adapting to the body's many movements through minute amounts of sliding and tilting motions in relation to each other. Too much play between vertebrae disrupts the integrity of the joint, resulting in tissue damage and potential nerve impingement.

Tests have shown that ligament damage can occur with as little as 15 pounds of force placed on a spinal joint.[2] The spinal column must be able to absorb several hundred pounds of force; such an amount is easily generated during broad, strenuous movements. The support required to brace the spinal joints against this kind of stress is provided primarily by the paraspinal muscles, which connect the vertebrae as described above, along with other stabilizing muscles of the trunk.

Besides providing secondary support, one of the major functions of the disks and ligaments is to sense the positions of the vertebrae through a feedback connection with the nervous system.[5] When stress is placed on a spinal joint and the vertebrae are close to moving beyond a safe proximity to each other, messages from the nervous system activate stabilizing muscles to support the areas of the spine that are under duress. The most important stabilizing muscles of the spine are the multifidi, transverse abdominus, quadratus lumborum, and psoas.

Trauma placed on the spine, as well as the normal wear and tear of age, can damage disks and ligaments, interfering with their ability to send position-sensing information to the nervous system. When this occurs, the stabilizing muscles do not activate, creating spinal instability and its related problems. Lack of support from the stabilizing muscles causes the outer layer muscles that control large movements of the spinal column (the erector spinae muscles) to forcibly contract, resulting in a protective splinting action to prevent further damage to the weakened area. This phenomenon is commonly known as a muscle spasm.

Traditional rehabilitative therapy for back pain has focused on strengthening the erector spinae muscles, primarily in an attempt to provide support for the spine and to prevent future stress. Recent research has revealed that a focus on isolating and strengthening the middle layer support muscles, especially the multifidi and transverse abdominus muscles, is much more effective in reducing back pain and minimizing incidents of future spinal stress.[6] Programs that target awareness and control of the stabilizing muscles as well as provide educational information about proper spinal mechanics have been very effective in promoting long-term relief of back pain.

Possible Causes of Spinal Trauma

- Improper standing and sitting postures contribute to strain in the soft tissues around the spine. Many people wear shoes with high heels, which throw the body forward of the line of gravity. To remain upright, the upper back is brought backward, causing an increased lumbar curve with resulting compression in the soft tissues.
- Sitting in a slumped position with the low back rounded is a common habit. This position eliminates the proper lumbar curve. The vertebrae are no longer aligned, placing stress on the surrounding ligaments and muscles.

- Incorrect lifting techniques are a major cause of back strain. The spine should always maintain its integrity as a unit during any kind of lifting activity. The only flexing of the upper body that should occur during lifting is at the hip joints. Many people bend at the waist when reaching to pick up something. Bending at the waist throws a tremendous amount of pressure onto the disks and soft tissues of the low back, which are not designed to pull heavy weights when bringing the spine upright. To lift properly, persons should always bend from the legs rather than from the low back, bring the object as close to the body as possible before lifting it, and then push up to a standing position using the thigh muscles and keeping the back straight.
- Lack of exercise causes weakness in the abdominal muscles, which help to support the low back. If the psoas muscle is tight, it will also cause tightness and compression in the low back. Short, restricted hamstring muscles pull the pelvis downward, which reduces the lumbar curve and places stress on the ligaments of the low back.
- A sudden, unexpected movement or force, such as slipping on a wet floor or even sneezing (particularly if the back is already in a weakened condition), can result in muscle spasms and tears. Unfortunately, most furniture is not designed to position the spine properly. Most people find themselves slumping in it, which again compromises the lumbar curve and weakens the low back.

■ CONDITIONS

1. *Scoliosis* is a lateral curve, or curves, of the spine.
   a. Functional scoliosis originates from factors other than structural deformity in the spinal column itself. Imbalances in the feet and legs, such as a pronated foot or one leg being shorter than the other, can cause a lateral pelvic tilt, which leads to lateral spinal curvature. Unequal degrees of strength in the right and left psoas muscles will cause them to pull on the pelvis unevenly, resulting in pelvic rotation, which also leads to lateral spinal curvature. Muscular asymmetry as a result of dominant handedness also creates scoliosis. Functional scoliosis disappears when the factors that are distorting to the spine are eliminated.
   b. Structural scoliosis is a permanent condition that indicates a bony deformity, usually congenital. In severe cases, the vertebrae rotate, causing the rib cage to distort. The curvature remains no matter what position the person assumes.

   There may or may not be pain accompanying scoliosis. If the curve is long-standing, the person's musculature has probably adapted to the condition. Muscles on the concave side of the curve will be shortened.

Muscles on the convex side of the curve will be stretched.

2. *Kyphosis* is an exaggerated posterior thoracic spinal curve causing a rounded or humpbacked look in the upper back. The myofascial tissues of the upper back tend to become hardened and adhere to each other as a result of chronic compression. Contributing factors can include poor postural habits, poor nutrition, osteoporosis, or systemic disorders causing a deterioration of the spine.

3. *Lordosis* is an abnormal curvature in the lumbar portion of the spine. It results in compression of the lumbar intervertebral disks and the surrounding musculature. Some contributing factors are wearing high-heeled shoes, having shortened iliopsoas muscles, and having tight rectus femoris muscles. Most children exhibit a degree of lordosis that they outgrow.

4. *Damage to the intervertebral disks* can result from a variety of causes. Structural imbalances, such as leg length differences, pelvic rotation, and scoliosis, may lead to wear and tear on the disks. Muscle imbalance, poor posture, incorrect lifting habits, excess weight, and trauma resulting from accidents are other common causes of disk problems. Disk injury is accompanied by pain that can be sudden or gradual in onset. Progressive weakness on one side of the body in muscles that control the lower limb along with sensations of tingling, numbness, or pain are characteristic of disk injury.

Some common types of disk injury include:

a. *Degeneration*. This is a deterioration of the material of the disk. It is often caused by dehydration as a result of chronic squeezing of the disk and inadequate intake of water.

b. *Rupture*. This condition is also referred to as a herniated or protruding disk. It means that either the internal nucleus or the surrounding fibers of the disk have moved out of position. The lay term for this condition is slipped disk.

5. *Muscle spasm*. This is a protective reaction to, rather than a cause of, damage in the back. Causative factors can include torn ligaments, damage to disks, muscle sprain (refers to injury to muscle fibers), or stretching of the joints. Left untreated, muscle spasm will contribute to back pain. Treatment includes massage, application of ice, and mild stretching.

Please refer to Indications/Contraindications Box 6-4 for a list of other indications and contraindications.

■ POSTURAL EVALUATION

The client is standing and facing away from the therapist so that the back may be observed.

1. Imagine a vertical line running down the spine, or have the person's spine lined up to a plumb line, dividing the back into left and right segments.
   - Check for balance of the musculature on the right and left sides.
   - Observe underdevelopment and/or overdevelopment of muscles.
2. Check for exaggeration or underdevelopment of the spinal curves.
   - Sacral
   - Lumbar
   - Thoracic
   - Cervical
3. Note if any vertebrae are protruding or sunken. This is determined by observing or palpating the spinous processes.
4. Check for evenness in the height of the iliac crests.
5. Look for scoliosis. Lack of symmetry in the musculature on the left and right sides may be an indication of this condition. To confirm this, run your fingers down

---

BOX 6-4 INDICATIONS/CONTRAINDICATIONS

Conditions Affecting Back Massage

INDICATIONS	CONTRAINDICATIONS
Tension	Inflammation
Chronic back pain	Sunburn
Scoliosis	Rashes
Pelvic tilt	Recent trauma
Back injury	Severe hypertension
Back surgery	High fever
Open heart surgery	Severe bruises
Fatigue	

As mentioned previously, the spine is the major support structure of the body. Strength of character is often judged by the degree of strength exhibited by the back.

We speak of a courageous, forthright person as "having a strong backbone." Someone who is considered to be weak or cowardly is labeled as "spineless."

A baby's spine is extremely flexible, because the muscles around it have not yet developed the strength to support it and the balancing spinal curves have not yet formed.

Newborn infants are almost completely helpless. They cannot sit up or hold the weight of the head and thorax through the spine. Children's early movements of kicking and squirming are necessary to develop the musculature of the pelvis and low back. By exploring and exerting themselves through movement, infants gradually develop the core strength of support. Even the actions of crying and screaming are important in building up the muscles that will stabilize the necessary lumbar curve so that the child can hold the head up and, eventually, be able to sit and stand without aid.

When lying on the abdomen, a very young baby cannot lift his or her head off the floor. It is a great accomplishment when infants can finally pull the trunk up and be able to look around. As they survey the world around them, they are beginning the first stages of asserting themselves as individuals. Contractions of the extensor muscles control the lift and arching motion of the spine. The stance of opening the chest and stretching the arms back is associated with joy, expansion, and self-expression. Moshe Feldenkrais[7] called the extensor muscles the happy muscles, because their use tends to elicit a happy response in individuals throughout life.

When the body is open and lifted, we make ourselves available to receive and interact with the world around us. On the other hand, contraction of the flexor muscles causes the body to be pulled forward and the spine to flex. This position tends to produce feelings of withdrawal, fear, and lack of initiative. Opening and lifting the spine through deep tissue massage can do much to improve a person's self-esteem and tends to improve his or her outlook in general.

It is hoped that as a child develops and grows, the spine and the muscles around it will become strong and supple. The child will then gain a sense of independence and self-reliance. Dr. Ida Rolf[8] referred to the spine and its intrinsic support muscles as the inner core of the body. This core represents our sense of security and our will. When the spine and its associated muscles are weak, there may be a feeling of not being able to stand up for one's self or a lack of trust that one has the inner resources to handle all the conflicts or problems that may arise in life.

The low back acts as a bridge between two solid bony structures, the pelvis and the thorax. It is responsible for mediating feelings between these two areas. Having no bony protection around it, the lumbar spine is rather vulnerable. Pain and tightness in this area may reflect areas of vulnerability within a person. When weakness and degeneration in the lumbar spine are present, it may be beneficial to look at areas in one's life where security and support are not present. This could relate to a person's finances, job, home life, or relationships.

The upper back has a direct structural relationship to the shoulders. Feelings of anger or even rage can lodge in this segment. We tend to "hold back" aggressive actions of the arms, like punching, with the upper back muscles. The thoracic curve corresponds to the heart center. It is usually when the heart center is shut down that hostile and resentful feelings arise.

---

the back, over the spinous processes, and check for lateral deviations.

Refer to Table 6-2 for a description of abnormal spinal curvatures and muscles that are possibly involved.

■ EXERCISES AND SELF-TREATMENT

Deep Breathing on All-Fours

This exercise emphasizes the stabilizing action of the transverse abdominus and multifidus muscles. It may be incorporated during the exercises on the ball described below (Fig. 6-21).

Position—Kneel on your hands and knees, with the spine in a neutral position parallel to the floor.

Execution—Inhale deeply, allowing the chest to expand and the abdomen to relax. Exhale, lifting the navel toward the spine and allowing the abdominal wall to partially contract. Do not alter the position of the spinal column. Maintain this lift of the navel for 5 to 10 breaths. If low back pain is present, focus on contracting the multifidus muscles attaching to the vertebrae at the level of the injury. Try to keep the other multifidus muscles relaxed. This precise muscular isolation is difficult to achieve but with practice can be accomplished.

TABLE 6–2	Body Reading for the Back
Conditions	**Muscles That May Be Shortened**
Scoliosis	Muscles on concave sides of the spinal curves:
	Erector spinae
	Paraspinal muscles
	Check for lateral imbalances in:
	Iliopsoas
	Quadratus lumborum
	Biceps femoris
Kyphosis	Capital extensors
	Neck extensors
	Pectoralis minor
	Anterior deltoid
Lordosis	Iliacus
	Psoas major
	Rectus femoris
	Quadratus lumborum

FIGURE 6-21 Exhaling in the all-fours position, isolating the transverse abdominus and affected multifidus muscles.

Exercises Using a Ball

Incorporating a fitness ball into a back training program is beneficial because the act of maintaining the ball in a stable position during the exercises engages the primary stabilizing muscles that support the spine.

- *One-leg raise* (Fig. 6-22)

    Position—Sit on top of the ball with both feet planted on the ground. Imagine the crown of your head being pulled up toward the ceiling by a thread. Allow your arms to hang at your sides with the hands resting against the ball.

    Execution—Inhale deeply, maintaining an elongated spine. Exhale, raising the right leg several inches off the floor while the navel pulls toward the front of the spine. Inhale, lowering the right foot back to the floor. Repeat the lift with the left leg. Perform 5 to 10 sets.

- *Rear leg lift* (Fig. 6-23)

    Position—Lie prone on top of the ball with both hands touching the floor in front and both legs extended in back with the toes tucked under, making contact with the floor.

    Execution—Exhale, raising the right leg straight off of the floor with the toes pointed. Inhale, lower the right leg back to the starting position. Repeat the lift with the left leg. Perform 5 to 10 sets.

- *Side stretch for the abdominal muscles and quadratus lumborum* (Fig. 6-24)

    Position—Sit on top of the ball with your arms at your sides and the palms of the hands against the ball.

    Execution—Inhaling, raise the right arm overhead. Exhaling, shift your hips to the right as you extend

FIGURE 6-22 Single leg raise.

FIGURE 6-23 Rear leg lift.

FIGURE 6-24 Side stretch while sitting on the ball.

your right arm toward the left, bringing your navel toward the front of the spine. Use your left hand to brace yourself from sliding off the ball. Hold the stretch for several breaths. To release the stretch, bring the right arm back to your side as you center your pelvis back on top of the ball. Repeat the stretch on the left side.

- *Spinal lift* (Fig. 6-25)

  Position—Lying on your back with your arms on the floor at your sides, place your feet on the ball.

  Execution—Inhale, pressing your palms against the floor. Exhale, raise your pelvis several inches off the floor as you press into the ball with your feet. Pull your navel in toward the front of the spine. Inhaling, lower your hips back down to the floor. Repeat the pelvic lift several times.

- *Forward bend* (Fig. 6-26)

  Position—Sit on the floor with your legs extended in front of you and the ball placed in between them. Place the palms of both hands on the ball.

  Execution—Inhale, elongating the spine toward the ceiling. Exhale, rolling the ball forward with your hands as you flex the torso forward over your extended legs. Draw the navel in toward the front of your spine. Remain in the stretch for several breaths as you visualize extending the crown of the head forward toward the ball.

Release for the Back Muscles

Place two tennis balls under your back, one on either side of the spine, beginning between the shoulder blades. Take deep breaths, allowing the muscles to sink into the balls and visualizing the tension melting. Reposition the balls farther down the spine, and repeat the procedure. Continue, down to the sacrum.

FIGURE 6-25 Spinal lift.

FIGURE 6-26 Stetch for spinal muscles.

CASE STUDY 4 The Back

 The client is a 29-year-old man named Clint, who works in real estate. He has received massage treatments from different therapists on an irregular basis over several years. His goal is to relax and relieve tension in tight neck, shoulder, and back muscles. Clint is tall and muscular. He used to lift weights but quit 4 years ago because he strained his low back and found that weight lifting put stress on his neck muscles. Recently, he has felt the need to return to exercising and has just begun to work out again. He is in good health. His only physical problem is residual tightness in low back muscles from the weight-lifting injury 4 years ago.

Clint's upper body is more developed than his lower body. His shoulders and arms carry more bulk, relatively speaking, than his hip and thigh muscles do. He exhibits a small degree of posterior pelvic tilt. His erector spinae muscles are very pronounced, particularly on the right side. He used to play baseball regularly and exhibits the right side–left side muscular imbalance that one-handed sports generate. His neck appears short as a result of contracted trapezius muscles as well as other shortened head and neck extensors. The focus of this session will be to elongate the spinal column by releasing the erector spinae and deep paraspinal muscles.

During the session, initial work on the back revealed that the superficial musculature was fairly relaxed.

However, the deep muscles along the spine were extremely contracted. The client requested very deep pressure on these muscles. He barely felt any sensation in the deep paraspinal muscles regardless of the depth of pressure. These muscles seemed to be numb. Deep pressure applied with the elbow did not cause the contractions in the muscles to yield. The lack of feeling and response from these muscles seemed to indicate that the tension may be psychologically based. In other words, the client may contract these muscles on a subconscious level to prevent certain feelings from arising to conscious awareness, which is known as armoring.[9]

Although the client wanted very deep pressure applied to these muscles so that he could feel something there other than numbness, the tissues were guarding against the invasion by contracting further. It was explained to the client that this deep, invasive pressure was being counterproductive, and so the pressure was decreased. Although the client could not feel anything in the deep muscles, these muscles relaxed to a small degree when the pressure was lessened.

The session continued with deep tissue strokes applied to the muscles along the entire spinal column. Then, the client turned supine so that balancing work could be applied to the anterior neck and chest areas. Shiatsu compression moves were performed on the legs, and the session was completed with massage of the spinal reflex points on the feet.

After the session, the client described himself as high strung and unable to relax. This description matched the assessment of the condition of the soft tissues of the back. It was suggested that, if interested, he should participate in a yoga class, where he could learn slow, sustained stretching movements along with coordinated deep breathing to begin to relieve some of the deep-seated stress in his intrinsic muscles. Regular yoga practice, along with deep tissue therapy sessions, would help to uncover and release the tightly held tension that had accumulated along his spinal column. The client appreciated the suggestion and added that he had wanted to start taking yoga and this session had been a good incentive for him to follow through on it.

CASE STUDY 4 *(continued)*

Topics for Discussion

1. Describe a viable course of treatment for a client experiencing low back pain, assuming that pain is muscular in origin.
2. What other areas of the body should be included in a session focusing on the spine to achieve an even distribution of forces along the vertebral column?
3. How would you approach a client who cannot feel any response in his back muscles, no matter how much pressure you apply?
4. What self-care suggestions might you give to a client who is experiencing back strain?
5. What are some visual indications of exaggerated curvatures of the spine (kyphotic, scoliotic, or lordotic) in a client who is lying in a prone position?

◼ BACK AND SPINAL COLUMN ROUTINE

Objectives

- To relax the back area, which tends to hold excessive tension
- To lengthen the spine by releasing the muscles that control the position and movement of the vertebrae
- To release the posterior breathing muscles
- To balance the weight segments along the spine (head, thorax, and pelvis)
- To treat tissues that have been strained by back injuries and/or poor postural habits

Energy

POSITION

- The client is lying prone on the table. A bolster may be placed under the ankles and/or the pelvis.

POLARITY

Contact the sacrum and occiput with the palms of your hands. Imagine the spine decompressing and lengthening between your hands. Hold for at least 30 seconds.

SHIATSU

Cat's Paws

With your hands placed on either side of the spine at the level of the upper back, alternately press your palms down

the back, as if walking on your hands. When you reach the iliac crests, bring your hands back to the shoulders, and perform the sequence again, only this time with the hands wider apart (Fig. 6-27).

Swedish/Cross Fiber

1. Perform basic effleurage strokes on the musculature of the back.
2. Stand at the side of the table, and face the client's back. Perform the swim stroke by rolling and spreading your forearms across the back muscles, avoiding pressure on the spinous processes.

FIGURE 6-27 Cat's paws.

3. Apply cross fiber strokes to the erector spinae muscles with the heel of the hand or the knuckles.

Connective Tissue

MYOFASCIAL MOBILIZATION TECHNIQUE

Using the fingers or the palms, roll the muscles of the back over the underlying ribs and vertebrae. Use the myofascial spreading technique on areas of tissue that do not easily slide over the bones.

Deep Tissue/Neuromuscular Therapy

SEQUENCE

1. Erector spinae group
2. Deep paraspinal muscles (the lamina groove) 💿
3. Iliac crest
4. Sacral ligaments
5. Intercostals

Ⓧ Trigger points may be located in any of the musculature of the back, particularly where injuries have occurred and tissues have been damaged. Observe the client's posture and movement patterns. Note where bending and reaching are initiated along the spine. These are stress points and likely candidates for trigger point formation and connective tissue build-up.

1. Erector Spinae Group (Spinalis, Longissimus, Iliocostalis)

Origin: **Iliocostalis lumborum**—external lip of the iliac crest, posterior surface of the sacrum. **Iliocostalis thoracis**—upper borders of ribs 12–7. **Longissimus thoracis**—transverse processes of L1–L5 vertebrae. **Spinalis thoracis**—spinous processes of T11–T12 and L1–L2 vertebrae.

Insertion: **Iliocostalis lumborum**—angles of ribs 6–12. **Iliocostalis thoracis**—transverse process of C7, angles of ribs 1–6. **Longissimus thoracis**—accessory processes of L1–L3 vertebrae, transverse processes of T1–T12 vertebrae, between the tubercles and angles of ribs 2–12. **Spinalis thoracis**—spinous processes of T1–T4 vertebrae.

Action: **Iliocostalis lumborum and thoracis; longissimus thoracis**—extension and lateral flexion of the vertebral column, depression of the ribs. **Spinalis thoracis**—extension and rotation of the vertebral column.

Ⓧ The longissimus and iliocostalis muscles are the most likely sites for trigger point activity. Trigger points in the iliocostalis thoracis at its upper level tend to refer along the scapular border and between the shoulder blades. In the lower portion of the muscles, pain may be referred downward, into the lumbar and hip region and into the abdomen.

Strokes
- Perform elongating strokes down the back and parallel to the spine, beginning at the level of T1 and ending at the iliac crest. Use the base of the palm, forearm, or knuckles (Fig. 6-28). Cover each of the three erector spinae muscles.
- Using the elbow or thumbs, stroke along the borders of the muscles. Begin at the level of T1, and end at the iliac crest.

2. Deep Paraspinal Muscles (Semispinalis, Multifidi, Rotatores)

Origin: **Semispinalis thoracis**—transverse processes of T6–T10 vertebrae. **Semispinalis cervicis**—transverse processes of T1–T5 vertebrae. **Semispinalis capitis**—transverse processes of C4–C7 and T1–T6 vertebrae. **Multifidi**—sacrum to S4 foramen, erector spinae aponeurosis, posterior superior iliac spine, posterior sacroiliac ligaments, mammillary and transverse processes of T1–T12 vertebrae, articular processes of C4–C7 vertebrae. **Rotatores**—transverse process of all vertebrae.

Insertion: **Semispinalis thoracis**—spinous processes of C6–C7 and T1–T4 vertebrae. **Semispinalis cervicis**—spinous processes of C2–C5 vertebrae. **Semispinalis capitis**—occiput, between superior and inferior nuchal

FIGURE 6-28 Elongation stroke on the erector spinae muscles using the base of the palm.

lines. **Multifidi**—spinous process of two to four vertebrae above origin. **Rotatores**—base of spinous process of next highest vertebra.

Action: Extend and rotate vertebral column.

 Trigger points in the semispinalis thoracis often register as a continuous, aching sensation. In the next lower layer, the multifidi, the referral pattern tends to be across the vertebra at the level of the trigger point. At the lowest level, the rotatores, trigger points may be found along the entire length and often create a band of pain across the back at the level of involvement.

Strokes

- Perform elongating strokes down the spine in the space between the spinous processes and the transverse processes of the vertebrae, from T1 to the sacrum (Fig. 6-29). Use the thumbs or the elbow.
- Use static compression and/or short spreading techniques in muscular areas that feel dense, fibrous, or unyielding.
- Place the thumbs end to end at C7 (Fig. 6-30). Do an elongating stroke along the lamina groove of the cervical spine to the occiput. Repeat, using the side to side strokes, along the muscle fibers.

3. Iliac Crest, Iliolumbar Ligament

Position

- Place a pillow under the client's pelvis for the next three sections (iliac crest, iliolumbar ligament, sacral ligaments).

Superior Border of the Iliac Crest

Strokes

- Trace the edge of the iliac crest using the thumbs or the elbow. Feel for congested areas of tissue and/or tender spots.
- Use static compression on tender spots. Do the side to side spreading technique across the congested tissues to release them.

Thoracolumbar Fascia

 This broad band of fascia, covering the low back, attaches to the iliac crest and covers the sacrum. Examine it carefully, because trigger points may be formed anywhere.

FIGURE 6-29 Placement of the thumbs next to the spinous processes to release the deep paraspinal muscles.

David Rini

FIGURE 6-30 Hand placement for releasing the cervical paraspinal muscles.

Iliolumbar Ligament

Strokes

- Find the junction formed by the lumbar spine and the pelvis. Place your elbow into it, pressing inward and downward, at approximately a 45° angle toward the iliac crest (Fig. 6-31).
- Hold, with static compression. Perform short cross fiber strokes.

4. Sacral Ligaments

Strokes

- Warm up the sacral area by applying fingertip friction over the entire sacrum.
- Using the thumbs or fingers, do all the deep tissue spreading techniques over the sacrum (up-down, side-side, and combination) (Fig. 6-32).

FIGURE 6-31 Elbow position for contacting the iliolumbar ligament.

FIGURE 6-32 Directions of strokes on the sacrum.

FIGURE 6-33 Direction of strokes on the intercostal muscles.

5. Intercostals

Strokes

- Stand on the opposite side of the table from the section of ribs on which you are working. Place your fingers just below the inferior angle of the scapula. Moving your fingers back and forth and up and down, feel for the spaces between the ribs.
- Using short back and forth motions, feel for restricted areas in the soft tissues between the ribs (i.e., knots, strings, lumps) (Fig. 6-33). Check for trigger point

activity. The thumbs or a knuckle may be used in the intercostal spaces, where more pressure is required.
- Continue to the 12th rib.

STRETCH

1. Bring the client's knees to his or her chest. Either holding the client's knees with your hands or by pressing your forearm against them, slowly lean forward, flexing the thighs to the chest (Fig. 6-34). This stretches the client's low back muscles.
2. Reaching across the table, press down on the client's shoulder to stabilize it against the table. With your other hand, slowly pull the client's knees toward you and down toward the table, creating a twist for the spine and back muscles (Fig. 6-35).
3. Have the client hold the knees to the chest. Standing at the head of the table, hold the client's head in your hands. Traction the neck very slightly by drawing the head toward you, then by lifting the head off the table and bringing the forehead toward the knees. This stretches the upper back muscles.

ACCESSORY WORK

1. *Occipital Release.* Sitting at the head of the table, slide your fingers under the client's occipital ridge and lift the head slightly (Fig. 6-36). Wait for the muscles to soften and for the sensation of an even pulse on both sides of the occiput.

FIGURE 6-34 Stretching the client's low back.

David Rini

FIGURE 6-35 The spinal twist.

David Rini

FIGURE 6-36 Hand position for the occipital release.

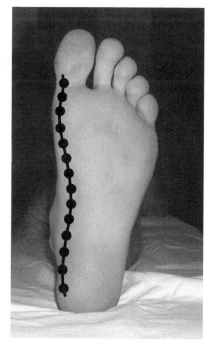

FIGURE 6-37 The spinal reflex zone.

2. *Spinal Reflex Points on the Foot.* With your thumb, press points along the medial border of the foot, beginning at the big toe and working down to the heel. The curves of the instep correspond to the curves of the spine (Fig. 6-37). Hold sensitive spots for 8 to 12 seconds.

CLOSING

Sitting at the foot of the table, lightly hold the heels of the client's feet in your hands for 30 to 60 seconds. Remove your hands slowly.

REFERENCES

1. Benjamin BE. Are you tense? The Benjamin system of muscular therapy: tension relief through deep massage and body care. New York: Pantheon Books, 1978: 10.
2. Kogan G, ed. Your bodyworks: a guide to health, energy and balance. Berkeley, CA: Transformation Press, 1981: 34.
3. Heller J, Henkin W. The body as a tensegrity structure. In: Bodywise. Berkeley, CA: Winbow Press, 1991: 47–52.
4. Jemmet R. Spinal stabilization: the new science of back pain. 2nd edition. Halifax, Canada: Novont Health, 2003: 7.
5. Jemmet R. Spinal stabilization: the new science of back pain. 2nd edition. Halifax, Canada: Novont Health, 2003: 10.
6. Jemmet R. Spinal stabilization: the new science of back pain. 2nd edition. Halifax, Canada: Novont Health, 2003: 14.
7. Feldenkrais M. Body and mature behavior. New York, NY: International Universities Press, 2005.
8. Rolf IP, Feitis R, ed. Rolfing and physical reality. Rochester, VT: Healing Arts Press, 1990: 211.
9. Greene E, Goodrich-Dunn B. The psychology of the body. Baltimore, MD: Lippincott Williams &Wilkins, 2004: 9.

7

Aligning the Upper Extremity

The Shoulder, Arm, and Hand

■ GENERAL CONCEPTS

The shoulder, arm, forearm, and hand form the upper extremity. This is an extremely important area, because it is largely through the shoulder–arm complex that we express ourselves bodily and make contact with the world. The ways in which individuals hold their shoulders and arms say much about their attitudes and characters in general.

Functionally, the pectoral girdle forms a base of support for the arms that allows almost unlimited range of motion. It also protects the lungs and heart from damage as a result of impact stress arising from use of the arms by diverting force away from the chest cavity.

The pectoral girdle and pelvic girdle share a similar function: They both support and anchor the limbs. The major difference between the two is that the pelvis is a more rigid structure. Unlike the pectoral girdle, all of its bones are joined together, limiting its movement. The shoulder girdle is open in the back, because the scapulae do not connect to each other. This design allows the arms much greater freedom of individual motion at the shoulder joints than the legs are capable of at the hip joints.

For proper balance and integration of the body, the pectoral girdle and pelvis need to be aligned with each other. The muscles of the pectoral girdle and arms should be free to adjust to weight shifts that occur from movements in the lower body. By design, the pectoral girdle acts like a yoke suspended over the rib cage by muscles attaching to the neck and head. The arms should hang loosely from the shoulder joints, with freedom to swing. Tension in the muscles of the shoulders produces rigidity in the upper

back and neck that contributes to imbalance and stress throughout the body.

When the muscles of the upper extremity are working in a coordinated fashion, the centers of the shoulder joints will be directly at the sides of the body, creating maximum width in the upper torso. According to Dr. Ida Rolf, as the arms hang to the sides, the lateral aspects of the elbows should turn out slightly and the palms of the hands face posteriorly. Rolf's opinion that the hands should face in a posterior direction in a properly aligned body is controversial. She claimed that this position affords the greatest width across the shoulder girdle. Illustrations of her views on correct vertical standing alignment can be found on page 72 of her book, *Rolfing*.[1]

When all the joints of the upper extremity are balanced, a force applied through the fingers and hand will pass cleanly through the wrist, up the forearm and humerus, and through the scapula to the spine. From there, the force will pass down the vertebrae to the sacrum and flare out across the ilium to the hip joints. Then, it will pass down the bones of the legs to the ankles and across the feet. In this way, forces are transferred smoothly through the body, eliminating strains caused by soft tissues having to brace uneven forces around misaligned joints.

Integrated deep tissue therapy on the shoulder girdle, arms, and hands helps to remove uneven pulls on the scapula and clavicle and balances the humerus in the shoulder joint. Soft tissue reorganization at the shoulder girdle improves movement of the arms, increases breathing capacity, and reduces the risk of injury to the area.

■ MUSCULOSKELETAL ANATOMY AND FUNCTION

See Essential Anatomy Box 7-1 for a summary of musculoskeletal anatomy and function.

The Shoulder

The shoulder girdle consists of the clavicles, the scapulae, and the humerus bones (Fig. 7-1). It does not attach to the spine; its only connection to the rest of the skeleton is where the clavicles attach to the sternum. The lateral ends of the clavicles join the scapulae via the acromioclavicular joint. The clavicles support the shoulder joints and keep the scapulae away from the chest wall so that they may move freely and independently. In maintaining this distance from the thorax, the clavicle prevents the shoulder girdle from interfering with the important functions of circulation and respiration, and it protects the nerves passing through the upper ribs. It also absorbs shocks coming through the shoulder and arm, protecting the sternum and ribs from the force of direct impact.

The humerus and scapula are joined via a ball-and-socket type joint. The rounded head of the humerus fits into a concave depression on the side of the scapula, called the glenoid fossa. This fossa is shallow, and it does not fit around the humerus as the acetabulum of the pelvis does with the femur. The humerus is held in the joint by a ligamentous capsule and supporting muscles.

This design allows for greater range of motion than is possible at the hip. When the arms no longer have to function solely for support of body weight, as they do in most animals, they become free to develop other capabilities. Early humans learned to fashion tools with their hands, which allowed them to rise far above the rest of the animal kingdom.

The motions of the arms are controlled by a series of muscles attached around the shoulder joint and along the humerus (Fig. 7-1A). These muscles form a wheel-like design, fanning out from the shoulder joint to connect to the skeleton over a broad area. Thus, the action of the arms depends on coordination of movement coming through the trunk and legs. Isolated movement of the arms, without support of the body, creates strain that can lead to injury.

The muscles that control the movements of the arm include those that must also stabilize the scapula. It is important that the scapula is free to move in combination with all movements of the humerus, but it must also remain anchored to the body wall through muscular action to provide leverage for the head of the humerus.

In the back, the **trapezius** and rhomboids help to support the scapulae (Fig. 7-1A). The upper trapezius, with assistance from the lower trapezius, elevates the shoulders. The trapezius can become strained when the arms are held in elevated positions for long periods, as when carrying a bag of groceries home.

A tender point that frequently develops near the attachment point of the **levator scapula** muscle on the superior angle of the scapula is often attributed to holding the shoulders in an elevated position. More likely, however, this soreness is caused by a chronic forward head position. When the head is held forward, the levator scapulae are constantly active, drawing the neck posterior to bring the head back toward the vertical axis of gravity. The scapulae must be held steady to stabilize the pulling action of the

---

BOX 7-1 ESSENTIAL ANATOMY   The Shoulder and Arm Routines

MUSCLES	BONES AND LANDMARKS
Trapezius	Scapula
Supraspinatus	Spine of scapula
Infraspinatus	Acromion process
Teres minor	Humerus
Teres major	Olecranon process
Latissimus dorsi	Olecranon fossa
Deltoid	Deltoid tuberosity
Biceps brachii	Lateral epicondyle
Triceps brachii	Medial epicondyle
Brachialis	Ulna
Forearm extensors and flexors	Radius
Hand muscles	Carpals and metacarpals
	Phalanges

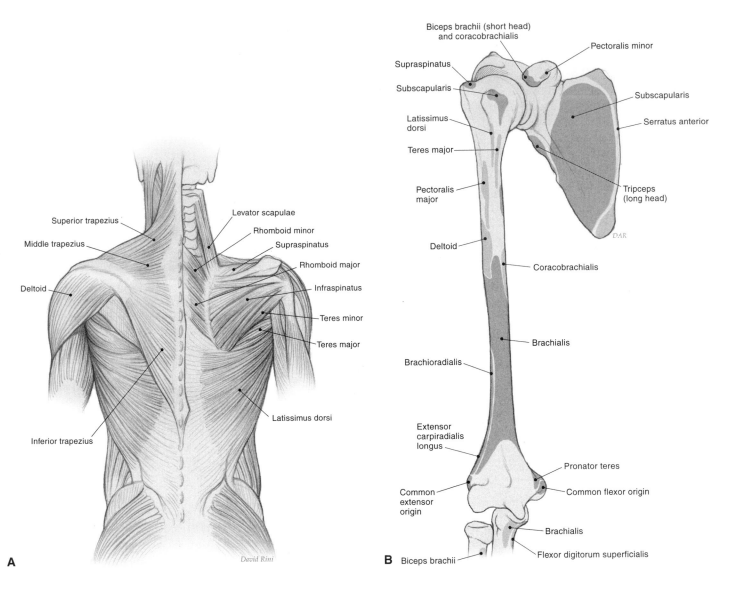

FIGURE 7-1 A. Muscles of the scapula and arm, posterior view. **B.** Attachment sites of the muscles of the scapula and arm, anterior view.

muscles, causing the scapular attachments of the levator scapulae to become strained.[2] The stress on these muscles is relieved by properly positioning the head on the neck, thus reducing the pulling action by the levator scapulae.

The **rhomboids**, which retract the scapulae, are opposed by the **serratus anterior** muscles, which protract them. When the musculature controlling the placement of the scapulae is balanced, the rhomboids lie on the horizontal plane along with the clavicles (e.g., when a man is standing with his arms at his sides). When the rhomboids are weak, they cannot fix the vertebral borders of the scapulae to the body wall, and the lower portion of the scapulae will lift away from the back, or wing.[1]

Several large muscles emanating from the spine, sternum, and ribs contribute to arm movements. These muscles include the trapezius, latissimus dorsi, and pectoralis major. This arrangement is advantageous, because it distributes forces generated from the arms throughout the length of the spine, helping to stabilize the spine against large, peripheral motions.

The ligamentous capsule surrounding the head of the humerus is quite loose, allowing increased range of motion for the arm. Because of this laxity of the capsule, it cannot maintain the head of the humerus in the joint. Instead, this support is accomplished by the tendons of four muscles positioned around the shoulder joint, known as the rotator cuff. The muscles that comprise the rotator cuff are the **supraspinatus, infraspinatus, teres minor**, and **subscapularis**. They are joined in their function of reinforcement by the tendon of the long head of the **biceps brachii** on the top of the joint and the long head of the **triceps brachii** on the underside of the joint. The

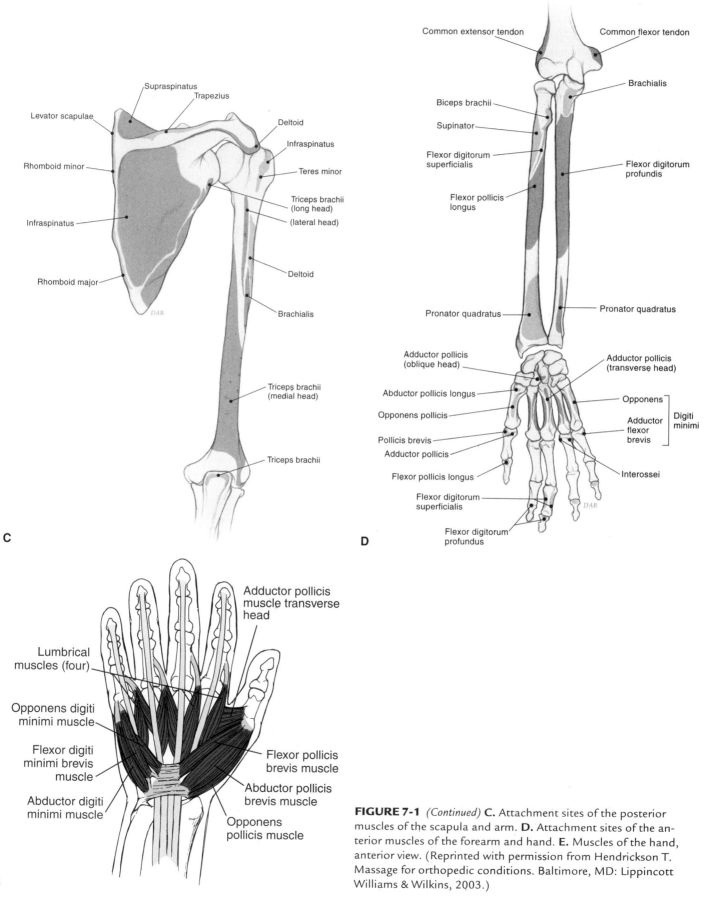

C

D

E

FIGURE 7-1 *(Continued)* **C.** Attachment sites of the posterior muscles of the scapula and arm. **D.** Attachment sites of the anterior muscles of the forearm and hand. **E.** Muscles of the hand, anterior view. (Reprinted with permission from Hendrickson T. Massage for orthopedic conditions. Baltimore, MD: Lippincott Williams & Wilkins, 2003.)

balance of all these muscles is crucial to proper positioning of the humerus in the shoulder joint.

The primary abductors of the humerus are the **deltoids**. Because of their position at the superior end of the humerus, however, they lack the leverage to initiate abduction when the arm is against the side of the body. Instead, the supraspinatus muscle initiates abduction, which is taken over by the deltoids when the arm is abducted about 12 inches from the side of the body.

The infraspinatus muscle is responsible for external rotation of the humerus. It is opposed by the subscapularis, which internally rotates the arm. Both muscles help to stabilize the humerus in the glenoid fossa, and they are easily strained by swinging the arm forward or backward from a horizontal position. Sleeping on one's side with full body weight resting on the folded underneath arm can also aggravate strain in both muscles. Placing a small pillow under the side of the head takes some weight off the arm when lying on one's side.

The teres minor assists the infraspinatus in external rotation and stabilization of the head of the humerus against the scapula. The **teres major** assists the **latissimus dorsi** in internal rotation and extension of a flexed arm. The teres major and latissimus dorsi muscles form the posterior axillary fold, which is the back of the armpit.

The **pectoralis minor** 🔊 connects the scapula to the anterior side of the rib cage. It brings the scapula forward, downward, and medial. Shortened pectoralis minor muscles are characterized by rounded or stooped shoulders. The lateral bundle of nerves of the **brachial plexus** and the axillary artery pass underneath the pectoralis minor. When this muscle is chronically contracted, it may impinge blood flow and nerve supply to the arm when that arm is abducted and externally rotated. In this position, the pectoralis minor is unable to lengthen, and it presses against these structures. The most common symptom of this form of impingement is numbness in the forearm and on the palmar side of the first 3.5 digits of the hand.

The Forearm and Hand

The forearm consists of two bones, the ulna and the radius (Fig. 7-1D). The radius is capable of rotation around the ulna at its proximal end via a ligamentous ring that joins the two bones. This ring also prevents the radius from being pulled away from the ulna by the biceps muscle as it supinates the forearm and hand and flexes the elbow. The radius and ulna are tied together by an interweaving interosseus membrane. This gives additional strength to the forearm while keeping it much lighter than if it were composed of one large bone.

The **brachialis** is deep to the biceps, and of the two, it is the stronger flexor of the forearm. Both muscles are opposed by the triceps, which extends the forearm. The triceps is usually much weaker than the biceps and brachialis, and it is prone to overuse injuries from actions that require repetitive flexing and straightening of the forearm (e.g., hammering). It often requires strengthening to balance movement at the elbow joint.

The hand connects to the forearm by the wrist joint, which is formed between the radius and ulna and the eight small carpal bones. The number of small gliding joints that this design creates allows great mobility and flexibility at the wrist. A unique feature of the human hand is that the thumb is opposable, meaning it is capable of touching each of the fingers. This allows for an oppositional type grip and a superior degree of control and refinement of movement.

Most of the muscles that control the hand lie along the forearm. The extensor muscles merge at the **common extensor tendon**, which attaches on the lateral epicondyle of the humerus. The flexor muscles merge at the **common flexor tendon**, which attaches on the medial epicondyle of the humerus.

■ CONDITIONS

Shoulder

1. *Bursitis.* This is an inflammation of the bursal sac, which is a cushioning, fluid-filled sac in the shoulder joint. Bursitis is characterized by achiness and pain when lifting the arm.
   a. *Acute bursitis* can be an extremely painful condition that usually starts mildly and progressively worsens over a period of days. A blow to the shoulder can cause the bursal sac to become irritated and then swell to a much larger than normal size. Pain in the shoulder will be intense for days or weeks, making it extremely difficult to lift the arm or lie on the shoulder. Massage and exercise are contraindicated, because both will worsen the condition. Rest is the treatment of choice.
   b. *Chronic bursitis,* although not nearly as debilitating as acute bursitis, can still be an annoyance. Lifting the arm to shoulder height becomes painful because of compression and irritation to the bursal sac within the humeral joint. As the arm is lifted overhead, the pain diminishes, because pressure on the sac is relieved. Pain comes in bouts, lasting anywhere from weeks to years if untreated. Massage is contraindicated. Cortisone injections are effective.
2. *Arthritis.* This is a general term covering a broad range of ailments. Osteoarthritic conditions indicate a degeneration of the joint, either from a deformation of the bones or an irritation caused by shrinkage or compression of the soft tissue components of the joint. Arthri-

tis can be brought on by chronic misuse of the arm or by misalignment of the shoulder. It also may be aggravated by trauma to the shoulder, resulting in irritation to the joint capsule.

Another common form of arthritis is rheumatoid arthritis, a chronic, systemic disease believed to be related to an antigen–antibody reaction that leads to crippling deformation of joints. Rheumatoid arthritis is characterized by periods of painful, inflammatory flare-ups of joints. Massage is contraindicated during these times. A physician can prescribe anti-inflammatory compounds that may be helpful. Light massage can be performed on the muscles between periods of flare-up, but affected joints should always be avoided.

Proper assessment of the cause of the arthritis is necessary for correct treatment. Stretching or corrective movement work may be indicated. Massage of irritated tissues is contraindicated.

3. *Injuries to Muscles and Tendons.* It is often difficult for a client to tell exactly where a shoulder injury is originating. To pinpoint injury sites in this area, the therapist should apply resistive tests to the suspected muscles. Once located, the injured muscle or tendon may be treated with a combination of ice and massage. If massage treatments are not helping, they should be discontinued; ice and rest should then be recommended.
4. *Shoulder Separation.* The source of this injury is usually a tear in the ligament that binds the clavicle and the acromion. It is caused by trauma to the joint, such as a fall. Massage is contraindicated. Initial treatment should be rest, followed by stretching exercises when the injury begins to heal.
5. *Shoulder Dislocation.* The humerus is held in place at the glenoid fossa, mainly through ligamentous binding. It is fairly easy to knock the humerus out of the socket, which is painful and results in irritation and possible chronic stretching of the ligaments. The injury tends to be repeated as the ligaments lose their integrity. Surgery to tighten the ligaments may be the only solution.

Forearm and Hand

1. *Tennis Elbow.* This term describes an injury to the extensor tendon that connects the extensor muscles of the hand to the elbow. It may be caused by incorrect form when swinging a tennis racquet or a baseball bat—or during any action that involves use of the wrist extensor muscles. Rest and ice are appropriate treatments. Massage to the forearm to increase blood flow to the injured tendon is indicated.
2. *Carpal Tunnel Syndrome.* This is a painful condition in the wrist area caused by a compression of the median nerve. The site of irritation is usually the carpal tunnel through the wrist, which forms a passage for the nerve and the tendons of the hand muscles. If these tendons swell as a result of overuse or improper use of the hand, they will put pressure on the median nerve. The result is pain and, perhaps, a numbing sensation in the thumb and index finger. Other causes of the tunnel becoming restricted include fracture of the wrist, endocrine disorders (e.g., diabetes), menopause, tumors, and body fluid retention. Treatment consists of rest, ice, elevation of the arm, and massage to the forearm.
3. *Painful Weak Grip.* This is a condition in which a person loses the ability to close the hand powerfully. It is attributed to overuse and trigger point development in the extensor carpi radialis longus, extensor carpi radialis brevis, and extensor digitorum muscles.[3] Activities that involve grasping with the hand (e.g., gripping a steering wheel, digging with garden tools, or holding a hammer) aggravate the condition. Massage and trigger point deactivation are the recommended treatment protocols. If inflammation is present, the client should apply ice and rest the affected muscles and not attempt massage therapy until the inflammation subsides.

Please refer to Indications/Contraindications Box 7-2 for an additional list of indications and contraindications for the upper extremity.

BOX 7-2 INDICATIONS/CONTRAINDICATIONS Conditions Affecting Shoulder

INDICATIONS
Pain in the shoulder
Limited range of motion
Subacute injuries
Poor posture
Headaches
Carpal tunnel syndrome
Fatigue in arms and hands

CONTRAINDICATIONS
Inflammation
Bursitis
Acute injury
Bad bruising
Broken bones

By design, the shoulder girdle is similar to an old-fashioned yoke, which was a weight-carrying device that was balanced across the shoulders. A yoke consisted of a broad piece of wood with ropes or chains attached at either end for hanging buckets or bundles of some sort. Although in the Western world we no longer use yokes to carry things, the shoulders themselves often continue to serve that function psychologically: In our minds and emotions, we often carry heavy loads across our shoulders.

The muscles of the shoulder girdle often receive the brunt of our concerns and worries about our ability to carry all the responsibilities and burdens that accompany us in life. It is not uncommon to see a person literally stooped over, as if weighted down by some tremendous, invisible load.

As explained previously, the position of the shoulders is dependent, perhaps more than any other joint, on muscle action. Because muscles are controlled by the nervous system, which ultimately is controlled by the mind, there is an obvious relationship between the way a person positions the shoulders and his or her beliefs and attitudes in general. An interesting experiment is to stand in front of a mirror and put your shoulders and arms into different poses. Observe how the way you feel and the image you project change based on your body posture.

The shoulders and arms reflect how we interact with the world. The arms can act as a barrier, pushing people away, or they can draw people in with an embrace. Being on the same plane as the heart center, the arms physically manifest the state of the heart's energy. The hands give and receive energy. It is through the medium of the hands that healing therapeutic touch is administered. The Chinese qi gong and Indian yoga systems both refer to the existence of energy centers in the hand. The Bill Moyers PBS series *The Healing Mind* (available on video) includes a demonstration of a qi gong master's ability to move a candle flame utilizing qi directed from his hand.

■ POSTURAL EVALUATION

1. Check the position of the clavicles. How close are they to being horizontal?
2. Compare the height of the right and left shoulders. Observe the distance from the shoulder to the ear.
3. Compare the length of both arms. Where do the fingertips reach on the thigh?
4. Make note of any hollow spaces around the clavicles.

5. Have the client raise the arms to the sides. Do the arms move independently of the shoulder girdle? (They should.)
6. Note any areas of restriction or muscle tension around the shoulder girdle.
7. How do the arms hang?
   - Are the arms straight or flexed at the elbow?
   - In what direction do the hands face?
   - What is the distance of the arms from the sides of the body? Is it the same on both sides?
8. From a side view, observe the alignment of the tip of the shoulder to the ear, hip, knee, and ankle.
9. From the posterior view, check the position of the scapulae.
   - Protracted?
   - Retracted?
   - Depressed?
   - Elevated?
   - Upward or downward rotation?
   - Relaxed and properly positioned?
10. Observe the condition of the musculature affecting the scapulae.

Refer to Table 7-1 for a description of common distortions of the shoulder girdle and possible muscles involved. Table 7-2 lists the muscles responsible for various actions of the upper extremity.

■ EXERCISES AND SELF-TREATMENT

Shoulders

1. *Stretch for Pectoralis Minor and Clavicular Division of Pectoralis Major.* Standing in a doorway, extend your arms upward, and open them slightly wider than shoulder width. Placing your palms against the top of the door frame, and lean your body forward, leading with the hips and chest, until you feel a stretch in the shoulders. Hold for a few seconds as you breathe deeply into the stretch.
2. *Stretch for Anterior Deltoid and Sternal Division of Pectoralis Major.* Stand in front of a dresser or table, and face away from it. Reach your arms behind you with the elbows flexed, and place your palms on top of the flat surface, with the fingers facing you. Squeezing your shoulder blades and elbows toward each other, slowly flex your knees, and sink down as if sitting into a chair until you feel a stretch in the shoulder area. Hold as you breathe deeply, and focus on releasing tension in the shoulders.
3. *Exercises from a Seated Position.* The following shoulder exercises may be performed from a seated position:
   - *Strengthen Upper Trapezius.* As you inhale, raise both shoulders toward your ears. Hold for a few sec-

TABLE 7–1	Body Reading for the Shoulder Girdle
Conditions	**Muscles That May Be Shortened**
Raised shoulder(s)—one or both shoulders are elevated	Scalenes Upper trapezius Lower trapezius
Rounded shoulders—shoulders are rotated medially	Trapezius Pectoralis major Pectoralis minor Anterior deltoid Teres major Serratus anterior
Retracted shoulders—shoulder blades are pulled back, scapulae winged	Rhomboids Trapezius Teres minor Infraspinatus Latissimus dorsi

onds. Light weights may be held in the hands to increase resistance.

- *Stretch for Upper Trapezius.* Exhaling, lower your shoulders slowly, feeling the tension flowing out of the muscles.
- *Contract Rhomboids.* Inhaling, draw both shoulders back, squeezing the vertebral borders of the scapulae toward each other.
- *Stretch for Rhomboids.* Exhaling, press the outside edges of the shoulders forward, feeling the space between the scapulae stretching.
- *Stretch for Rotator Cuff.* Slowly circle the shoulders. Inhale for half of the circle, and exhale for half of the circle. Repeat a few times, and then reverse the direction of the circle.

4. *Stretch for Rotator Cuff Muscles, Pectoralis Major, and Latissimus Dorsi.* Lie on your side with both knees flexed. Your head may rest on the arm closest to the floor. The uppermost arm is straight and placed on the floor in front of your chest, with the palm facing downward. Slowly circle the arm around your body, tracing the circle on the floor with your fingers. As the arm moves overhead, allow it to rotate naturally so that the palm is facing upward. Pause in positions that feel tight or restricted, and imagine breathing into the shoulder. Repeat a few times, and then reverse the direction of the circle. Turn onto your other side, and repeat the entire exercise.

Arms

1. *Strengthen Biceps, Brachialis, and Triceps.* Stand facing a wall with your arms extended so that your palms are against the wall. Lean into the wall, flexing only your arms, like doing a push-up. Keep your body straight. Vary the speed of the push and the degree of lean to strengthen the arm muscles effectively. Repeat several times.

Wrists

1. *Strengthen Wrist Flexors and Extensors.* To strengthen your wrists, hold a broom handle out in front of you as if shaking hands with it. Slowly raise the broom upward and downward with the motion of your wrist. To work with less weight, hold the broom closer to the broom head. To use more weight, hold the broom closer to the end of the handle.
2. *Stretch for Wrist Flexors.* Sitting cross-legged on the floor, lean forward slightly from the hip joints. With your arms fully extended in front of you, place the palms on the floor with the fingers turned toward your ankles. Gently press the heel of the palm toward the floor. Hold for at least 10 seconds.
3. *Stretch for Wrist Extensors.* In the same position as above, place the back of the hands on the floor, and press down very gently until you feel a mild stretch in the back of the wrist. Hold for 5 to 10 seconds.

Hands

1. *Alternately Strengthen and Stretch the Muscles of the Hand.* Exhaling, squeeze the fingers and thumbs of both hands into fists. Inhaling, slowly open them all the way against resistance as if a rubber band were wrapped around the fingers.

TABLE 7–2	Range of Motion (ROM) for the Shoulder and Arm
Action	**Muscles**
Shoulder	
Flexion (ROM 170°)	Anterior deltoid
	Biceps brachii
	Pectoralis major
	Coracobrachialis
Extension (ROM 60°)	Posterior deltoid
	Teres major
	Latissimus dorsi
	Triceps brachii
Abduction (ROM 170°)	Supraspinatus
	Deltoids
	Biceps brachii
Adduction (ROM 50°)	Biceps brachii
	Pectoralis major
	Teres major
	Coracobrachialis
	Latissimus dorsi
	Triceps brachii
Medial rotation (ROM 70°)	Anterior deltoid
	Pectoralis major
	Subscapularis
	Teres major
	Latissimus dorsi
Lateral rotation (ROM 90°)	Infraspinatus
	Teres minor
	Posterior deltoid
Elbow	
Flexion (ROM 150°)	Biceps brachii
	Brachialis
	Brachioradialis
	Extensor carpi radialis
	Pronator teres
	Flexor carpi ulnaris
	Flexor carpi radialis
Extension (ROM 0°)	Triceps brachii
	Anconeus
Forearm	
Supination (ROM 90°)	Biceps brachii
	Brachioradialis
	Supinator
Pronation (ROM 90°)	Brachioradialis
	Pronator teres
	Pronator quadratus
Wrist	
Flexion (ROM 80°)	Flexor carpi radialis
	Flexor carpi ulnaris
Extension (ROM 70°)	Extensor carpi radialis
	Extensor carpi ulnaris

CASE STUDY 5 (The Shoulders and Arms)

The client is a 43-year-old massage therapist named Doris. She has been practicing massage therapy professionally for 10 years. For the past several months, she has been experiencing tightness and pain in her neck, shoulders, and upper back. The tightness is exacerbated by giving a massage. During the previous 2 weeks, she has begun to experience sharp pains in her right forearm muscles. It is becoming increasingly difficult for her to administer pressure with her right arm; the pain in her forearm becomes intense when she pushes with her right hand.

Doris is a frail-looking woman. She is small-boned and does not have well-developed musculature. She is somewhat stooped over, with a slight kyphosis in her upper back. Her scapulae are protracted, with her arms medially rotated and her upper chest collapsed. She also exhibits a forward position of the head. Based on observing her posture and listening to the description of her arm complaint, the likelihood that she may be lacking in body mechanics skills is being considered. She probably tries to push too much with her arm and back muscles, rather than leaning forward and distributing force throughout her entire body, when applying pressure during massage strokes.

This and future deep tissue sessions will focus on releasing the muscles of the scapulae and relieving tension in the neck, around the clavicles, in the serratus anterior and pectoralis minor muscles, and throughout the muscles of the forearms and hands. She will obviously require a series of deep tissue sessions to address all the problems arising from her poor posture and lack of proper body mechanics.

Because of the protraction of the scapulae, collapse of the chest, and medial rotation of the arms, her serratus anterior, pectoralis major and minor, and anterior deltoid muscles were emphasized during the session. Numerous trigger points were encountered, particularly in the lateral section of the pectoralis minor. Working on the right forearm, the common extensor tendon was found to be very tender and perhaps inflamed. It was recommended that the client apply ice to it regularly. The borders of the forearm muscles were carefully traced and separated. The client found that the degree of mobility in both hands was greatly increased following the session. The muscles of the thenar eminence were tender on both hands but on the right side in particular.

After the session, the likelihood that she is favoring her right arm and hand while performing massage was discussed. Doris is also overusing her arm and hand muscles to apply pressure instead of allowing the weight of her body to flow through her arm and supply the force needed for the massage strokes. It was suggested that she diminish her workload of massage clients until the strain in her muscles from incorrect body mechanics is reduced. In addition to receiving deep tissue therapy treatments twice a week for the next month, she is going to engage in daily stretching of the chest, shoulder, arm, and hand muscles. She will also receive coaching in proper body mechanics. Once the initial trauma to the upper body muscles is reduced and better alignment of the shoulder girdle achieved, she will begin a very mild weight-training program to build strength and acquire more kinesthetic awareness of her entire body.

Topics for Discussion

1. Based on the client in the case study above, describe some specific exercises that would help to counteract muscular weaknesses and postural distortions.
2. What suggestions regarding body mechanics would you offer to a muscular, male massage therapist who relies exclusively on his strong shoulder and arm muscles to perform massage strokes?
3. Describe the position and movement capabilities of well-aligned shoulders and arms in relation to the rest of the body.
4. List several examples of postural deviation from proper alignment of the shoulders and arms. Which muscles are overly contracted and weakened in each deviation?
5. How would you treat a client who describes difficulty gripping the steering wheel while driving?

■ SCAPULA ROUTINE

Objectives

- To balance the scapula in relation to the clavicle and humerus
- To release tension in muscles affecting the scapula
- To help alleviate painful conditions in the scapular region arising from dysfunction and imbalance
- To explore movement patterns and habits that might be generating stress in the scapular muscles

Energy

POSITION

- The client is lying prone on the table. A bolster may be placed under the ankles.
- The therapist is standing at the side of the table next to the client's shoulder.

POLARITY

Contact the superior angle of the scapula with the index finger of one hand (negative pole on the hand) and the inferior angle of the scapula with the middle finger of the other hand (positive pole on the hand). Envision the scapula floating freely over the underlying ribs. Allow any subtle movements of the scapula to occur. Hold the position for 30 seconds or longer.

SHIATSU

1. Press points along the vertebral border of the scapula with the thumbs or elbow. The outer branch of the bladder channel runs slightly medial to the border of the scapula.
2. With your outside hand holding the shoulder, place the fingers of your inside hand along the lower portion of the vertebral border of the scapula near the inferior angle. The palm of your hand is facing upward. As you circle the shoulder with your outside hand, slide the fingers of your inside hand under the border of the scapula, and point them toward the shoulder joint (Fig. 7-2). Attempt this move only if the musculature feels fairly relaxed.

Swedish/Cross Fiber

1. Use a three-stroke effleurage pattern over the scapula. Beginning at the upper thoracic region of the spine, stroke outward over the upper, middle, and lower scapular region. Alternate hands with each stroke.
2. Apply cross fiber strokes over the upper back and shoulder area using fingertips and the broad side of the thumb.

David Rini

FIGURE 7-2 Shiatsu scapula release.

Connective Tissue

1. In the myofascial mobilization technique, slide the muscles of the upper back, using the fingers or palms, over the scapula and ribs. Note areas that are not moving freely.
2. Apply the myofascial spreading technique to tight, unyielding musculature.

Deep Tissue/Neuromuscular Therapy

SEQUENCE

1. Trapezius (upper, middle, and lower)
2. Levator scapula (attachment)
3. Rhomboids
4. Subscapularis 💿
5. Pectoralis minor
6. Serratus anterior

1. Trapezius

Upper Trapezius
Origin: Medial third of the superior nuchal line and external occipital protuberance, ligamentum nuchae, and the spinal processes of C1–C5 vertebrae.
Insertion: Lateral third of the clavicle.
Action: Elevation and upward rotation of the scapula, capital extension.

Trigger points are best located using the sifting technique. Flexing the client's head in the direction of the side being examined may make palpation of the muscle fibers easier. Trigger points may be found along the border of the muscle, slightly above the lateral portion of the clavicle. Pain is referred up the posterior neck to the mastoid process. Trigger point activity in this muscle is a major source of tension headaches. Complementary trigger points may be located in the supraspinatus and levator scapulae muscles.

Strokes
- Using the fingers, perform an elongation stroke down the posterior portion of the neck from the occiput to C7. At the base of the neck, switch to the knuckles or heel of the hand, and continue stroking outward to the acromioclavicular joint (Fig. 7-3).
- Sift the upper trapezius by grasping the belly of the muscle between the thumb and fingers, and roll the fibers, feeling for taut bands. Treat any trigger points that are found (Fig. 7-4).

Middle Trapezius
Origin: Interspinous ligaments and spinous processes of C6–T3 vertebrae.
Insertion: Acromion and superior lip of the spine of the scapula.
Action: Adduction (retraction) of the scapulae.

 A commonly occurring trigger point in the middle trapezius may be located on the superior edge of the spine of the scapula near the acromion process. It shoots pain to the top of the shoulder.

FIGURE 7-3 Elongation stroke on the upper trapezius from the occiput to the acromion process.

FIGURE 7-4 Sifting the upper trapezius to locate trigger points.

Strokes
- Stand at the side of the table, facing the client's shoulder that is to be treated. Perform an elongation stroke using the knuckles.
- Covering the space between T1 and T3, stroke laterally across the middle trapezius, and end on the lateral edge of the superior lip of the spine of the scapula.

Lower Trapezius
Origin: Interspinous ligaments and spinous processes of T4–T12 vertebrae.
Insertion: Tubercle on the medial end of the spine of the scapula.
Action: Depression and upward rotation of the scapula.

 The lateral border of the middle and lower trapezius should be examined carefully for trigger points. Trigger points in these muscles are best located by rubbing the fibers over the underlying ribs.

Strokes
- Stand at the side of the table, and face toward the client's head. Perform a series of elongation strokes using the forearm. Beginning at T4, stroke diagonally upward to the medial end of the spine of the scapula.
- Repeat the stroke, covering the muscles in strips. The final stroke begins at T12. Cover the muscle completely (Fig. 7-5).

2. Levator Scapula (Insertion)

Origin: Posterior tubercles of the transverse processes of C1–C4 vertebrae.
Insertion: Vertebral border of the scapula between the superior angle and the root of the spine.

FIGURE 7-5 Elongation strokes on the middle and lower trapezius from origins (T1–T12) to insertion (spine of the scapula).

Action: Elevation and adduction of the scapula, rotation causing the lateral angle to move downward.

To find a trigger point, palpate the fibers slightly lateral to the superior angle (0.5 inch). This trigger point is one of the most common, and it is usually very tender. It refers pain to the surrounding area of the neck.

Strokes

- Sit or stand at the head of the table. The client's arm is flexed at the elbow, with the palm resting against the table next to the shoulder. Using your outside hand, hold the client's elbow. Place the thumb of your other hand against the inferior end of the edge of the superior angle of the scapula.
- Draw the client's arm toward the head of the table. This lifts the superior angle of the scapula. Apply cross fiber strokes with your thumb pad to the attachment of the levator scapula, just inferior to the superior angle, palpating the tendon for tenderness (Fig. 7-6).

FIGURE 7-6 Cross fiber stroke on the insertion of the levator scapula (superior angle of the scapula).

3. Rhomboids

Rhomboid Minor

Origin: Ligamentum nuchae and spinous processes of C7–T1 vertebrae.

Insertion: Medial border of the scapula at the root of the spine.

Action: Adduction of the scapula; elevation of the scapula; rotates the scapula so that the lateral angle faces downward.

Rhomboid Major

Origin: Supraspinous ligament and spinous processes of T2–T5 vertebrae.

Insertion: Medial border of the scapula below the root of the spine.

Action: Adduction of the scapula; elevation of the scapula; rotates the scapula so that the lateral angle faces downward.

 To locate trigger points, check just medial to the vertebral border of the scapula. The pain pattern for these trigger points is local, along the edge of the scapula.

Strokes

- Using thumbs or elbow, do short, up and down strokes along the origin of the rhomboids at the sides of the spinous processes of C7–T5 (Fig. 7-7A).
- Perform an elongation stroke with the knuckles along the belly of the muscle, from the upper thoracic spine to the vertebral border of the scapula (Fig. 7-7B). Cover the area from C7–T5.
- Face the client's scapula from the opposite side of the table. The scapula may be raised by placing the client's forearm across the back or by sliding a folded towel under the shoulder of the arm being massaged. Using the thumbs or an elbow, do short, up and down strokes on

FIGURE 7-7 Strokes on the rhomboids. **A.** Origin (C7–T5). **B.** Belly (spinous processes to the vertebral border of the scapula). **C.** Insertion (vertebral border of the scapula).

the insertion of the rhomboids (Fig. 7-7C) along the vertebral border of the scapula. Release any trigger points that are found.

4. Subscapularis

Origin: Subscapular fossa along axillary margin of the anterior surface of the scapula.

Insertion: Lesser tuberosity of the humerus and anterior capsule of the shoulder joint.

Action: Medial rotation of the shoulder; stabilizes the shoulder (glenohumeral) joint by keeping the head of the humerus in the glenoid fossa.

Position
- The client is resting in side posture, with the bottom leg extended and the top leg flexed 90° at the hip and knee. A bolster is placed under the knee. A small pillow or folded towel may be placed under the side of the head.
- The therapist is standing behind the client at shoulder level.

The lateral fibers are the most likely to contain trigger points. These trigger points send pain into the posterior part of the shoulder and, sometimes, down the arm.

Strokes
- To reach the muscle on the client's right side, place the fingers of your right hand on the ribs just in front of the medial side of the scapula, with your left hand grasping the client's upper forearm near the elbow. Pull the client's arm upward to protract the scapula, exposing more of the medial surface (Fig. 7-8). Reverse hand positions for the left side.

David Rini

FIGURE 7-8 Contacting the subscapularis along the lateral anterior surface of the scapula.

- Move the fingers posteriorly along the ribs until the anterior surface of the scapula is felt. Apply short, side to side strokes with the fingers along the bone, seeking out tender areas. These fibers often have painful spots, so move slowly, and elicit client feedback often.

⚠️ **Move slowly, and stay close to the edge of the scapula. The axilla contains several arteries and nerves that are not well protected by muscle, including the axillary, brachial, and cephalic arteries and nerves of the brachial plexus.**

- This muscle can also be treated with the client supine. The humerus is abducted 90°, with the forearm flexed 90°. Slide your fingers posteriorly along the ribs until the medial surface of the scapula is felt. Slowly press the fingers into the front side of the scapula, and apply short, side to side and up and down strokes to treat the subscapularis muscle.

5. Pectoralis Minor

Origin: Upper and outer surfaces of ribs 3–5.

Insertion: Coracoid process of the scapula.

Action: Protraction of the scapula (moves the scapula forward, with a downward tilt); elevation of the ribs in forced inhalation, with the scapulae fixed.

Position
- The client's top arm rests over a bolster placed in front of the chest.
- The therapist stands behind the client at chest level.

Trigger points will most likely be found in the section of the pectoralis minor that attaches to rib 5. This is the easiest portion of the muscle to palpate. The referral zone is the anterior deltoid. When trigger points are found in this muscle, complementary trigger points almost always are located in the pectoralis major.

Strokes
- To relax the pectoralis major, perform circular friction with the fingers on the muscle.
- Position your fingers under the pectoralis major muscle, and palpate the ribs (Fig. 7-9). Slide along the length of the muscle, from its origins on ribs 3–5 to its insertion on the coracoid process. Move slowly, and pause at painful areas with static pressure. Lift the client's arm that is resting on the bolster, and hold it in your nonworking hand to gain better access to the muscle.

6. Serratus Anterior

Origin: Outer surfaces of ribs 1 to 8 or 9.

Insertion: Anterior (costal) surface of the vertebral border of the scapula.

FIGURE 7-9 Reaching the pectoralis minor from underneath the pectoralis major.

Action: Abduction (protraction) of the scapula; upward rotation of the scapula; fixes the medial border of the scapula to the thoracic wall.

Position
- The client's top arm rests on a bolster placed in front of the chest or is extended overhead.
- The therapist stands behind the client.

Examine the section of the muscle that lies over the fifth and sixth ribs, in an approximate line with the nipple. The pain referral zone is surrounding the trigger point. Expect much tenderness in this muscle, even when trigger points are not present.

Strokes
- Use the heel of the hand over the side of the chest when applying pressure during massage strokes.
- Perform an elongation stroke with the heel of the hand from the axillary border of the scapula to the muscle's insertion on the ribs (ribs 1–8). Repeat the stroke several times to cover the entire muscle.
- Perform short, up and down and side to side strokes on the fibers of the muscle over the ribs (Fig. 7-10).
- Pause to treat trigger points.

STRETCH

Position
- The client is supine.
- The therapist stands at the side of the table facing the client's shoulder.

1. Hold the client's arm on the upper forearm, just below the elbow. Place the client's arm perpendicular to the table, with the forearm at a right angle to the humerus and facing across the client's chest (Fig. 7-11).
2. Pull up on the arm, protracting the scapula. The humerus may be adducted to stretch the scapular muscles.

ACCESSORY WORK

1. Shiatsu in the chest region (fingertip compression in the intercostal spaces).
2. Trigger point work on the pectoralis major muscle.
3. Circumduction of the arm in both directions.

CLOSING

Sitting at the foot of the table, lightly hold the heels of the client's feet in your hands for 30 to 60 seconds. Remove your hands slowly to complete the session.

■ SHOULDER AND UPPER ARM ROUTINE

Objectives

- To relieve muscular pulls that may be causing misalignment of the shoulder
- To achieve full range of motion of the humerus in the shoulder joint

FIGURE 7-10 Contacting the serratus anterior over ribs 1–8.

FIGURE 7-11 Stretch for the scapular muscles.

- To reduce stress caused by poor posture and movement
- To reduce or eliminate pain resulting from soft tissue damage/dysfunction

Energy

POSITION

- The client is lying supine on the table, with his or her arms at the sides of the body.
- The therapist is standing at the side of the table next to the client's shoulder.

POLARITY

Place the right palm (positive pole) on the posterior side (negative pole) of the shoulder joint; place the left palm (negative pole) on the anterior side (positive pole) of the shoulder joint. Align the two hands along the vertical axis that passes through the center of the shoulder joint. Sense any subtle movements or adjustments that occur in the shoulder, and allow your hands to follow them. Hold for 1 minute or longer.

SHIATSU

Wrap the hands around the upper arm at the shoulder. Compress the arm, and roll it slightly medially, from the shoulder to the wrist (Fig. 7-12). This procedure stimulates the yin channels (lung, pericardium, and heart) and the yang channels (large intestine, triple heater, and small intestine) of the arm.

Swedish/Cross Fiber

1. Perform effleurage strokes on the arm, from the wrist to the shoulder.

2. Perform pétrissage strokes from the elbow to the shoulder.
3. Perform circular friction with the heel of hand on the shoulder area.

Connective Tissue

MYOFASCIAL SPREAD

Place the client's upper arm slightly away from the body. Wrap your hands around the upper arm, just above the elbow, with the base of the palms at the midline of the arm. Slowly slide the palms apart as the fascia softens, spreading the tissues of the arm with the heels of the hand. Continue, in horizontal strips, to the top of the shoulder.

Deep Tissue/Neuromuscular Therapy

SEQUENCE

1. Deltoids
2. Supraspinatus
3. Infraspinatus
4. Teres minor
5. Teres major and latissimus dorsi
6. Triceps brachii
7. Biceps brachii
8. Brachialis

POSITION

- The shoulder sequence is performed with the client in side posture. Place a pillow between the client's knees and a small support under the side of the client's head. The top arm rests along the client's side.
- The therapist stands at the head of the table and cups both hands around the client's shoulder (Fig. 7-13).

FIGURE 7-12 Shiatsu compression of the upper arm.

FIGURE 7-13 Beginning hand position for releasing the deltoids (posterior, medial, and anterior).

1. Deltoids

Posterior Deltoid

Origin: Lower lip of the posterior border of the spine of the scapula.

Insertion: Deltoid tuberosity on the lateral midshaft of the humerus.

Action: Extension and lateral rotation of the humerus.

 To locate trigger points, check along the posterior portion near the border of the muscle. The referral zone is throughout the posterior deltoid and, sometimes, down the arm.

Strokes

• Apply elongation strokes with the knuckles or the heel of the hand from the inferior border of the spine of the scapula to the deltoid tuberosity on the humerus. The hand on the front of the shoulder provides stability and support.

• To palpate trigger points, stand behind the client's shoulder. Grasp the shoulder using both hands, with the fingers in front and the thumb tips touching each other at the level of the posterior deltoid (Fig. 7-14). Perform short, back and forth and side to side strokes along the entire length of the muscle to seek taut bands.

Medial Deltoid

Origin: Lateral border of the acromion process.

Insertion: Deltoid tuberosity on the lateral midshaft of the humerus.

Action: Abduction of the humerus.

 This muscle does not develop trigger points as commonly as the other two deltoid muscles do. Trigger points may be found in the upper portion, just below the acromion.

Strokes

• Stand at the head of the table, and cup both hands around the shoulder. Using the knuckles or the heel of the hand, stroke down the middle of the upper humerus, from the acromion process to the deltoid tuberosity.

• To palpate trigger points, the hands should remain cupped around the shoulder, with the sides of the thumbs touching. Perform short, back and forth and side to side strokes along the entire length of the muscle, from the acromion to the deltoid tuberosity (Fig. 7-15).

Anterior Deltoid

Origin: Anterior surface of the lateral third of the clavicle.

Insertion: Deltoid tuberosity on the lateral midshaft of the humerus.

Action: Flexion and medial rotation of the humerus.

 Check for trigger points in the front portion of the muscle, high up, where the muscle covers the head of the humerus. Pain can refer over the anterior and medial deltoid and down the arm.

Strokes

• Apply elongation strokes with the heel of the hand, from the lateral third of the clavicle to the deltoid tuberosity.

• To palpate trigger points, stand in front of the client's shoulder. Grasp the shoulder using both hands, with the fingers wrapped around the back and the thumb tips touching in front, over the anterior deltoid (Fig. 7-16). Perform the techniques to search for trigger points over the entire length of the muscle.

FIGURE 7-14 Locating trigger points in the posterior deltoid along the medial border.

FIGURE 7-15 Locating trigger points in the medial deltoid.

FIGURE 7-16 Locating trigger points in the anterior deltoid beginning along the anterior border.

FIGURE 7-17 Elongation stroke on the supraspinatus from origin to insertion.

2. Supraspinatus

Origin: Supraspinous fossa of the scapula.

Insertion: Superior facet of the greater tuberosity of the humerus, capsule of the shoulder joint.

Action: Abduction of the shoulder; stabilizes the head of the humerus in the shoulder joint.

Position

- Stand at the head of the table, and face the client's shoulder. Cup your hands around the shoulder near the base of the neck. The thumbs are placed against the superior border of the spine of the scapula, with one thumb on top of the other to reinforce it.

 Search for trigger points along the superior border of the spine of the scapula. These trigger points refer pain into the medial deltoid and down the side of the arm. A trigger point is often located in the space between the clavicle and scapula, just before they meet at the acromioclavicular joint. The pain referral zone is over the deltoid.

Strokes

- Perform an elongation stroke along the superior border of the scapula to the acromioclavicular joint (Fig. 7-17). With the thumbs placed slightly superior to the spine of the scapula, repeat the stroke.
- Palpate trigger points in the muscle using the strokes to seek trigger points. Treat any that are found.

3. Infraspinatus

Origin: Infraspinous fossa of the scapula.

Insertion: Middle facet of the greater tuberosity of the humerus, capsule of the shoulder joint.

Action: Lateral rotation of the shoulder; stabilizes the head of the humerus in the shoulder joint.

 Trigger points tend to accumulate readily in this muscle. Pay close attention to the fibers that run about 0.5 inch below the spine of the scapula. These trigger points refer pain to the deltoid and down the arm. Another trigger point is found about halfway down the vertebral border of the scapula; it refers pain along the medial edge of the scapula.

Strokes

- Using the knuckles or elbow, perform an elongation stroke, from the vertebral border of the scapula to the head of the humerus. The stroke is repeated several times, in strips, over the body of the scapula to cover the entire muscle. Place your nonworking hand on the front of the client's shoulder to provide stability (Fig. 7-18).
- A bolster can be placed in front of the client's chest to prevent the upper body from rolling forward when pressure is applied to the infraspinatus muscle.
- To locate trigger points more effectively, turn the client to the prone position, with the upper arm abducted 90° and the forearm hanging off the table. Use thumb strokes to palpate and treat trigger points.

4. Teres Minor

Origin: Upper two-thirds of the dorsal surface of the axillary border of the scapula.

Insertion: Lowest facet of the greater tuberosity of the humerus, capsule of the shoulder joint.

Action: Lateral rotation of the humerus; weak adduction of the shoulder; stabilizes the humeral head in the shoulder joint.

David Rini

FIGURE 7-18 Elongation stroke on the infraspinatus from origin to insertion.

Position
- The client is lying in side posture, with the side to be treated uppermost.
- The therapist stands at the side of the table, behind the client's shoulder. If treating the right side of the client, the therapist's right thumb is placed along the axillary border of the scapula, and the left thumb is over the top of the client's right shoulder. (When working on the left side, hand positions are reversed.)

X This muscle is often clear of trigger points. Trigger points are more likely to form in the synergistic muscle to the teres minor, the infraspinatus.

Strokes
- Beginning with the thumb one-third of the way up along the axillary border, stroke along the edge of the bone, following the muscle fibers out to the head of the humerus (Fig. 7-19).
- Pause at tender areas, and treat.

5. Teres Major and Latissimus Dorsi

Teres Major
Origin: Dorsal surface of the scapula near the lateral side of the inferior angle.
Insertion: Medial lip of the bicipital groove of the humerus.
Action: Medial rotation, adduction, and extension of the arm.

X Easily confused in palpation with the latissimus dorsi, the teres major is closer to the border of the scapula and more medial. Trigger points are usually close to the scapular border. The pain referral zone is over the posterior deltoid and the long head of the triceps.

FIGURE 7-19 Elongation stroke on the teres minor from origin to insertion.

Latissimus Dorsi

Origin: Spinous processes of T6–T12 vertebrae, spinous processes of L1–L5 vertebrae and sacral vertebrae, supraspinal ligament, posterior one-third of the iliac crest of the ilium, ribs 9–12, inferior angle of the scapula.

Insertion: Floor of bicipital groove of the humerus.

Action: Extension, adduction, and medial rotation of the arm (most powerful when arm is in the overhead position); active in strong inspiration and expiration.

 When using the sifting technique, the latissimus dorsi is the most superficial muscle that is felt. Check the upper portion, particularly near the posterior deltoid. This trigger point, which is found in the axillary fold, refers pain to the midback region.

Strokes

- Standing behind the client's shoulder, grasp the muscles along the posterior border of the axilla, with your thumbs on the surface and your fingers underneath, in the axilla.
- Sift the muscle fibers thoroughly, and feel for taut bands and adhered tissues (Fig. 7-20). Treat any trigger points that are found.

STRETCH

The client is in side posture. Lift the client's arm overhead so that the upper arm is resting along the ear, with the forearm flexed. Holding the arm near the elbow, rotate the humerus medially, and allow the forearm and hand to hang off the back of the table (Fig. 7-21). If further stretch is needed, press down on the humerus until an adequate stretch is felt.

6. Triceps Brachii

Origin: Long head—infraglenoid tuberosity of the scapula. **Lateral head**—upper half of the posterior shaft of the humerus. **Medial head**—lower half of the posterior shaft of the humerus.

Insertion: Posterior surface of the olecranon process of the ulna.

Action: Extension of the forearm; when the arm is abducted, the long head aids in adduction.

Position

- The client is placed in prone position. The arm to be worked on is abducted 90°, with the forearm hanging off the side of the table.
- The therapist is standing at the side of the table, next to the client's shoulder.

 Trigger points may be found along the lateral border of the triceps near the elbow. A trigger point that contributes to the pain of tennis elbow is located in the medial portion of the muscle, from 1.5 to 2.5 inches above the lateral epicondyle. Using the thumb, snap across a taut band in that area to find the trigger point. Pain is referred to the lateral epicondyle and may continue down the radial side of the forearm.

FIGURE 7-20 Sifting the latissimus dorsi and teres major.

David Rini

FIGURE 7-21 Stretch for the teres major and minor, latissimus dorsi, and subscapularis.

Strokes

- Using the heel of the hand or knuckles, apply elongation strokes from the elbow to the head of the humerus.
- With the thumbs, stroke up the middle of the triceps, between the heads of the muscle (Fig. 7-22).
- Grasp the edges of the triceps between the thumb and fingers. Lift the muscle away from the bone and squeeze. Check for trigger points along its length.

7. Biceps Brachii

Origin: Short head—apex of the coracoid process of the scapula. **Long head**—supraglenoid tubercle of the scapula.

Insertion: Radial tuberosity of the radius, bicipital aponeurosis fusing with the deep fascia over the forearm flexors.

Action: Flexion and supination of the forearm; weak flexion of the arm at the shoulder joint when the forearm is fixed.

Position

- The client is placed in the supine position. The arm to be treated is resting, with the palm supinated, on the table next to the client's side.
- The therapist is standing at the head of the table, superior to the client's shoulder.

FIGURE 7-22 Direction of strokes on the triceps from the insertion (olecranon process) to origin (upper portion of the humerus).

rior deltoid. These trigger points are most easily palpated by stretching the biceps fibers. Hold the client's arm at the wrist, and extend it slightly off the table, keeping the forearm fully extended. With your other hand, feel for taut bands in the biceps muscle.

Strokes

- Using the heel of the hand or the knuckles, apply elongation strokes from the elbow to the shoulder joint.
- With the thumbs, stroke up the center of the biceps, between the two heads (Fig. 7-23).
- Grasp the edges of the biceps, between the fingers and thumb. Lift the muscle away from the bone, and squeeze. Check for trigger points along its length.

8. Brachialis

Origin: Lower two-thirds of the anterior shaft of the humerus.
Insertion: Tuberosity and coronoid process of the ulna.
Action: Flexion of the forearm.

Position

- The client is supine, with the arm to be worked on flexed at the elbow about 45°.
- The therapist stands at the side of the table and holds the wrist of the flexed arm.

DAR

FIGURE 7-23 Direction of strokes on the biceps from insertion (tuberosity of the radius) to origin (coracoid process of the scapula).

 The lower third of the biceps brachii may contain a trigger point in each head. They may refer pain throughout the biceps and upward into the ante-

 Trigger points are usually located in the distal portion of the brachialis, near the elbow. They refer pain chiefly to the base of the thumb.

David Rini

FIGURE 7-24 Contacting the brachialis deep to the biceps brachii.

FIGURE 7-25 Stretch for the triceps muscle.

FIGURE 7-26 Stretch for the biceps brachii.

FIGURE 7-27 Reflex zone for the shoulder.

Strokes
- The brachialis muscle is deep to the biceps. To reach it, slide your fingers under the biceps brachii muscle, on the medial side of the humerus, about halfway down the upper arm (Fig. 7-24).
- Do the side to side stroke, with your fingers along the muscle fibers to the elbow, allowing the muscle to lengthen and relax.

STRETCH

Position
- The client is lying supine.
- The therapist is standing at the head of the table.

1. *Triceps.* Lift the client's arm overhead, with the humerus next to the ear and the forearm hanging over the end of the table. Holding the humerus near the elbow, press the arm toward the table while the client flexes the forearm further by reaching the palm toward the underside of the table (Fig. 7-25).
2. *Biceps and Brachialis.* The client slides to the edge of the table. Bring the client's straight arm off the side of the table, and holding at the wrist, extend it downward, toward the floor, as the client reaches down and back with the hand (Fig. 7-26).

ACCESSORY WORK

1. Circumduct the shoulder, hip, and ankle joints on both sides of the body to help balance the muscles acting on the joints.

2. With your thumb tips, press the shoulder line on the feet (Fig. 7-27). It runs horizontally across the foot at the base of the toes.

CLOSING

Sitting at the foot of the table, lightly hold the heels of the client's feet in your hands for 30 to 60 seconds. Remove your hands slowly to complete the session.

◼ FOREARM AND HAND ROUTINE

Objectives

- To reduce stress and pain in the muscles of the forearm and hand brought about by extended use of the hand in work-related and other activities
- To improve dexterity and coordination skills of the hand
- To promote relaxation through the reflexive effects of hand massage

Energy

POSITION

- The client is lying supine, with the arms to his or her sides.
- The therapist stands at the side of the table and faces the client's forearm.

POLARITY

Lightly contact the wrist and elbow with the palms of the hands. Envision the forearm lengthening and relaxing. Hold for at least 30 seconds.

SHIATSU

1. With both hands, grasping the client's forearm just below the elbow joint, and compress the forearm from the elbow to the wrist. This move stimulates the same meridians as the upper arm shiatsu procedure.
2. Flex the client's forearm 90°. Interlace your fingers with your client's fingers. Holding the client's forearm slightly inferior to the wrist with your other hand, flex, extend, and circumduct the hand in both directions (Fig. 7-28). Opening up the wrist area stimulates the flow of energy (qi) through the arm channels.

Swedish/Cross Fiber

1. Perform effleurage strokes from the wrist to the elbow.
2. Perform thumb gliding on the palm and the back of the hand.

David Rini

FIGURE 7-28 Hand position for performing shiatsu wrist movements.

3. Perform pétrissage strokes on the muscles of the forearm.
4. Perform cross fiber strokes with the broad side of the thumb on the hand and forearm muscles.

Connective Tissue

MYOFASCIAL SPREAD

1. Grasping both sides of the client's hand, curve your fingers, and press them into the center of the palm. Slowly slide the fingers of each hand away from each other, stretching the tissues of the palm.
2. Flex the client's forearm 90° at the elbow. Place your hands around the forearm at the wrist, with the fingers sinking into the midline of the palmar side of the forearm. Slowly spread the fingers away from the midline, stretching the fascia. Continue, in horizontal strips, to the elbow. Repeat on the other side of the forearm.

Deep Tissue/Neuromuscular Therapy

SEQUENCE

1. Palm—superficial muscles, lumbricales, interossei
2. Thenar eminence—adductor pollicis brevis, flexor pollicis brevis, opponens pollicis

3. Fingers—digital flexors and extensors, ligaments, retinacula
4. Dorsal surface of the hand—extensor digitorum tendon, interossei
5. Wrist—flexor tendons and retinaculum, extensor tendons and retinaculum, pronator quadratus
6. Forearm
   a. Anterior surface—pronator teres, flexor carpi radialis, palmaris longus, flexor carpi ulnaris, flexor digitorum superficialis, flexor pollicis longus, flexor digitorum profundus, and brachioradialis.
   b. Dorsal surface—extensor carpi radialis longus, extensor carpi radialis brevis, extensor carpi ulnaris, extensor digitorum, extensor digiti minimi, supinator, abductor pollicis longus, extensor pollicis brevis, extensor pollicis longus, and extensor indicis.
7. Elbow
   a. Lateral epicondyle—attachments of extensor carpi radialis longus and brevis, extensor digitorum, and supinator.
   b. Medial epicondyle—attachments of the common flexor tendon, brachialis, and pronator teres.

1. The Palm

Position
- The client is lying supine, with the arm to his or her side and the palm supinated.

- The therapist is standing at the side of the table, next to the client's hand.

Interossei Muscles

a. Palmar

Origin:

First—entire ulnar side of second metacarpal

Second—entire radial side of fourth metacarpal

Third—entire radial side of fifth metacarpal

Insertion:

First—index finger at base of proximal phalanx on ulnar side

Second—ring finger at base of proximal phalanx on radial side

Third—entire radial side of fifth metacarpal

Action: Adduction of index, ring, and pinkie fingers toward middle finger

b. Dorsal

Origin:

First—lateral head: first metacarpal of thumb on proximal half of ulnar border, medial head: second metacarpal of index finger on entire radial border

Second—adjacent sides of metacarpals of index and middle fingers

Third—adjacent sides of middle and ring fingers

Fourth—adjacent sides of metacarpals of ring and pinkie fingers

Insertion:

First—radial side of index finger at base of proximal phalanx

Second—radial side of proximal phalanx of middle finger

Third—ulnar side of proximal phalanx of middle finger

Fourth—ulnar side of proximal phalanx of ring finger

Action: Abduction of fingers away from middle finger

FIGURE 7-30 Contacting the lumbricales muscles between the finger tendons.

To locate trigger points, have the client spread the fingers wide apart to separate the metacarpal bones. Using your thumb and index finger, squeeze the spaces between the bones. Nodules are often found around active trigger points in these muscles. Pain usually refers into the finger of the adjacent tendon.

Strokes

- Perform an elongating stroke with the fist, lengthwise, from the base of the palm to the fingers, and then horizontally across the palm, from the pinkie side to the thumb side (Fig. 7-29).
- For the lumbricales, perform an elongating stroke along the sides of the finger tendons using the thumb or tip of the index finger (Fig. 7-30).

FIGURE 7-29 Elongation stroke from the fifth metatarsal to the first metatarsal.

FIGURE 7-31 Deep tissue strokes on the thenar eminence.

2. Muscles of the Thenar Eminence

Adductor Pollicis Brevis, Flexor Pollicis Brevis, and Opponens Pollicis

Strokes

- Using your thumb, apply up and down and side to side strokes over the mound, checking for tenderness and taut bands (Fig. 7-31).

Adductor Pollicis

Origin: Oblique head—bases of second and third metacarpals, capitate, trapezoid. **Transverse head**—distal two-thirds of the palmar side of the third metacarpal.

Insertion: Base of the thumb at the ulnar side of the proximal phalanx.

Action: Adduction of the thumb.

 Trigger points may be located in this muscle by squeezing the webbing between the thumb and index finger. The referral zone is on the thumb, particularly on the lower outside edge near the wrist.

Flexor Pollicis Brevis

Origin: Flexor retinaculum and trapezium, first metacarpal bone.

Insertion: Base of the proximal phalanx of the thumb.

Action: Flexion of the metacarpophalangeal joint of the thumb.

 Place the tip of your thumb against the head of the metacarpal bone. As the client flexes the thumb several times, feel for the tendon, and press. The referral zone is local, around the trigger point.

Opponens Pollicis

Origin: Flexor retinaculum, tubercle of the trapezium.

Insertion: Entire radial side of the first metacarpal bone.

Action: Draws the first metacarpal bone forward and medial, bringing the thumb into opposition to the other fingers.

 Using the thumb tip, roll across the muscle fibers on the thenar eminence, feeling for taut bands and tenderness. Pain is referred to the inside portion of the thumb and to a spot on the radial side of the wrist.

3. Fingers

Preparation

Begin the following sequence at the base of the proximal phalanx of the thumb. Continue to the tip of the thumb, and then repeat, sequentially, on each of the four fingers.

Strokes

- Grasp the digit with the tip of the thumb on one side and the tip of the index finger on the other side. Alternately move the thumb and index finger up and down along the sides of the bone between the joints.

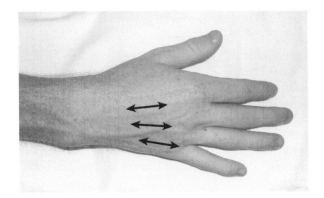

FIGURE 7-32 Direction of strokes on the dorsal interossei.

- Repeat the stroke, grasping the front and back of the bone.

4. Dorsal Surface of the Hand

Strokes

- Apply the fanning stroke with the thumbs over the entire dorsal surface of the hand.
- Perform short, up and down strokes with the tip of the index finger on the interosseus muscles between the tendons of the extensor digitorum muscle (Fig. 7-32).

5. Wrist (Tendons of Flexor and Extensor Muscles of Fingers)

Strokes

- Apply the fanning stroke, with the thumbs on the palmar and dorsal surfaces of the wrist (Fig. 7-33A).
- With the sides of your thumbs touching, do short, up and down and side to side strokes on the palmar and dorsal surfaces of the wrist (Fig. 7-33B).

FIGURE 7-33 A. Fanning and **B.** up and down strokes on the tendons of the finger flexor muscles at the wrist.

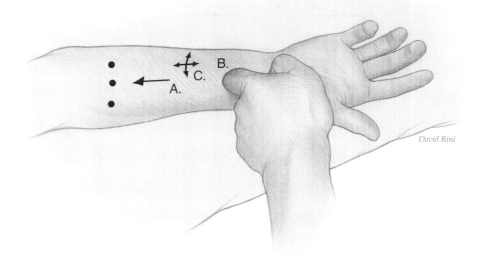

FIGURE 7-34 Location and direction of strokes on the hand and finger flexor muscles along the forearm.

6. Forearm

Hand and Finger Extensor Muscles

 Trigger points will lodge in the distal portion of the muscles, near the elbow. Pain is referred to the lateral epicondyle and down the forearm to the wrist and hand area.

Hand and Finger Flexor Muscles

 Trigger points tend to be located in a line across the muscles, about one-third of the way down the forearm from the elbow. They are best palpated with cross fiber strokes, feeling for taut bands in the fibers. They refer pain to the wrist and into the fingers.

Strokes
- Using the knuckles, perform elongation strokes from the wrist to the elbow (**A** in Fig. 7-34). Work in strips, with the palm supinated and then pronated, to cover the forearm thoroughly.
- Separate the muscles of the forearm by stroking between them with a thumb, knuckle, or elbow (**B** in Fig. 7-34).
- Using the thumbs or the elbows, perform short, up and down and side to side strokes on the bellies of the muscles (**C** in Fig. 7-34). Treat areas of tenderness and trigger points.
- Turn the client's forearm so that the thumb side of the hand is up. Grasp the brachioradialis muscle between the thumb and fingers, on the forearm, below the lateral epicondyle of the elbow. Roll the muscle fibers, checking for tenderness and trigger point activity (Fig. 7-35).

7. Elbow

Supinator

Origin: Lateral epicondyle of the humerus, radial collateral ligament of the elbow joint, annular ligament of the radioulnar joint, supinator crest of the ulna on the dorsal surface of the shaft.

Insertion: Dorsal and medial surfaces of the upper one-third of the radial shaft.

Action: Supination of the forearm and hand.

 A trigger point may be located near its attachment on the lateral epicondyle. The referral zone is the lateral epicondyle. Pain may also shoot to the webbing of the thumb.

Pronator Teres

Origin: Humeral head—distal supracondylar ridge, medial epicondyle of the humerus.

Ulnar head—coronoid process of the medial ulna.

FIGURE 7-35 Rolling the fibers of the brachioradialis muscle.

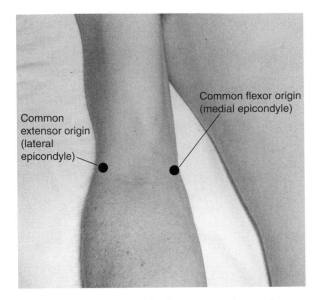

FIGURE 7-36 Location of the forearm muscle attachments.

Insertion: Pronator tuberosity on the lateral surface of the radius.

Action: Pronation and flexion of the forearm.

> A trigger point may be located near its attachment on the medial epicondyle. Pain is felt deep in the radial side of the wrist and may spill over into the forearm.

Strokes

- With the thumb, apply up and down, side to side, and static compression strokes around the lateral epicondyle. Treat the attachments of the extensor carpi radialis longus and brevis, extensor digitorum, and supinator muscles (Fig. 7-36). Having the client extend the hand makes these tendons easier to palpate.

> ⚠ **Because of the close proximity of the radial nerve, be careful when treating these attachments. If the client experiences a sharp, radiating sensation that is characteristic of nerve stimulation, release the pressure immediately, and shift the location of your thumb.**

- With the thumb, apply up and down, side to side, and static compression strokes around the medial epicondyle. Treat the attachments of the common flexor tendon, brachialis, and pronator teres muscles. Having the client flex his or her hand makes these tendons easier to palpate. Because of the position of the median nerve at the medial epicondyle, use the same caution as above.

STRETCH

1. With both hands facing each other in front of him or her, the client cups the palms and spreads all the fingers. Touching the tips of the fingers of both hands together, the client begins to push the hands toward each other, keeping the fingers apart and resisting somewhat with the cupped palms. The client continues to press the hands toward each other until a stretch is felt in the fingers and palms. The stretch is held for a minimum of 10 seconds.
2. Place your palm across the palmar surface of the client's fingers, and extend the client's hand until a stretch is felt in the flexor muscles of the fingers and hand (Fig. 7-37). (This and the following stretch are more effective if the client's arm is kept fully straight.)
3. Place your palm across the dorsal surface of the client's fingers, and flex the client's hand until a stretch is

David Rini

FIGURE 7-37 Stretch for the flexor muscles of the fingers and hand.

FIGURE 7-38 Stretch for the extensor muscles of the fingers and hand.

felt in the extensor muscles of the fingers and hand (Fig. 7-38).

ACCESSORY WORK

1. "Snapping off" the fingers (a shiatsu technique) will help to draw off accumulated energy that has built up from release of the hand and forearm muscles. An indication of this build-up is sweaty hands. To perform the move, hold the anterior and posterior sides of the client's finger at the base between your index and middle fingers. Gently slide down the finger, gliding straight off at the tip (Fig. 7-39). Begin with the thumb, and continue with each finger in succession to the pinkie.
2. A thorough foot massage is a good accompaniment to hand and forearm work. It gives the client a sense of integration between the upper and lower extremities.

CLOSING

Sitting at the foot of the table, lightly hold the heels of the client's feet in your hands for 30 to 60 seconds. Remove your hands slowly to complete the session.

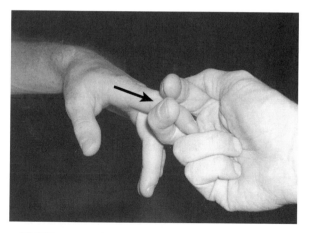

FIGURE 7-39 The shiatsu technique, "snapping off."

REFERENCES

1. Rolf IP. Rolfing: re-establishing the natural alignment and structural integration of the human body for vitality and well-being. Rochester, VT: Healing Arts Press, 1989.
2. Meyers T. Body 3: hanging out with the shoulder. Massage Magazine January/February 1999.
3. Travell JG, Simmons DG. Myofascial pain and dysfunction: the trigger point manual, volume 1. 2nd edition. Baltimore, MD: Lippincott Williams & Wilkins, 1999: 699.

Establishing a Firm Foundation

The Foot, Leg, and Knee

■ GENERAL CONCEPTS

The legs and feet are responsible for efficiently transferring weight from the upper body to the ground with minimal stress. They are also the locomotive structures of the body, providing the means for its movement through space. To perform the multiple tasks of weight transfer and movement, the knees and feet are necessarily complex in design. A balance of muscle, tendon, and ligament in the lower extremity is essential to enable its effective operation without breakdown. The focus of deep tissue work on the knees, lower legs, and feet is to re-establish the precise integration of muscle action with correct bony alignment. Lack of harmony among these body parts results in tension and instability throughout the rest of the body.

The feet form a horizontal platform on which the entire weight of the vertical body rests. The feet are small in proportion to the load they carry, which can create problems for effective weight distribution and support. This dilemma is solved by a series of arches that are located throughout the feet. Architecturally, the arch is used to distribute weight evenly from a smaller, concentrated area over a broad surface. In the case of the feet, the body forms a vertical column whose weight is focused at the ankle joints and then spread out through the feet and transferred to the ground.

When the body's weight is properly balanced on the foot, it radiates out from the talus through the bones of the foot. This even distribution of weight can be observed in the symmetrical shape of a footprint in the sand. (Photographs of footprints in the sand demonstrating various patterns of weight distribution can be found in Rolf.[1]) When the arches break down, the body's weight is more concentrated on the outside or the inside of the foot. This

causes a distortion in the footprint and an uneven wearing down of the soles of the shoes. Whether the initial breakdown occurs in the foot itself or further up in the body, it results in a redistribution of weight throughout the body segments in an effort to compensate for the lack of balance. This creates stress and pain around joints, particularly the knee, and loss of full function in the muscles.

The arches of the foot are supported and stabilized by muscles of the lower leg, which attach in various places along the bottom of the foot. These muscles pull up on the plantar surface of the foot, acting as guy wires that suspend the arches from above.[2] Ineffective support of the foot through muscular weakness is evident in legs that lack shape and proportion. Abnormal thickening in the legs denotes lack of fluid flow, which results from the inefficient pumping action of toneless muscles. As effective neuromuscular patterns of action are taught to the leg muscles through integrated deep tissue therapy, diminished arches can be effectively strengthened and raised. (Additional exercises for strengthening the feet can be found in Franklin.[3]) This re-education of the foot and leg muscles results in better-coordinated action throughout the body.

The joints of the legs are meant to operate in a relay fashion. In other words, the hip, knee, and ankle should all flex together and extend together during most leg movements. Although these three joints are not all technically hinges, they can be thought of in that way when working as a unit. They should be positioned so that they are aligned directly over each other in flexion movements, with the hinge at each joint forming a horizontal platform in relation to the vertical standing body. This alignment allows the muscles of the leg to store power when the joints flex, as in a preparation to jump, and to release that power effectively when the joints extend. Deep tissue work can help to restore this balanced alignment.

■ MUSCULOSKELETAL ANATOMY AND FUNCTION

See Essential Anatomy 8-1 for a summary of musculoskeletal anatomy and function.

The Foot

The ankle and foot should be thought of as a unit, because their functions are interdependent. Structurally, they are similar to the wrist and hand, and they are potentially capable of many of the same movements. The foot is organized as a series of arches that are meant to distribute weight. The foot also acts as a springboard to push the body away from the ground and propel it through space. To accomplish these functions, the foot must be both strong and mobile. It is composed of 26 bones, 31 joints, and 20 intrinsic muscles (Fig. 8-1). The bones of the foot are connected by a series of more than 100 ligaments. These ligaments reinforce the arches and limit movement at the joints so that the foot can maintain its integrity.

The foot has three major arches. The inner longitudinal arch is largely responsible for pushing the foot forward in locomotor movements. It is made up of the inner portion of the calcaneus, the talus, the navicular, the three cuneiforms, and the first three metatarsals and phalanges. The outer longitudinal arch is more weight-bearing and weight-distributing. It supports the inner arch by supplying lift and balance, and it is formed by the calcaneus, the cuboid, and the fourth and fifth metatarsals and phalanges. When the outer longitudinal arch is col-

lapsed, the weight of the body is thrown too much onto the outer portion of the foot, and the integrity of the balance of the lower limb is lost.

The third arch is actually a series of transverse arches crossing the foot. They are formed by the relationship of the tarsal and metatarsal bones with the surrounding muscles and ligaments. All the arches of the foot depend on strong muscular stability and action as well as on ligamentous support. The majority of these muscles attach on the tibia or fibula, providing a long lever of support. The long and short plantar ligaments are crucial in maintaining the shape of the arches. They connect the bones that form the ends of the longitudinal arches, like the string of a bow, and prevent them from sliding too far apart when weight is placed on the foot.

The superficial intrinsic muscles on the plantar surface of the foot are the **extensor hallucis brevis**, **abductor hallucis**, **flexor digitorum brevis**, and **abductor digiti minimi** (Fig. 8-1*B*). The only intrinsic muscle on the dorsal surface of the foot is the extensor digitorum brevis. Overall, these muscles serve to stabilize the foot when a person is balancing on one leg, and they are used in walking and running. Flexor digitorum brevis is responsible for clutching actions of the foot, where the toe joints are flexed and the person appears to be grasping the ground with the feet. This stance is indicative of tension and instability higher up in the body. Sore feet and pain when walking may indicate the presence of trigger points in the intrinsic foot muscles.

The deep intrinsic muscles consist of the **quadratus plantae and lumbricales**, **flexor hallucis brevis**, **adductor hallucis**, **flexor digiti minimi brevis**, and the **interossei** (Fig. 8-1*E*). Their primary function is to align and stabilize the bones of the foot during propulsion. They guide and move the toes, providing a balanced pulling action on the bones so that the foot tracks forward properly, with the

---

BOX 8-1 ESSENTIAL ANATOMY The Foot, Leg, and Knee Routines

MUSCLES
Toe tendons
Insertion points of flexor hallucis longus, flexor hallucis brevis, and abductor hallucis
Muscles of the plantar surface of the foot
Muscles of the dorsal surface of the foot
Ankle retinaculum
Flexor digitorum longus
Lateral leg muscles—tibialis anterior, extensor hallucis longus, extensor digitorum longus, and peroneals
Gastrocnemius
Soleus
Knee—ligaments and tendons

BONES AND LANDMARKS
Bones of the foot—phalanges, metatarsals, cuboid, navicular, talus
Tibia
Lateral malleolus
Medial malleolus
Tibial tuberosity
Fibula
Head of fibula
Patella

FIGURE 8-1 A. Muscles that move the foot and toes, superficial layer—anterior view. (Reprinted with permission from Hendrickson T. Massage for orthopedic conditions. Baltimore, MD: Lippincott Williams & Wilkins, 2002.)
B. Attachment sites of muscles of the leg and foot—anterior view.

A

B

FIGURE 8-1 *(continued)* **C.** Muscles that move the foot and toes, superficial layer—posterior view. (Reprinted with permission from Oatis CA. Kinesiology: the mechanics and pathomechanics of human movement. Baltimore, MD: Lippincott Williams & Wilkins, 2003.) **D.** Attachment sites of muscles of the leg and foot—posterior view.

FIGURE 8-1 *(continued)* **E.** Third layer of muscles on the plantar surface of the foot. (Reprinted with permission from Hendrickson T. Massage for orthopedic conditions. Baltimore, MD: Lippincott Williams & Wilkins, 2003.) **F.** Attachment sites of muscles on the plantar surface of the foot.

Adductor hallucis (transverse head)

Adductor hallucis (oblique head)

Flexor hallucis brevis

Opponens digiti minimi

Flexor digiti minimi

E

Flexor digitorum longus

Flexor digitorum brevis

Flexor longus

Adductor flexor brevis   Hallucis

Abductor flexor brevis

Abductor digiti minimi

Flexor digiti minimi

Peroneus longus

Adductor hallucis

Tibialis anterior

Flexor digiti minimi

Tibialis posterior

Quadratus plantae

DAR

Abductor digiti minimi

Flexor digitorum brevis

Plantar aponeurosis

F

toes not spread too far apart or overlapping each other. Restricted movement or hypermobility of the toes, as well as calluses on them, may indicate tension in the deep intrinsic muscles.

The Ankle

The ankle joint consists of the articulation of the tibia over the talus bone. The medial malleolus, which is a projection on the tibia, and the lateral malleolus at the lower end of the fibula form the sides of a cavity that fits over the talus, creating a pure hinge joint.

The talus articulates with the calcaneus bone below it, transferring weight to the calcaneus from the tibia and forming another joint capable of inversion and eversion (the lifting and lowering of the medial side of the foot). This joint is extremely important in maintaining the integrity of the foot, because the strength of the arches is largely dependent on the position of the calcaneus. When the calcaneus slides out to the side from underneath the talus, it causes the inner arch to fall and the tibia to rotate medially. In the case of an abnormally high medial arch, the calcaneus has pulled inward under the talus, decreasing the length of the foot and throwing weight to the outside of the foot. An overly high arch inhibits flexibility in the foot, causing the ankle to become looser, because it has to accommodate adjustments that normally would be made by a more flexible foot.

The Leg

The bones of the leg are the tibia and fibula. The tibia supports more weight than the femur, yet the tibia is smaller. The fibula attaches to the tibia via an interosseus membrane. It reinforces the tibia, giving increased elasticity and flexibility to the leg, and it provides attachment points for important muscles of the lower extremity.

The following groups of muscles control movements of the foot but have their origins on various places on the leg (Fig. 8-1*B*). The **extensor hallucis longus dorsiflexes** the big toe and foot, while the **extensor digitorum longus** flexes the other four toes. Both muscles are important in preventing the entire foot from dropping hard against the ground during walking. Night cramps of the toes are caused by spasms in these muscles.

The **flexor hallucis longus plantar flexes** the big toe and ankle, **inverts** the foot, and assists support of the medial arch. The **flexor digitorum longus** plantar flexes the four toes and ankle and also provides support for the arches. Both muscles provide stability when a person is standing on tiptoe.

The **tibialis anterior** is the strongest **dorsiflexor** of the foot and inverts the foot (Fig. 8-1*A*). It is highly active during running and jumping movements. Attaching on the base of the first metatarsal bone and the medial cuneiform, the tibialis anterior supports the medial arch. Overuse of this muscle is one of the primary causes of shin splints. Driving a car for long periods with the foot held on the accelerator pedal in a dorsiflexed position can also be stressful to the tibialis anterior muscle. Regular stretching of the gastrocnemius and soleus, the antagonist muscles on the back of the leg, helps to keep tibialis anterior in proper balance.

The **peroneus longus** and **peroneus brevis** are responsible for plantar flexion, **eversion** of the foot, and support of the lateral arch (Fig. 8-1*A*). They oppose the tibialis anterior in their actions. The coordinated action of these muscles is crucial in preventing sideways rolling of the foot.

The **gastrocnemius** crosses the ankle and knee joints (Fig. 8-1*C*). When the knee is extended or slightly flexed, it is a strong plantar flexor of the ankle. This muscle also flexes and medially rotates the knee. When the knee is flexed, the gastrocnemius is too slack to be effective as an ankle flexor.

The **soleus** is deep to the gastrocnemius. The two muscles act as a unit in their action at the ankle, merging at the Achilles tendon. The soleus attaches broadly on the tibia and fibula. Both muscles act to prevent overflexion of the knee during walking by stabilizing the ankle.

The Knee

The articulation of the tibia and femur forms the knee joint. The two convex condyles of the femur fit into the two concave condyles of the tibia, allowing flexion, extension, and slight rotation movements at the beginning of flexion because of the uneven size of the condyles. The femur moves on the tibia with a combination of rolling and gliding movements. It is prevented from sliding off the tibia through the reinforcement of strong muscles and ligaments.

Eight ligaments reinforce the knee joint. The four primary ligaments are the anterior and posterior cruciate ligaments and the lateral and medial collateral ligaments. Two other ligaments, known as the menisci, are ring-shaped structures of cartilage that are formed at the top of the tibia. They provide cushioning, even distribution of weight, and shock absorption between the femur and tibia.

The patella is a small, triangular-shaped bone in front of the knee joint that is formed within the quadriceps tendon. It protects the knee, and it provides greater leverage for the action of the quadriceps muscle by acting as a pulley.

Twelve muscles directly affect movement at the knee. Eight of these muscles are two-joint muscles, meaning that they cross two joints; the remaining four muscles are one-joint muscles (the popliteal and three of the quadricep -muscles). Six of the two-joint muscles affect the movements of the femoral and knee joints. They are the three hamstring muscles (biceps femoris, semimembranosus, and semitendinosus), the rectus femoris, sartorius, and gracilis. The other two affect movements of the knee and ankle joints. They are the gastrocnemius and the plantaris. These eight muscles need to be balanced and coordinated for proper function of the knee to occur. All eight muscles should be examined in conjunction with the muscles controlling the arches of the foot to assure stress-free movements of the knee.

CONDITIONS

Feet and Ankles

1. To help a *fallen medial arch*:
   - Have the client perform exercises to build the arch (e.g., picking up marbles with the toes).
   - Release the peroneal muscles, because the foot will be overly everted.
2. A *callus* indicates too much strain or wear on that section of the foot, resulting from misalignment or improperly fitted shoes. Releasing the muscles that are pulling the toes or metatarsal out of position will sometimes reduce the callus.
3. *Plantar fasciitis* is an inflammation of the plantar fascia, often caused by overuse of the foot through walking, running, or jumping. Ice packs may be applied. Massage is contraindicated.
4. With a *sprained ankle*, ligaments will be damaged and at least partially torn. Damage can also be more severe. Apply ice immediately. Have the ankle checked by a physician. Massage work may be indicated after the initial swelling has subsided. Range of motion assessment can indicate more specifically which ligaments have been damaged.

Leg

1. *"Shin splints"* is a vague term describing a variety of strain conditions that affect the lower leg. Any of the muscles along the lower leg that move the foot may be subject to slight tearing away from the bone when overused or fatigued, resulting in pain and inflammation. Treatment consists of rest, application of ice, and mild massage to bring blood to the area. Left untreated, shin splints may result in stress fractures to the tibia.
2. *Achilles tendinitis* is an inflammatory condition brought about by overuse of the gastrocnemius and soleus muscles. Rest and ice are the appropriate treatment. Shortness of the gastrocnemius muscle is a common cause of strain in the Achilles tendon. Regular massage and stretching of this muscle is an excellent preventive measure (see exercises for calf muscles).
3. *Muscle cramps* occur frequently in the gastrocnemius muscles. To relieve cramping, stretch the muscle by dorsiflexing the foot and holding it for at least 30 seconds. If the cramp does not subside, rest and ice are appropriate treatment.

Knees

1. *Pain around the knee* may be caused by poor alignment of the leg. Pain on the medial side can be an indication of shearing actions. Pain in the patellar ligament below the knee can be caused by overly deep, forward-lunging actions or hyperextension of the knee, which is often accompanied by pain in the ligaments at the back of the knee.
2. *Chondromalacia* is a softening or roughening of the underside of the patella. It can be caused by a blow to the knee or by poor muscle tone around the knee, and it is accompanied by a grinding or creaking sound when the knee is flexed. Strengthening the quadriceps muscles is recommended.

Please refer to Indications/Contraindications Box 8-2 for an additional list of indications and contraindications for massage of the foot and leg.

BOX 8-2 INDICATIONS/CONTRAINDICATIONS Conditions Affecting Foot and Leg Massage

INDICATIONS	CONTRAINDICATIONS
Uneven weight placement on feet	Acute shin splints
Collapsed arches	Stress fracture
Bunions	Broken bones
Misalignments of toes	Varicose veins
Muscle strain	Phlebitis
Muscle cramps	Spreadable rashes or fungus
Well-healed foot surgery	
Knee problems	

TABLE 8-1 | Body Reading for the Feet

Conditions	Muscles That May Be Shortened
Pigeon-toed—legs rotate medially, feet turn in; a valgus alignment of the knees	Adductors Gluteus medius and minimus Tensor fascia latae
Duck feet—legs rotate laterally, feet turn out; a varus alignment of the knees	Gluteus maximus Iliopsoas Piriformis, deep lateral rotators
High insteps	Tibialis anterior Tibialis posterior
Fallen arches	Peroneal muscles
Hammer toes	Toe flexor muscles

TABLE 8-2 | Range of Motion (ROM) for the Knee and Ankle

Action	Muscles
Knee	
Flexion (ROM 135°)	Biceps femoris Semitendinosus Semimembranosus Sartorius Gracilis Gastrocnemius Plantaris Popliteus
Extension (ROM 0°)	Quadriceps Tensor fascia latae
Internal rotation (ROM 10°)	Semitendinosus Semimembranosus Popliteus Gracilis Sartorius
External rotation (ROM 10°)	Biceps femoris
Ankle	
Dorsiflexion (ROM 10°)	Tibialis anterior External digitorum longus Peroneus tertius Extensor hallucis longus
Plantar flexion (ROM 65°)	Gastrocnemius Soleus Plantaris Peroneus longus Peroneus brevis Tibialis posterior Flexor hallucis longus
Inversion of the foot (ROM 5°)	Tibialis anterior Tibialis posterior
Eversion of the foot (ROM 5°)	Peroneus tertius Peroneus longus Peroneus brevis

the **mind body** *connection*

The feet and ankles support and move the entire body. They are also our physical connection to the ground beneath us. Any form of imbalance or distortion in this area may be reflected as a sense of insecurity. How can we take a strong stance in life, or move with grace and fluidity, if we are unsure of our self at our foundation? A person who takes solid steps, who is trusting of firm support underneath his or her feet, exudes a sense of confidence. Such persons know their places and stand their ground.

A close examination of the feet not only reveals structural imbalances higher up in the body but also provides a map of how an individual might be compensating for feelings of insecurity. The way a person's feet relate to the earth mirrors the way that individual relates to the issues of contact and grounding. For example, a person with flat feet is making a fuller contact with the ground. Such a person may need the feeling of knowing that he or she is supported or held up by external influences. Someone with extremely high arches is making minimal contact with the earth. That person may experience a sense of disconnection with the ground or the kind of diminished mental clarity associated with a lack of grounding.

The ankle joints are essential for moving the feet. They express, as do all joints, the ability to adapt and change direction. Inflexible ankles prevent the feet from pointing in various directions and stepping on different paths, limiting the number of choices a person may feel he or she is able to make in life. Ankles that are weak and buckle under prevent individuals from feeling they can stand up fully and carry their own weight.

The knees are important joints for weight support and transfer. They tie in with a wide variety of emotions. We tend to collapse and shake at our knees in response to a number of emotional stimuli. Fear can cause a person to feel weak in the knees, as can powerful joy and excitement.

When the knees, ankles, and feet are aligned through the vertical axis, with the feet pointing straight forward, energy is able to flow freely through the lower extremity. The feet relate to the root chakra, dealing with issues of survival and sustenance of the physical body. Interpretations of body stances are subjective, with many possible nuances of meaning, and these interpretations should only be used as indicators, not as blanket categorizations of personality or behavior.

■ POSTURAL EVALUATION

1. Check the alignment of the legs.
   - How does the line of gravity flow from the knee to the foot?
   - What is the shape of the legs: straight, bowed, knock-kneed?
2. Observe where the body's weight is concentrated on the feet. Is it forward, back, medial, or lateral?
3. Compare the directions in which the right and left feet are facing.
4. Observe the arches.
   - Are they high?
   - Are they collapsed?
5. Describe the shape and configuration of the toes.
   - Are they squeezed together?
   - Are they spread apart?
   - Are they curled under?
   - Does the big toe pull inward?
6. Check for bunions, calluses, and blisters on the feet, which indicate stress points on the feet.
7. Observe imbalance and/or weakness in the ankles. Compare the right and left ankles. Are the ankle joints on the same horizontal plane?
8. Look at the shape of the lower legs.
   - Are the muscles toned?
   - Is there swelling?
9. Describe the positioning of the knees.
   - Are they locked or hyperextended?
   - Are they flexed?
   - Are the patellae drawn up?
   - Are there bulges on the medial side of the knees, indicating a bracing of the soft tissues against gravity?
10. Examine the shape and muscle tone of the posterior legs.
    - What is the muscular condition of the calves? Are they large, underdeveloped, of equal size and shape on both sides? Are there differences between the right and left legs?
    - Are the Achilles tendons on both legs vertical, or is one (or both) pulling to the side?

Refer to Table 8-1 for a description of common distortions of the feet and possible muscles involved. Refer to Table 8-2 for the range of motion for the knee and ankle.

■ EXERCISES AND SELF-TREATMENT

Feet and Ankles

Lie down on your back, with both knees flexed. Both feet are on the floor and parallel to each other. Bring the right knee to the chest. Place both hands around the knee to stabilize it (Fig. 8-2).

FIGURE 8-2 Body position for performing foot exercises.

1. *Foot circles* (alternately stretches and strengthens all the muscles that move the ankle joints). Rotate the foot slowly in a full circle, as if tracing the face of a clock. Inhale during the first half of the circle; exhale while completing the circle. Repeat the movement three times in each direction (Fig. 8-3).
2. *Flexing* (alternately stretches and strengthens the intrinsic muscles of the foot and the plantar and dorsiflexor muscles of the ankle). Begin the exercise with the right foot fully flexed. Slowly, and with resistance, point the foot, articulating each joint. Reverse the motion, bringing the foot back to full dorsiflexion. Repeat the movement two more times (Fig. 8-4).
3. *Toe clutching* (alternately stretches and strengthens the flexors and extensors of the toes). Begin with the foot dorsiflexed. Imagine a pencil placed behind the toes. On exhalation, imagine squeezing the pencil with the toes, making a fist with the foot (Fig. 8-5). Inhaling, release the flexion of the toes. Repeat the movement three times.
4. Repeat the above three exercises on the left side.

Calf Muscles

Stack two telephone books against the base of a wall. Stand facing the wall, with the balls of your feet on the edge of the telephone books. Put your hands against the wall for support.

1. *Toe raises* (strengthens the gastrocnemius, soleus, tibialis posterior, peroneus longus and brevis, and flexor hallucis longus). Slowly raise up onto the balls of the feet. Hold for three counts. Lower your feet until the heels are parallel to the top of the telephone books. Repeat the movement several times.
2. *Calf stretch* (stretches the gastrocnemius, soleus, tibialis posterior, and other plantar flexor muscles). Slowly lower your heels toward the floor, until you feel a stretch in the calf muscles. Hold the stretch for a minimum of 20 seconds.

■ FOOT, LEG, AND KNEE ROUTINE

Objectives

- To balance the muscles that control the foot so that weight placement and walking patterns can be improved
- To relieve stress and uneven pulls on the muscles of the foot so that the formation of bunions, calluses, and other manifestations of foot dysfunction are minimized
- To balance muscular action around the knee, allowing the knee to track properly and thus eliminating strain on the soft tissue components of the joint
- To help relieve painful conditions that manifest in the muscles of the leg, such as spasms, shin splints, and trigger points

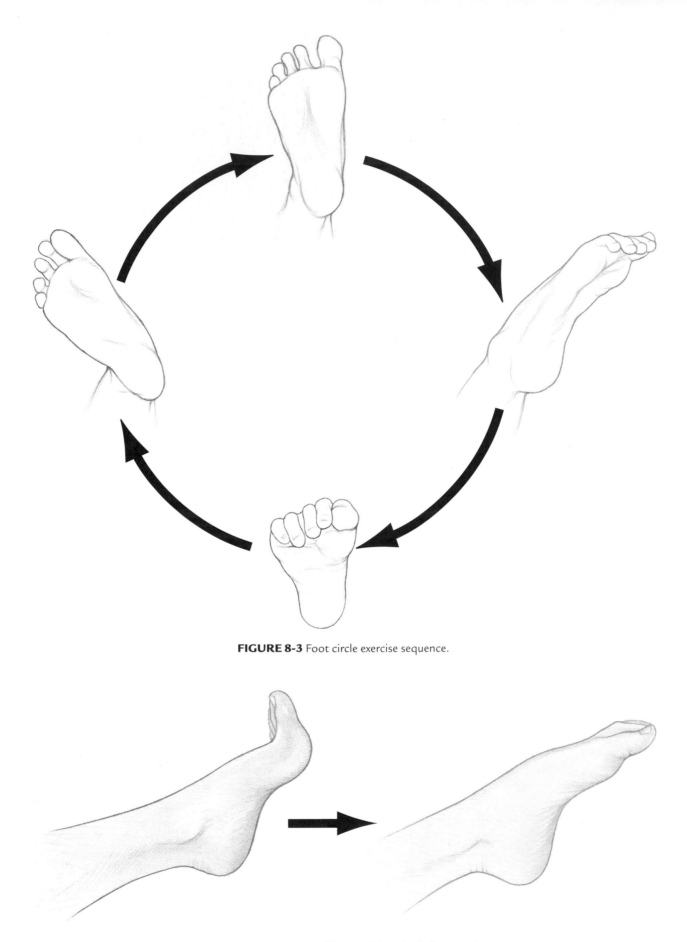

FIGURE 8-3 Foot circle exercise sequence.

FIGURE 8-4 Sequence of foot positions in flexing exercise.

FIGURE 8-6 Shiatsu compression of the foot.

FIGURE 8-5 Toe clutching to strengthen the arches of the foot.

Energy

POSITION

- The client is lying supine on the table. A bolster under the knees is optional.
- The therapist is standing at the foot of the table.

POLARITY

Hold the toes of each foot between the thumb and index finger for 10 seconds each, beginning with the fifth toe and ending with the big toe. According to polarity theory, the tip of each toe is the culmination point of a vertical line of force that runs through the body from head to toe. These energy currents stimulate proper physiologic and psychological functioning. Moving from the fifth toe to the big toe, the energy currents are labeled earth, water, fire, air, and ether, respectively, in accordance with ayurvedic terminology. Holding each toe assists in clearing any blockages along these five energetic pathways.

SHIATSU

1. Compress the leg with both hands from the knee to the ankle. This stimulates the flow of qi through the channels that flow through the leg. The yang channels on the outside of the leg are the gallbladder and stomach.

The yin channels on the inside portion of the leg are the spleen, liver, and kidney.
2. Squeeze down the sides of the foot to the toes (Fig. 8-6).

Swedish/Cross Fiber

1. Alternately apply effleurage strokes down the dorsal and plantar surfaces of the foot.
2. Perform knuckle kneading on the plantar surface of the foot.
3. Perform thumb gliding on the dorsal surface of the foot.
4. Perform effleurage and draining strokes from the ankle to the knee.
5. Reach the fingers of both hands underneath the calf, and place the fingertips between the heads of the gastrocnemius muscles. Rake outward, drawing the hands away from each other. Cover the entire calf, from several inches above the ankle to the knee.
6. Perform thumb gliding around the knee.

Connective Tissue

MYOFASCIAL SPREADING TECHNIQUES

1. Facing the dorsal side of the client's foot from the side of the table, place the hands around the sides of the foot, with the fingertips touching at the midline of the plantar surface. Sink in with the fingers, and spread from the midline to the outside edges of the foot.
2. Standing at the foot of the table, place the fingers on the dorsal surface of the foot at the base of the toes. Sink into the tissues, and slowly glide toward the ankle.

CASE STUDY 6 The Foot and Leg

 The client is a 50-year-old man named Eugene, who is the head manager of a fast-food franchise. The duties of his job require that he stand all day. He is constantly moving around the store to ensure the smooth operation of the business. He sought out deep tissue therapy because his feet and legs are becoming extremely sore and swollen, especially by the end of the workweek. Because he is so uncomfortable, it has become increasingly difficult for him to carry out the functions of his job.

Postural evaluation revealed that Eugene has flat feet. This causes the medial side of the knees to fall inward, creating stress on the medial collateral ligaments. He exhibits a high degree of lordosis, and his scapulae are depressed. His clavicles angle downward, and his arms hang forward of his sides. Eugene also exhibits a forward head position, with his chin held abnormally high.

To deal fully with the problems in his lower body, a series of deep tissue sessions was commenced to align the entire body. Isolated massage to his feet and legs would not resolve the problems in his feet, because they are reflective of postural imbalances throughout the entire body. Massage to the feet was performed in every deep session. The current case study, however, details the fourth session performed, during which the muscles of the lower limb were emphasized.

Eugene's feet are very stiff and immobile. There is limited movement in the ankles and throughout the joints of the foot. After the first session, he was shown foot exercises to practice at home to begin to alleviate some of the inflexibility of the foot muscles.

The session focusing on the feet began with work on the intrinsic muscles of the foot. The deep tissue strokes revealed tiny, granular-feeling lumps accumulated along the toe tendons and extreme sensitivity to pressure in many areas on the plantar surface of the foot. Sustained, therapist-assisted flexion and extension of the toes was administered to stretch the muscles and fascia of the foot, along with plantar flexion, dorsiflexion, inversion, and eversion movements.

Low medial arches force both feet into eversion while the client is standing. Therefore, the peroneal muscles, which evert the foot, are extremely contracted. Eugene's

feet like concrete. Slow, deep strokes with the elbow were performed on these muscles. A high degree of softening of the peroneal longus and brevis was achieved. To balance the release of the peroneals, the client was taught an exercise to strengthen the tibialis anterior muscle, which lifts the medial arch. Its action counterbalances that of the peroneal muscles. The lesson took place after the session. Eugene was taught to sit in a chair with his leg flexed at the hip, knee, and ankle. He was to hang a petite-size gift bag containing two soup cans from his flexed foot. He would then slowly invert his foot (turn the plantar surface inward) and hold for 3 seconds. This movement was to be repeated 10 times on the right and left sides.

The gastrocnemius and soleus muscles were also massaged. The heads of the gastrocnemii were sensitive to touch. Extensive Swedish pétrissage and friction strokes were used to relax the muscles. Cross fiber strokes were incorporated rather than deep tissue elongation strokes, because the muscles were too sensitive to withstand sustained direct pressure. All the muscle attachments around the knee were treated. The muscle attachments of the pes anserinus were particularly sensitive.

Deep tissue therapy to the legs and feet was followed by shoulder, neck, and cranial massage to complete the session. To supplement the foot exercises, additional home care suggestions (including elevation of the legs following a long day at work and regular foot soaks in warm water with epsom salts) were made.

Topics for Discussion

1. Describe the likely configuration of the legs and pelvis in a client with fallen medial arches.
2. A client stands with the majority of weight on the backs of the heels. Which muscles of the legs and feet are probably shortened?
3. How would you explain to a client the importance of taking care of the feet?
4. What are some important features of a well-designed shoe to provide support and comfort to the foot?
5. What are some possible indications that a client has plantar fasciitis?

3. Place the heels of the hands at the midline of the leg, above the ankle. Slowly spread the hands apart. Work in horizontal strips to the knee.

Deep Tissue/Neuromuscular Therapy

SEQUENCE

1. Tendons of the toes
2. Insertion points of flexor hallucis longus, flexor hallucis brevis, and abductor hallucis 💿
3. Muscles of the plantar surface of the foot
   a. First layer—abductor digiti minimi, flexor digitorum brevis, abductor hallucis
   b. Second layer—flexor hallucis longus, flexor digitorum longus, four lumbricals, quadratus plantae
   c. Third layer—flexor digiti minimi, adductor hallucis, flexor hallucis brevis
   d. Fourth layer—three plantar and four dorsal interossei; tendons of peroneus longus and tibialis posterior
4. Muscles of the dorsal surface of the foot
   a. Tendons—tibialis anterior, extensor hallucis longus, extensor digitorum longus, peroneus tertius
   b. Muscles—interossei, extensor hallucis brevis, extensor digitorum brevis, abductor digiti minimi
5. Retinaculum of the ankle—anterior portion
6. Medial leg muscles—flexor digitorum longus, soleus, gastrocnemius
7. Lateral leg muscles—tibialis anterior, extensor hallucis longus, extensor digitorum longus, peroneus longus, peroneus brevis, peroneus tertius, soleus
8. Retinaculum of the ankle—posterior portion
9. Gastrocnemius
10. Soleus and deep posterior leg muscles
11. Knee—ligaments and tendons

1. Tendons of the Toes

- Standing at the foot of the table, grasp the base of the proximal phalanx of the big toe, front and back, with the thumb and index finger (Fig. 8-7). Do short, up and down strokes on the flexor and extensor tendons. Repeat on the distal phalanx.
- Repeat the above stroke on each of the other four toes, moving in sequence from the base of the second toe to the fifth toe.

2. Insertions of Flexor Hallucis Longus, Flexor Hallucis Brevis, Abductor Hallucis, and Adductor Hallucis

Flexor Hallucis Longus
The attachment point is located at the center of the base of the distal phalanx of the big toe, just above the joint, on the plantar surface of the foot.

Strokes
- Do static compression and cross fiber friction on the attachment with the tip of your thumb or index finger.

Flexor Hallucis Brevis
The medial part inserts on the medial side of the base of the proximal phalanx of the hallux. The lateral part inserts on the lateral side of the base of the proximal phalanx of the hallux.

Abductor Hallucis
The abductor hallucis inserts on the medial side of the base of the proximal phalanx of the hallux.

David Rini

FIGURE 8-7 Contacting the flexor and extensor tendons of the toes.

Adductor Hallucis

The adductor hallucis inserts on the lateral side of the base of the proximal phalanx of the hallux.

Strokes

- To contact these attachments, hold the base of the big toe on both sides between your thumb and index finger. Feel for the tender spots on either side of the toe.
- Apply static compression and cross fiber friction on tender areas.

3. Muscles of the Plantar Surface of the Foot

Position

- The therapist sits at the foot of the table, with the non-working hand holding the client's foot around the toes and maintaining a dorsiflexed position.

Flexor Hallucis Brevis

Origin: Medial portion of the cuboid bone, lateral cuneiform bone.

Insertion: Base of the proximal phalanx of the hallux on the medial and lateral sides.

Action: Flexes the proximal phalanx of the hallux.

Abductor Hallucis

Origin: Tuberosity of the calcaneus, flexor retinaculum, plantar aponeurosis.

Insertion: Medial side of the base of the proximal phalanx of the hallux.

Action: Abduction of the hallux.

 Trigger points tend to collect in the flexor hallucis brevis and abductor hallucis, which are muscles that insert at the medial side of the base of the big toe. The referred pain zone for the flexor hallucis brevis is the region of the head of the first metatarsal and perhaps into the big toe. Trigger point pain from the abductor hallucis can run across the ball of the foot. Check carefully along the toe tendons as well.

Strokes

- Using a **soft fist**, stroke down the plantar surface of the foot from the base of the toes to the heel (Fig. 8-8).
- To reach the lumbricales muscles, stroke along the sides of each of the toe muscle tendons with the knuckle of the index finger or the thumb, from the base of the toes to the heel (Fig. 8-9). Maintain static compression on tender spots.

4. Muscles of the Dorsal Surface of the Foot

Extensor Digitorum Brevis

Origin: Anterior and lateral surfaces of the calcaneus, lateral talocalcaneal ligament, and extensor retinaculum.

Insertion: Base of the proximal phalanx of the hallux, joins the lateral sides of the tendons of the extensor digitorum longus on toes 2, 3, and 4.

Action: Extends the hallux (big toe) and toes 2, 3, and 4.

FIGURE 8-8 Deep tissue stroke on the muscles of the plantar surface of the foot.

FIGURE 8-9 Stroking the lumbricales muscles between the toe tendons.

 To check for trigger points, feel for tenderness in the extensor digitorum brevis muscle, near the ankle crease. Pain from trigger points can radiate over the entire dorsal surface but will be most pronounced near the ankle.

Strokes
- With the knuckle of the index finger or the thumb, stroke along the sides of the toe tendons, from the base of the toes to the ankle (Fig. 8-10).

FIGURE 8-10 Direction of deep tissue strokes on extensor digitorum brevis.

David Rini

FIGURE 8-11 Directions of strokes on the retinaculum of the ankle.

5. Retinaculum of the Ankle—Anterior Portion

Strokes
- Place both thumbs at the midline of the ankle joint. Simultaneously move both thumbs in short, up and down strokes, sliding the retinaculum over the tendon sheaths.
- Separating the thumbs slightly, repeat the stroke (Fig. 8-11). Continue to the medial and lateral malleoli.

6. Medial Leg Muscles (Flexor Digitorum Longus, Soleus, and Gastrocnemius)

Position
- Stand at the side of the table, and place the fingers of both hands along the medial border of the tibia, behind the medial malleolus.

Strokes
- Perform circular friction strokes with the fingertips on the muscles medial to the edge of the tibia bone. Work from the medial malleolus to the knee.
- Perform short, up and down and side to side strokes with the fingertips on the borders of the muscles just medial to the edge of the tibia, from the medial malleolus to the knee (Fig. 8-12).

David Rini

FIGURE 8-12 Directions of deep tissue strokes on the medial leg muscles.

7. Lateral Leg Muscles (Tibialis Anterior, Extensor Hallucis Longus, Extensor Digitorum Longus, Peroneus Longus, Peroneus Brevis, Peroneus Tertius, and Soleus)

Tibialis Anterior
Origin: Lateral condyle and proximal two-thirds of the lateral surface of the tibia, interosseus membrane.
Insertion: First medial cuneiform on the medial and plantar surfaces, base of the first metatarsal.
Action: Dorsiflexion of the ankle at the talocrural joint; inversion (supination) of the foot at the subtalar and midtarsal joints.

 Trigger points are most often found in the upper third of the tibialis anterior muscle. The referred pain zone will be on the front of the ankle toward the medial side and over the entire big toe (hallux).
Note: It may be easier to work on the tibialis anterior muscle with the client in a supine position.

Peroneus Longus
Origin: Head and upper two-thirds of the lateral shaft of the fibula.
Insertion: Lateral plantar side of the base of the first metatarsal, lateral plantar side of the first cuneiform.
Action: Eversion of the foot; assists plantar flexion of the ankle; support of the transverse arch.

Check the fibers of peroneus longus approximately 1 inch below the head of the fibula. The trigger point referral zone is around the lateral malleolus, extending along the lateral side of the foot.

Peroneus Brevis
Origin: Distal two-thirds of the lateral surface of the shaft of the fibula.
Insertion: Tuberosity on the lateral surface of the fifth metatarsal.

Action: Eversion of the foot; assists plantar flexion of the ankle.

Peroneus Tertius
Origin: Distal third of the medial surface of the fibula.
Insertion: Dorsal surface of the base of the fifth metatarsal.
Action: Dorsiflexion of the ankle; assists foot eversion.

Strokes
- Trace the lateral side of the lateral malleolus with the knuckle or thumb to contact the tendons of the peroneal muscles. Perform the short, up and down strokes on the tendons.
- For the tibialis anterior, perform an elongation stroke with the elbow lateral to the shaft of the tibia from the ankle to the lateral condyle of the tibia (Fig. 8-13).

FIGURE 8-13 Elongation stroke on the tibialis anterior.

DAR

FIGURE 8-14 Elongation stroke on the peroneal muscles.

Position
- The client is turned onto his or her side so that the leg to be worked on is uppermost. The top leg is flexed 90° at the hip and knee.
- A bolster is placed under the leg so that the hip does not roll forward.

Strokes
- For the peroneal muscles, perform elongation strokes with the elbow from the lateral malleolus to the head of the fibula (Fig. 8-14).
- Using the elbow, separate the lateral leg muscles by stroking along their borders, from the ankle to the knee.
- A cross fiber motion with the elbow may be used to locate trigger points.

The Posterior Leg
Position
- The client is placed in the prone position; a bolster is placed under the ankle, if required.
- The therapist is standing at the side of the table next to the client's foot.

Strokes
- The therapist warms up the posterior leg muscles as described above for the anterior leg.

8. Retinaculum of the Ankle—Posterior Portion

Strokes
- Place the thumbs on either side of the Achilles tendon. Do short, up and down strokes on the retinaculum, sliding it over the underlying tendons.
- Separating the thumbs slightly, repeat the stroke. Continue to repeat the stroke, widening the distance between the thumbs, to the lateral and medial malleoli.

9. Gastrocnemius

Origin: Lateral head—lateral epicondyle and posterior surface of the shaft of the femur above the condyle. **Medial head**—popliteal surface of the femur above the medial condyle.
Insertion: Middle posterior surface of the calcaneus via the tendo calcaneus.
Action: Plantar flexion of the foot; assists in knee flexion.

 Clusters of trigger points may form symmetrically in the upper quadrant of the gastrocnemius, in the medial and lateral heads. The referred pain zone is for the most part local, radiating in the upper portion of the muscle and over the knee joint. A trigger point found just above the midline of the medial head of the muscle refers pain primarily to the instep of the foot and along the back of the calf on the medial side.

Strokes
- Perform an elongation stroke using the forearm or knuckles, from the calcaneus to midcalf region (**A** in Fig. 8-15).
- Reposition the forearm or knuckles directly over the lateral head of the gastrocnemius. Continue the elongation stroke to the knee. Repeat on the medial head (**B** in Fig. 8-15).

 Never stroke over the center of the back of the knee (popliteal fossa). Stay on the muscle by stroking on the side of the knee, maintaining your pressure on the muscle fibers of the gastrocnemius.

- Perform an elongation stroke with the thumbs up the midline of the posterior leg to separate the heads of the gastrocnemius (**C** in Fig. 8-15).
- Palpate trigger points in the bellies of the muscle using short, up and down and side to side strokes with the thumbs. Treat any trigger points that are found.

FIGURE 8-15 Sequence of strokes on the gastrocnemius.

10. Soleus and Deep Posterior Muscles

Soleus

Origin: Middle third of the medial side of the shaft of the tibia, proximal third of the shaft on the posterior surface and head of the fibula, fibrous arch between the tibia and fibula.

Insertion: Posterior surface of the calcaneus via the tendo calcaneus (along with the gastrocnemius).

Action: Plantar flexion of the foot; strong stabilizer of the body in standing position, prevents falling forward.

> **X** The best way to examine the soleus is to disengage the gastrocnemius by flexing the client's leg 90°. The most frequent trigger point that forms

in the soleus is found on the medial side, just above the Achilles tendon. It refers pain primarily into the Achilles tendon and heel, but pain may also radiate up into the medial side of the soleus.

Strokes

- Place thumbs or fingertips on both sides of the Achilles tendon. Working in small sections, apply up and down strokes lateral to the gastrocnemius muscle, from the ankle to the knee. Seek out areas of tightness and sensitivity to treat in the deeper layers of muscles.
- Trigger points in the soleus muscle may be palpated by pressing deeply through the gastrocnemius.

11. The Knee

Position

- The client is placed in a supine position, with a bolster under the knee.
- The therapist is standing at the side of the table next to the client's knee.

Strokes

Static compression as well as up and down and side to side strokes are used on the following attachment points (Fig. 8-16):

- **Pes anserinus** (insertion point of semitendinosus, sartorius, and gracilis)—on the head of the tibia, medial to the patella.
- **Biceps femoris and peroneus longus**—on the head of the fibula on the lateral side of the leg.

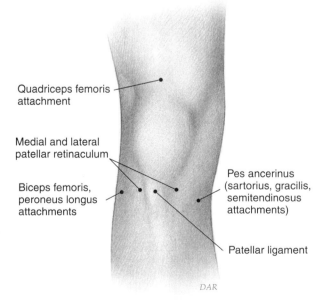

FIGURE 8-16 Muscle attachment sites at the knee.

- **Quadriceps femoris**—on the center of the head of the tibia, slightly superior to the tuberosity.
- **Patellar ligament**—place the thumbs just above the tuberosity of the tibia. Do short, up and down and side to side strokes on the ligament to the inferior border of the patella.
- **Medial and lateral patellar retinaculum**—place the thumbs on either side of the patellar ligament. Move up and down and side to side, sliding the retinaculum. Pause at tender points

STRETCH

1. Standing at the foot of the table, grasp the toes of the client's foot with one hand while holding the foot at the heel with the other. Flex and extend the toes several times.
2. Dorsiflex the foot, and hold for several seconds.
3. Plantar flex the foot, and hold for several seconds. (Stretches 2 and 3 above may be performed with the client lying in the supine or the prone position, with the leg flexed 90° at the knee.)
4. Sandwich the foot between the palms. Invert the foot, and hold for a few seconds. Evert the foot, and hold for a few seconds.

ACCESSORY WORK

1. Hand and forearm massage complement this session well, because these areas correspond reflexively to the foot and leg.
2. Neck and cranial massage will help to balance the upper pole of the body after this work.

CLOSING

Sitting at the head of the table, lightly cup the client's head in both your hands, and hold for at least 30 seconds, allowing the client to relax and assimilate the effects of the session.

REFERENCES

1. Rolf IP. Rolfing: re-establishing the natural alignment and structural integration of the human body for vitality and well-being. Rochester, VT: Healing Arts Press, 1989.
2. Meyers T. The foot: understanding the arches. Massage Magazine, September/October 1997.
3. Franklin E. Conditioning for dance: training for peak performance in all dance forms. Champaign, IL: Human Kinetics, 2004.

Stabilizing the Core

This chapter focuses primarily on re-establishing balanced action of the muscles that act on the pelvis. These include many of the thigh muscles as well as the abdominal and pelvic muscles. The thigh/hip and abdominal/pelvic regions are discussed separately to clarify anatomic and functional distinctions. Within the routines, however, these areas are integrated to promote coordination of all the muscles affecting pelvic placement and movement.

The four routines presented in this chapter should be viewed as a progressive unit. They should be performed in the prescribed order to achieve the maximum results and to prevent imbalance or trauma to the pelvic region. The deep-lying psoas and iliacus muscles should never be massaged until the surface abdominal muscles and thigh muscles have been released. Premature work on the iliopsoas can seriously disrupt the integrity of the pelvic core.

The four sessions should be scheduled at close intervals, with no more than 2 weeks between each one, so that the results from the previous session can be carried over effectively to the next. The therapist should teach the client the exercises described in the lessons to stretch the muscles that are worked on so that the client may better integrate the muscular release and increased core awareness achieved within the sessions.

The order of the routines is as follows:

1. The posterior thigh muscles and hip muscles
2. The abdominal muscles, including their attachments on the rib cage and pelvis
3. The lateral and medial thigh muscles and massage to the intestines
4. The anterior thigh muscles and hip flexors, including the rectus femoris and iliopsoas

The Thigh and Hip

■ GENERAL CONCEPTS

The thigh consists of the femur, which is the longest and strongest bone in the body, and the muscles that are attached to it. The hip is the articulation of the femur with the pelvis. It is a ball-and-socket joint capable of a broad range of movements, including flexion and extension, abduction and adduction, rotation, and circumduction. The thigh and hip are active in balancing the body while standing and in initiating movement of the lower limb. The muscles at the front of the thigh, the quadriceps, are among the most powerful in the body, and they are balanced by groups of muscles on the sides and back of the thigh.

A total of 22 muscles are involved in moving the femur at both of its joints. Twenty-one of these muscles have an origin at various places on the pelvis. In a standing position, the legs are fixed in their position over the feet. Therefore, when the thigh muscles are shortened, they tend to pull from their attachment on the pelvis, moving it out of position. One of the goals of deep tissue work on the thigh muscles is to balance their action so that the pelvis can sit freely over the heads of the femurs without being chronically pulled into a distorted alignment.

The hip joint is reinforced by strong ligaments and muscles. Because of its ball-and-socket design, the hip joint is capable of rotary and circular movements. In walking and running, however, its movement is limited by the hinge design of the knee and the ankle beneath it, which are capable of flexion and extension movements only. The femur must meet the challenge of absorbing and transferring a large number of stresses coming from various angles at both ends. Much stress is therefore placed on the knee, which must process the forces coming to it from the weight of the body above and the movements of the hip. It must also be able to absorb the shock from the impact of weight rising up to it from the ground below in walking and running movements.

In proper alignment of the thigh, a vertical axis passes from the center of the hip joint at the front of the thigh to the center of the knee joint (Fig. 9-1). This axis is distorted in both knock-kneed (**valgus** alignment of the knee) and bow-legged (**varus** alignment of the knee) conditions, adding additional stress to the joints of the legs (Fig. 9-2). The deep tissue therapist should be aware of this vertical axis when working on the thigh muscles and attempt to re-establish it by releasing uneven pulls in the musculature of the thigh.

A   Varus   **B**   Valgus

FIGURE 9-2 Varus and valgus alignment of the knee. **A.** In varus alignment of the knee, the angle formed by lines through the femur and tibia opens medially. **B.** In valgus alignment of the knee, the angle formed by lines through the femur and tibia opens laterally. (Reprinted with permission from Oatis, Carol A. Kinesiology—the mechanics and pathomechanics of human movement. Baltimore, MD: Lippincott Williams & Wilkins, 2004.)

■ MUSCULOSKELETAL ANATOMY AND FUNCTION

The proximal end of the femur consists of a rounded head, a neck, and two projections, called the greater and lesser trochanter. The head fits into a round cavity in the pelvis, called the acetabulum, that is formed by the junction of the ilium, pubis, and ischium. The entire circumference of the acetabulum is coated by a ring of cartilage, called the labrum. This ring holds onto the head of the femur, creating a snug fit for it in the hip joint. Extending from the labrum is a thick sleeve, or joint capsule, that encases the neck of the femur, reinforcing and protecting the joint. (See Essential Anatomy Box 9-1 for a summary of muscles, bones, and landmarks.)

Seven ligaments surround the hip joint, giving it additional strength and support (Fig. 9-3). The strongest of these is the iliofemoral or Y ligament. It attaches in front of the hip joint, at the anterior inferior iliac spine (AIIS), and in the space on the femur between the two trochanters. The ischiofemoral ligament is situated at the back of the joint, attaching to the ischium below the acetabulum and to the posterior femoral neck. These ligaments help hold the head of the femur firmly in the hip socket during movements of the thigh.

— Mechanical axis

FIGURE 9-1 The mechanical axis of the lower extremity aligns the centers of the hip, knee, and ankle joints. (Reprinted with permission from Oatis, Carol A. Kinesiology—the mechanics and pathomechanics of human movement. Baltimore, MD: Lippincott Williams & Wilkins, 2004.)

BOX 9-1 ESSENTIAL ANATOMY   The Thigh and Hip Routines

MUSCLES

Quadriceps—rectus femoris, vastus lateralis, medialis, and intermedius
Adductors—adductor brevis, longus, and magnus, gracilis, pectineus
Hamstrings—biceps femoris, semimembranosus, semitendinosus
Lateral rotators—piriformis, obturator internus, gemellus superior, gemellus inferior, obturator externus, quadratus femoris
Gluteus maximus, medius, minimus
Tensor fascia latae and iliotibial band
Sartorius

BONES AND LANDMARKS

Anterior superior iliac spine (ASIS)
Anterior inferior iliac spine (AIIS)
Sacrum
Coccyx
Ischial tuberosity
Femur
Greater trochanter
Lesser trochanter
Patella
Tibia
Tibial tuberosity
Fibula
Head of fibula

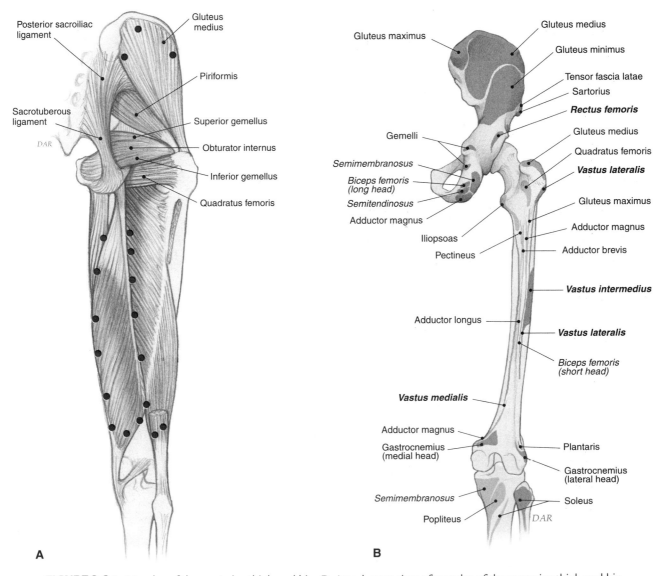

FIGURE 9-3 A. Muscles of the posterior thigh and hip. **B.** Attachment sites of muscles of the posterior thigh and hip.

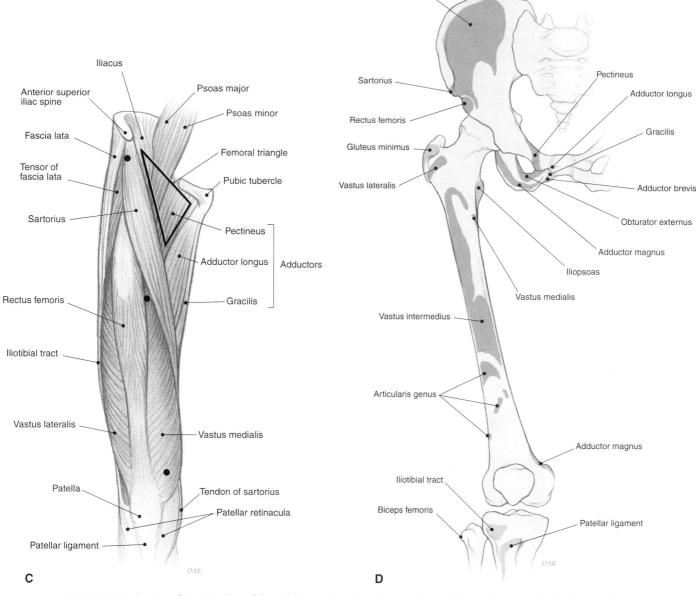

FIGURE 9-3 *(continued)* **C.** Muscles of the thigh, anterior view. **D.** Muscle attachment sites on the thigh and pelvis.

The neck of the femur extends diagonally upward from the shaft of the bone. Its design keeps the thigh clear of the pelvis, allowing for greater mobility of the pelvis over the legs. The disadvantage of the shape of the neck is that it is in the form of a bent lever, subjecting it to greater stress than a straight column would receive. It is potentially the weakest point on the thigh. Many older people break their leg at the neck of the femur.

The greater trochanter is the site of attachment for many muscles that initiate movements of the thigh. The six lateral rotators as well as the **gluteus medius** and **gluteus minimus** (the medial rotators) have their insertion there. These two sets of muscles oppose each other in rotation of the femur. They must all be in balance to allow the full range of movements of the head of the femur in the acetabulum. Muscular imbalance pulls the head of the

femur out of position slightly, and over time, this may result in arthritis of the hip joint. Movement restriction at the hip often has a relay effect, creating stress and imbalance at the knee and sometimes the ankle.

The muscles in front of the thigh, the flexors, move the leg forward in locomotor movements (Fig. 9-3, *C* and *D*). The primary hip flexors are the **iliopsoas** and the **rectus femoris**. The rectus femoris is also active in knee extension. Secondary flexors are the **sartorius** and **tensor fascia lata**. Of all these muscles, the iliopsoas is the most important. Because of its location at the body's core, it possesses the greatest power and leverage. It should be the foremost initiator of hip flexion. In a balanced body, walking motions are not initiated by the legs; rather, they are initiated in the trunk. The movement is then transferred to the legs by means of the psoas. The psoas muscle does not attach to the pelvis. It attaches instead to the anterior portion of the lumbar spine, and its insertion is on the lesser trochanter on the inner surface of the femur.

The psoas and rectus femoris muscles need to be in balance with each other for a smooth, coordinated walking action to occur. Often, the rectus femoris takes over hip flexion, and the psoas becomes shortened and weak, which tends to increase the lumbar curve and tips the rib cage both downward and forward. This causes misalignment in the body segments, with an inevitable breakdown in full-body movement integration.

When the psoas is functioning properly in hip flexion, the upper and lower body are coordinated around the lumbar spine. As a result of this integration, the sides of the pelvis will swing with each step rather than being held rigid by tight, inhibited muscles. In walking, the knees will swing forward and back, and the feet will roll like the base of a rocking chair, with the weight moving from heels to toes. This connected chain of movement through the body creates a gentle undulation of the spine, which helps to enhance physiologic processes through the increased pumping of fluids through the trunk, including the cerebrospinal fluid that flows through the spinal cord.

The opposing muscles to the hip flexors are the hip extensors, which include the three hamstrings ⦿ and the **gluteus maximus**. The hamstrings are two-joint muscles originating at the ischial tuberosity and inserting on the tibia. They also serve as knee flexors. Their movement is restricted by the presence of the iliofemoral ligament in the front of the hip, limiting pure extension to about 45°.

The primary hip abductors are the gluteus medius and minimus, with the tensor fascia lata assisting in abduction when the hip is flexed. The most important function of the tensor fascia lata is to maintain tension in the **iliotibial band**. ⦿ This band of fascia, which is located on the out-

side of the thigh, assists in absorbing tensile or stretching stresses acting on the femur. Bones are designed to absorb compression, or shortening stresses, better than tension, or lengthening stresses, which are absorbed by the muscles and fascia. Therefore, this additional support is crucial in strengthening the thigh.

The hip adductor muscles are the **pectineus, adductor brevis, adductor longus, adductor magnus**, and the **gracilis**. ⦿ The gracilis is the only two-joint muscle of this group, inserting on the medial surface of the shaft of the tibia.

■ CONDITIONS

1. *Muscle Strains.* These are common in thigh muscles. Rest and appropriately applied massage techniques are often adequate treatment.
2. *Varicose Veins.* These result from swelling of the veins caused by a breakdown of the one-way valves that prevent venous blood from flowing downward instead of toward the heart. The condition is caused by a weakening of the vein walls, which allows them to stretch and pull open the valves.

    There seems to be a genetic component in the tendency to develop varicose veins. Pregnancy can often trigger or exacerbate the condition. Certain dietary supplements may help to strengthen the vein walls. The client should consult a physician for guidance in this area. The best home care treatment is elevation of the legs for a period everyday, to assist the flow of blood out of the legs. Deep tissue massage is contraindicated.

Please refer to Indications/Contraindications Box 9-2 for an additional list of indications and contraindications for massage of the thigh and hip.

BOX 9-2 INDICATIONS/CONTRAINDICATIONS
Conditions Affecting Massage of the Thigh and Hip

INDICATIONS	CONTRAINDICATIONS
Fatigue	Varicose veins
Low back pain	Broken bones
Hip pain	Acute injury
Leg pain	Recent trauma
Pelvic misalignment	Severe bruises
Cellulite	Phlebitis
Muscle strain	Rashes
Muscle cramps	Burns
Poor circulation	
Polio and similar conditions	
Amputation	
Sciatica	

TABLE 9–1	Range of Motion (ROM) for the Hip	
Action	**Muscles**
Flexion (knee extended) (ROM 90°)	Psoas major Sartorius Pectineus Adductor longus Adductor brevis Adductor magnus (anterior) Sartorius Rectus femoris
Extension (ROM 45°)	Gluteus maximus Biceps femoris (long head) Semitendinosus Semimembranosus Adductor magnus Gracilis Pectineus
Abduction (ROM 45°)	Gluteus medius Gluteus minimus Iliopsoas Tensor fascia latae Sartorius
Adduction (ROM 25°)	Adductor brevis Adductor longus Adductor magnus Gracilis Pectineus
Internal rotation (sitting) (ROM 35°)	Gluteus medius Gluteus minimus Tensor fascia latae Pectineus Adductor—longus, brevis, magnus
External rotation (sitting) (ROM 40°)	Piriformis Gemellus superior Obturator internus Gemellus inferior Obturator externus Quadratus femoris Gluteus maximus

David Rini

FIGURE 9-4 Inner thigh lift.

the **mind body** connection

Like the leg and foot, the thigh is involved in moving the body. The muscles of the thigh, being closer to the core of the body, are more involved in initiating movement. The lower portion of the leg mirrors how we handle ourselves once we have completed our movement and planted our feet.

The thighs have been called the prime movers of the body. Observing their shape and tone indicates how a person moves through life. The quadriceps are thick, fiber-dense, and powerful muscles, potentially able to lift more weight than any other muscle group. The hamstring muscles, when chronically contracted, pull the ischial tuberosities of the pelvis downward, restricting pelvic movement and putting strain on the back of the knees.

These two muscle groups must be well-coordinated to orchestrate effectively the movements of flexion and extension at the knee joint and anterior and posterior tipping of the pelvis. The hamstrings are often weak in relation to the quadriceps, allowing the quadriceps to pull too strongly on the front of the knee, causing hyperextension of the joint.

Holding onto the adductor muscles often denotes a shielding or protective stance. Squeezing the inner thighs blocks access to the pelvic region. Constriction of the outer thigh often accompanies contraction of the gluteal muscles. These muscles tighten in an effort to contain feelings and sensations.

As the hip and thigh are released through deep tissue sessions, a client may experience a renewed surge to move ahead with life. Reconnecting with the ground gives a sense of sustenance and a feeling of belonging here on the earth. This, coupled with tapping into the vast reserve of personal power that we all contain, as represented by the thighs, is a powerful motivation to create positive changes in one's life.

■ POSTURAL EVALUATION

1. Check the overall alignment of the anterior thigh.
   - Does the line of gravity appear to fall in a straight line between the center of the hip joint in the front of the thigh and the center of the knee?
   - If not, how does the line of gravity deviate?
2. Observe the shape and muscular tone of the thighs.
   - What is the degree of muscular development? Bound, flaccid, well-toned?
   - Do the muscles appear to be pulling in any particular direction?
   - Note any differences between the right and the left thigh.

3. In what direction(s) are the thigh muscles pulling the pelvis? Which muscles are involved?
4. Check the alignment of the back of the thighs.
   - Where does the line of gravity fall through the back of the thighs?
   - Is the gluteal line at the base of the buttocks horizontal?
5. Observe the muscles of the posterior thigh and hip region (Table 9-1).
   - What is the muscular condition of the back of the thigh? Well-toned, weak, contracted?
   - What is the shape and tone of the gluteal region? Tight, loose, squeezed, overdeveloped, underdeveloped?
   - Are the tendons of the hamstrings prominent at the back of the knees? Do they appear even on the right and left legs?
   - Do the hamstrings appear to be pulling the pelvis downward?
   - Does the degree of muscularity match that of the front of the thighs?

■ EXERCISES AND SELF-TREATMENT

Adductors

1. Inner Thigh Lift (Strengthens Adductors)

Preparation
Lie on your right side. The right leg is fully extended along the floor, under you. The left leg is extended straight in front at hip level. Place your left hand on the floor in front of your chest for support. Hold your head in your right hand (Fig. 9-4).

Execution
Exhaling, lift the right leg straight up, keeping the instep parallel to the floor. Think of squeezing the right inner thigh against the left inner thigh. Inhale as you lower the leg. Repeat several times, then reverse the position to do the left side.

2. Inner Thigh Stretch (Stretches Adductors)

Preparation
Lying on your back, bring the soles of your feet together in front of you, close to your pelvis. Wrapping your hands around the outside edges of the feet, turn the knees outward (Fig. 9-5).

Execution
Exhaling, draw the heels toward you as you continue to turn the knees out until you feel a stretch in the adductor muscles. Hold for a minimum of 20 seconds.

FIGURE 9-5 Inner thigh stretch.

Abductors

1. Outer Thigh Lift (Strengthens Gluteus Medius, Gluteus Minimus, and Tensor Fascia Latae)

Preparation

The starting position is the same as for the inner thigh lift above, except that the bottom leg is flexed instead of straight. Medially rotate the leg extended in front of you at hip level so that the toes are pointing downward about 45° (Fig. 9-6).

Execution

Exhaling, lift the leg extended in front of you approximately 2 feet straight up in the air. Hold for a moment, then lower the leg as you inhale until the side of the big toe touches the floor. Repeat several times, then reverse your body position to do the exercise on the other side.

2. Outer Thigh Stretch (Stretches Gluteus Medius, Gluteus Minimus, Tensor Fascia Latae, and Piriformis)

Preparation

Lie on your back, with both legs extended and your arms out to your sides at shoulder level. Circle the right leg along the floor to the left side, bringing it in the direction of your left shoulder.

Execution

Reach down and take hold of the right ankle with your left hand. Slowly bring the leg toward your left shoulder until you feel a stretch in the outer thigh and hip of the right leg. Hold for 30 seconds. Repeat the stretch for the left leg.

Quadriceps

1. Quadricep Strengthener (Strengthens Vastus Lateralis, Vastus Medialis, Vastus Intermedius, and Rectus Femoris)

Preparation

Sit up tall, with the legs extended in front of you. Keeping the right leg extended and the right foot strongly flexed, slide the left thigh toward your chest, keeping the foot on the floor. Hold the left knee with both hands (Fig. 9-7).

Execution

Exhaling, lift the right leg straight up off the ground a few inches while pulling up on the patella. Hold for a few seconds. Inhaling, lower the leg to the floor. Adjust the position of your back, making sure it is straight, and repeat the leg lift a few more times. Reverse your position, then repeat on the left side.

FIGURE 9-6 Outer thigh lift.

FIGURE 9-7 Quadriceps strengthener.

FIGURE 9-8 Quadriceps stretch.

2. Quadricep Stretch (Stretches Vastus Lateralis, Vastus Medialis, Vastus Intermedius, and Rectus Femoris)

Preparation
To stretch your right thigh, lie on your left side. Place your head in your left hand. Flex both legs.

Execution
Lift your right leg, bringing the thigh toward the chest. Reach down and take hold of the top of the right ankle with your right hand. Slowly draw the thigh back until you feel a stretch in the center of your right thigh (Fig. 9-8). Hold for 20 seconds. Reverse the body position, then stretch the left thigh.

Hamstrings

1. Hamstring Strengthener (Strengthens Biceps Femoris, Semitendinosus, and Semimembranosus)

Preparation
Lie face down on the floor, and turn your head to one side. Flex your right leg at the knee. Place your left foot behind the right ankle (Fig. 9-9).

Execution
Try to draw the right heel toward your hip as you resist the movement by pressing against the right ankle with your

FIGURE 9-9 Hamstring strengthener.

FIGURE 9-10 Stretching the hamstrings using a belt.

David Rini

left leg. With resistance, flex the right leg toward the hip several times. Then, hold an isometric contraction of the right hamstring muscles for up to 30 seconds.

2. Hamstring Stretch (Stretches Biceps Femoris, Semitendinosus, and Semimembranosus)

Preparation
Have a belt or a tie handy. Lie on the floor on your back, with the left knee flexed and the left foot placed on the floor. Bringing your right thigh to your chest, loop the belt around the ball of the foot.

Execution
Exhaling, slowly extend the right leg toward the ceiling. Push upward with the heel as you flex the foot by pulling down on the sides of the belt (Fig. 9-10). Hold for 30 seconds.

Hips

1. Gluteal Strengthener (Strengthens Gluteus Maximus)

Preparation
Position yourself on your forearms and knees, with the right leg extended straight back and turned out so that the big toe is touching the floor.

Execution
Exhaling, lift the right leg straight up until you feel the gluteus maximus tighten (Fig. 9-11). Do not arch your

back. Lower the right leg, and repeat several more times. Reverse the leg position, and repeat the lifts with the left leg.

2. Gluteal Stretch (Stretches Gluteus Maximus and Piriformis)

Preparation
Sit cross-legged, with the right heel placed in front of the left. Leaning forward slightly from the hip joints, place both hands on the floor in front of the legs.

Execution
Exhaling, slide the hands forward, slowly folding the trunk toward the floor until you feel a stretch in the back of the right hip (Fig. 9-12). Make sure both hips are touching the floor. Hold the stretch for 30 seconds, then repeat with the left foot in front to stretch the left hip.

3. Hip Release

Preparation
Lying on the floor on your back, flex both knees, keeping the soles of the feet on the floor.

Execution
Bring your right thigh to your chest, and place both hands around the knee. Circle the thigh slowly as you imagine breathing into the right hip joint. Keep the thigh muscles totally relaxed. Let your arms guide the movement. Circle a few times in the other direction, then repeat the hip circles with the left leg.

FIGURE 9-11 Gluteal strengthener.

■ POSTERIOR THIGH AND HIP ROUTINE

Objectives

- To release restriction in the hamstring muscles and their attachments, which can contribute to low back problems and pelvic distortion.
- To open up the gluteal muscles, which are often a major site of stored tension.

- To release the deep lateral rotators, which helps to improve the walking pattern.
- To reduce sciatic pain generated by a tight piriformis muscle.
- To help heal injuries in the sacral ligaments, an overlooked contributor to low back pain.
- To bring balance to the soft tissues acting on the sacrum, allowing it to find its natural position. This brings greater ease throughout the body, as the upper and lower halves balance around the sacrum.

FIGURE 9-12 Position to stretch the gluteal and piriformis muscles.

This case demonstrates the pervasive effects that an injury can have on the soft tissues. The client is a 31-year-old homemaker named Mia, who is a former ballet dancer. She sustained an injury to her left hip while stretching in a dance class when she was 16 years old. At the time, she was sitting in a spread open-leg position on the floor, with her upper body flexed forward and her arms extended along the floor in front of her. After a few seconds in the stretch, she felt a shift of the left femur in the hip socket and a sharp pain running down the inside of her left thigh.

For several months after the injury, Mia experienced sharp pains extending down the inside of her left thigh. Over time, the pain has become less pronounced, but she still experiences a dull throbbing in that area. The most dramatic effect of the injury was a loss of full turn-out of the left leg, as a result of restriction of the femur in the hip socket. Mia found that this lack of turn-out on the left side affected her knee; it was difficult to plié (flex) the left leg while keeping the left knee properly aligned over the foot. She would experience pain and swelling in that knee after dancing.

The bracing of the muscles around the left hip has caused a build-up and hardening of connective tissue on the left side of the body, extending well up into the back. A hardened mass of connective tissue is found along the lateral border of the iliocostalis muscle under the 12th rib; this mass of connective tissue feels like another rib. Viewing the hips from the anterior position, the left hip appears to be narrower and posteriorly rotated. Mia walks with a small but noticeable limp on the left side.

The plan for the session was to attempt to improve the alignment of the muscles on the left side, which have been strained over the years in bracing the hip.

CASE STUDY 7 The Hip

These include the adductor muscles, gluteus medius and minimus, and erector spinae (particularly the iliocostalis). Deep tissue strokes along the borders of these muscles were incorporated extensively to relieve adhering of the muscles. Connective tissue spreading techniques and deep tissue elongation strokes were also applied to the muscles where a build-up of connective tissue was found. Deep tissue techniques were used to release the lateral rotator muscles of the posterior hip. Therapist-assisted stretches for the left hip included flexion, adduction, and abduction. The client was encouraged to continue to perform these stretches regularly between sessions.

A visit to a chiropractor or an osteopath was recommended to evaluate the condition of the hip. An adjustment to the left hip joint may alleviate some of the stress around the joint. Although the problem was not resolved by the deep tissue session (i.e., the left hip joint did not become unrestricted), the client felt much more range of motion in the left hip after the session and wishes to continue to receive deep tissue therapy. She feels that it will be of great benefit in halting the further build-up of connective tissue above the left hip.

Topics for Discussion

1. Describe several ways of evaluating restrictions in hip movement.
2. Design an exercise program to achieve greater lateral rotation of the thigh.
3. How would you explain to a client why connective tissue tends to accumulate around a misaligned joint?
4. If a client walks with both legs and feet laterally rotated, which muscles are probably short? Which muscles are weak?
5. Specify two functions of the gluteus medius muscle.

Energy

POSITION

- The client is lying prone on the table. A bolster may be placed under the ankles.
- The therapist is standing on the left side of the table and is facing the client's back.

POLARITY

Sacral Rock

1. The left hand contacts the C7–T1 area of the upper back. The palm of the right hand contacts the sacrum. Gently rock the sacrum with the right hand while stabilizing the upper back with the left hand. Continue for at least 30 seconds.

This procedure helps to mobilize the lumbar vertebrae by freeing constrictions around the joints as well as by relaxing the muscles of the pelvis. It also helps the client to experience a feeling of continuity throughout the length of the spinal column

2. The therapist's left hand (negative pole) contacts the client's sacrum (positive pole). The therapist's right hand (positive pole) rests on the back of the client's left knee (negative pole). This polarity procedure integrates the pelvis with the thighs.
   a. Rock the sacrum with the left hand.
   b. Place the right hand (positive pole) on the right knee (negative pole), and continue to rock the sacrum.

SHIATSU

1. Compress the back of the left thigh with both hands, from the hip to the knee. Repeat on the other leg. This shiatsu move stimulates qi flow through the bladder channel, which runs down the back of the leg.
2. Roll both fists across the muscles in the gluteal area. The bladder and gallbladder channels run through the back of the pelvis.

Swedish/Cross Fiber

1. Perform effleurage strokes on the posterior thigh and gluteal area.
2. Perform pétrissage strokes on the posterior thigh and gluteal area.
3. Perform friction strokes on the posterior thigh and gluteal area.
4. Using the broad side of the thumb and/or the heel of the hand, apply cross fiber strokes across the hamstrings and gluteal muscles.

Connective Tissue

Myofascial Spreading Techniques

1. Starting at the midline of the posterior thigh, spread outward, using the heels of both hands. Work in horizontal strips, from the knee to the hip.
2. Using the heels of the hand and/or fingertips, spread the gluteal muscles.

Deep Tissue/Neuromuscular Therapy

SEQUENCE

1. Hamstrings—bellies and attachments
2. Gluteus maximus, medius, and minimus
3. Lateral rotators—piriformis, obturator internus, obturator externus, gemellus superior, gemellus inferior, and quadratus femoris

4. Sacral ligaments—sacrotuberous and posterior sacroiliac

I. Hamstrings

Biceps Femoris

Origin: Long head—ischial tuberosity (inferior and medial aspects, sharing same tendon as semitendinosus), sacrotuberous ligament. **Short head**—entire length of the lateral lip of the linea aspera on the femur, proximal two-thirds of the lateral supracondylar ridge, lateral intermuscular septum.

Insertion: Lateral aspect of the head of the fibula, lateral condyle of the tibia.

Action: Knee flexion, knee external rotation. **Long head**—hip extension.

Semitendinosus

Origin: Ischial tuberosity (inferior medial aspect).

Insertion: Shaft of the tibia on the proximal medial side.

Action: Knee flexion, knee internal rotation, hip extension; assists hip internal rotation.

Semimembranosus

Origin: Ischial tuberosity (superior and lateral aspects).

Insertion: Medial condyle of the tibia on the posterior medial aspect, lateral condyle of the femur (posterior aspect via fibrous expansion, forming part of the oblique popliteal ligament).

Action: Knee flexion, knee internal rotation, hip extension; assists hip internal rotation.

Trigger points tend to cluster in the distal portion of all three hamstring muscles above the knee. Checking along the borders of the muscles will often reveal trigger points. Referral patterns can be up to the gluteal area, around the ischial tuberosity, and around the back of the knee.

Position

- The client is lying prone on the table. A bolster may be placed under the ankles.
- The therapist is standing at the side of the table next to the client's knees.

Strokes

- Flexing the client's knee, follow the tendons of the hamstrings across the knee joint to their insertions on the leg, and apply static compression and cross fiber techniques with your thumbs or fingers (Fig. 9-13).
- Perform an elongation stroke with your forearm from the knee to the ischial tuberosity. Repeat, covering each of the three hamstring muscles.
- Using the elbow, separate the three hamstring muscles. Follow the tendon of each muscle from the knee to find its border on the posterior thigh. Stroke from the knee to the ischial tuberosity along the edge of each muscle.
- Apply short, cross fiber strokes with your thumb or

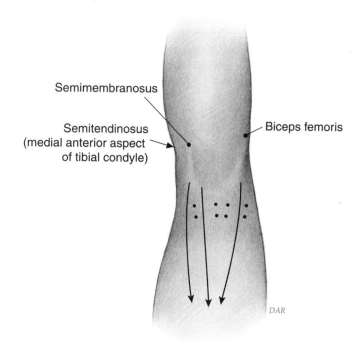

FIGURE 9-13 Origin of hamstrings and direction of deep tissue strokes.

knuckle to the origins of the hamstrings at the ischial tuberosity.

2. Gluteus Maximus, Medius, and Minimus

Gluteus Maximus

Origin: Posterior gluteal line and crest of the ilium, posterior surface of the sacrum and coccyx, aponeurosis of the erector spinae, sacrotuberous ligament.

Insertion: Iliotibial band of the fascia lata, gluteal tuberosity of the femur.

Action: Hip extension, lateral hip rotation, extension of trunk when insertion is fixed. **Upper fibers**—hip abduction. **Lower fibers**—hip adduction.

The most common trigger point in gluteus maximus is found in the fibers slightly above the ischial tuberosity. The referred pain zone can be over the entire gluteal region. Another trigger point can be located in the fibers next to the lower portion of the sacrum. Activity here can refer pain along the gluteal line at the base of the muscle. A third trigger point has been found in the most medial and inferior fibers of the muscle, near the coccyx. This third trigger point refers pain to the coccyx so that when active, people often mistakenly think they have a problem with the coccyx.

Strokes

- Standing at the side of the table next to the client's pelvis, perform elongation strokes with the forearm, fist, or heel of the hand. Work in strips, from the ilium and sacrum to the greater trochanter (Fig. 9-14).

FIGURE 9-14 Direction of deep tissue strokes on gluteal muscles.

- Taut bands may be palpated by rolling across the fibers of the muscle with the fingertips or elbow. Treat trigger points as they are found.

Gluteus Medius
Origin: Outer surface of the ilium inferior to the iliac crest.
Insertion: Oblique ridge on the lateral surface of the greater trochanter of the femur.
Action: Hip abduction. **Anterior fibers**—medial rotation of the hip. **Posterior fibers**—lateral rotation of the hip. The action of the gluteus medius prevents the pelvis from sliding laterally and tilting during the walking motion.

 The three most common trigger points in the gluteus medius are located along the iliac crest, each in one of the three portions of the muscle. The first trigger point is found along the underside of the crest, near the sacroiliac joint. The pain pattern is along the iliac crest and over the sacroiliac joint and sacrum. The second trigger point is at the center point of the iliac crest (dividing it in two equal portions, front and back) and just below the lip. It refers pain to the middle of the gluteal region and sometimes down the outside of the thigh. The third point is much less common than the other two. It is found near the anterior superior iliac spine (ASIS), again just below the lip of the iliac crest. Pain is referred along the iliac crest to the lower lumbar region and the sacrum.

Gluteus Minimus
Origin: Outer surface of the ilium between the middle and inferior gluteal lines.
Insertion: Anterior border of the greater trochanter of the femur.
Action: Hip abduction, medial rotation of the hip.

 Trigger point pain from the gluteus minimus is characteristically deep and quite severe. It projects down the leg more intensely than referred pain from the other gluteal muscles. There are two portions of the muscle. Trigger points in the anterior portion lie along the fibers vertically in a line to the greater trochanter. They refer pain to the lower buttock region and along the side of the thigh, sometimes all the way down to the ankle. Trigger points in the posterior portion accumulate in a fan-shaped pattern across the muscle, near its origin on the ilium. The pain pattern will cover the buttock and run down the back of the thigh, over the knee to the posterior calf region.

Strokes
- Perform elongation strokes with the forearm, elbow, or fist. Work in strips, from the lateral portion of the iliac crest to the upper portion of the femur just below the greater trochanter.
- Taut bands may be palpated by rolling across the fibers of the muscle with the fingertips or elbow. Treat trigger points as they are found.

3. Lateral Rotators (Piriformis, Obturator Internus, Gemellus Superior, Gemellus Inferior, Obturator Externus, and Quadratus Femoris)

Piriformis
Origin: Anterior surface of the sacrum, sacrotuberous ligament.
Insertion: Superior border of the medial aspect of the greater trochanter of the femur.
Action: Lateral rotation of the hip.

Obturator Internus
Origin: Margin of the obturator foramen on the pelvis, ramus of the ischium, inferior ramus of the pubis, pelvic surface of the obturator membrane.
Insertion: Medial surface of the greater trochanter of the femur.
Action: Lateral rotation of the hip.

Gemellus Superior
Origin: Gluteal surface of the ischial spine.
Insertion: Superior border of the greater trochanter.
Action: Lateral rotation of the hip.

Gemellus Inferior
Origin: Superior surface of the ischial tuberosity.
Insertion: Superior border of the greater trochanter.
Action: Lateral rotation of the hip.

Obturator Externus
Origin: Medial margin of the obturator foramen formed by the rami of the pubis and ischium.
Insertion: Trochanteric fossa of the femur.
Action: Lateral rotation of the hip.

Quadratus Femoris
Origin: Lateral border of the ischial tuberosity.
Insertion: Quadrate tubercle on the posterior aspect of the femur.
Action: Lateral rotation of the hip.

Strokes
- Apply short, side to side strokes with the elbow or thumbs next to the border of the sacrum to contact the medial portion of the piriformis near its origin on the anterior sacrum (**A** in Fig. 9-15).
- Perform an elongation stroke with the elbow, fist, or heel of the hand, from the border of the sacrum to the greater trochanter, following the length of the piriformis from origin to insertion (**B** in Fig. 9-15).

⚠ **Be careful while doing this move, because the piriformis covers the sciatic notch, where the sciatic nerve surfaces from the pelvis. Pressure on the sciatic nerve causes a shooting pain down the posterior thigh and should be avoided.**

- Roll across the fibers of the lateral rotator muscles with the fingertips or elbow, from the border of the sacrum

FIGURE 9-16 Contacting the sacrotuberous ligament.

to the greater trochanter. Treat trigger points as they are found.

- Using the elbow or thumbs, apply static compression and cross fiber strokes against the insertion points of the muscles on the greater trochanter (**C** in Fig. 9-15).

4. Sacral Ligaments

Sacrotuberous Ligament
Strokes

- Palpate the lateral edge of the sacrum just above the coccyx. Next, palpate the ischial tuberosity on the same side of the pelvis. The ligament runs between these two locations (Fig. 9-16).

FIGURE 9-15 Directions of strokes on the piriformis and the attachment sites of the lateral rotator muscles on the greater trochanter.

FIGURE 9-17 Contacting the posterior sacroiliac ligament.

David Rini

FIGURE 9-18 Hamstring stretch.

- Starting just lateral to the sacral edge, slide both thumbs under the gluteal muscles, then press up in a superior direction until you feel a dense, taut band of tissue.
- Move the thumbs slowly from side to side along the ligament, checking for tenderness. Hold painful areas with static compression for 8 to 12 seconds.

Posterior Sacroiliac Ligament

Injuries to this ligament will project pain across the low back and perhaps into the groin, thigh, and leg on the injured side.

Strokes

- Locate the posterior superior iliac spine with your thumbs. Press in and up on the underside of it with the thumb pads (Fig. 9-17). Perform short, cross fiber strokes against the edge of the bone.
- With your fingertips, do short, up-and-down and side-to-side strokes on the sacrum, covering the entire surface.

STRETCH

Position

- The client is lying supine, with the leg to be stretched extended along the table and the other leg flexed with the sole of the foot against the table.
- The therapist stands at the side of the table near the client's foot.

1. *Hamstrings.* Using your inside hand, hold the client's foot behind the heel, and lift the straight leg off the table. You may place the client's leg against your shoulder for additional support. Place your other hand on the client's anterior thigh. Stretch the leg by pressing forward and upward on the heel. Press against the anterior thigh with your other hand or forearm to encourage the knee to straighten (Fig. 9-18).
2. *Gluteus Maximus.* The client's knee is brought to his or her chest. The client and therapist both place their hands over the knee. As the client draws the knee toward his or her chest, lean forward to apply additional impetus to the stretch (Fig. 9-19).
3. *Gluteus Medius and Minimus.* Holding the client's ankle, bring the client's straight leg across his or her body to an adducted position. Rotating the leg laterally so that the toes and knee are facing upward, press the leg downward, in the direction of the table, until a stretch is felt in the gluteals (Fig. 9-20).
4. *Lateral Rotators.* The leg of the side to be stretched is flexed at the knee and hip. The other leg is also flexed at the knee and hip, with the sole of the foot against the table. Holding the client's knee and ankle, turn the knee out, and place the client's foot against the thigh of the client's other leg. As the foot rests there, take hold of the knee and ankle of the supporting leg, and bring it toward the client's chest, sandwiching the foot of the

FIGURE 9-19 Gluteus maximus stretch.

FIGURE 9-20 Stretch for gluteus medius and minimus.

FIGURE 9-21 Stretch for the lateral rotators.

stretched side between the client's chest and shoulder. Continue to bring the thigh toward the chest until a stretch is felt in the lateral rotator muscles (Fig. 9-21).

ACCESSORY WORK

1. This session is complemented with work on the rectus abdominus muscle, which, when shortened, contributes to posterior pelvic tilt along with shortened hamstrings.
2. Polarity balancing of the cranium and feet reinforces the release work that was done with the sacrum in this session.

CLOSING

Sitting at the head of the table, lightly cup the client's head in both of your hands, and hold for at least 30 seconds, allowing the client to relax and assimilate the effects of the session.

Move to the foot of the table. Lightly cup the client's heels with your hands. Hold for at least 30 seconds, then remove your hands slowly to complete the session.

The Pelvis and Abdomen

■ GENERAL CONCEPTS

The pelvis forms the body's core. Functionally, it is analogous to the hub of a wheel, with the spine and the limbs acting as spokes radiating from it. The pelvis serves four main purposes:

1. It houses and protects the vital organs.
2. It provides attachment sites for the muscles that control the trunk, legs, and arms.
3. It absorbs and distributes the shock that is transferred up the lower limbs in movement activities like walking.
4. It transfers the weight of the upper body to the legs and feet.

The pelvic bones create a series of arches and curves that, when joined together, form a bowl. This shape allows weight to be moved easily around and through the pelvis without jarring the bowl's contents. The pelvis is a highly mobile structure, able to alter its position to accommodate weight shifts brought about by the movement of the body segments above and below. The pelvis moves freely between the spine and the heads of the femora, with its position mostly determined by muscular action.

The muscles of the thigh and trunk that attach to the pelvis must be balanced for correct pelvic alignment. Chronic shortness in any of these muscles creates compensatory tightening in other muscles, ligaments, and fascia, leading to stress and dysfunction in the hips and low back. Releasing chronic muscular tension patterns in the pelvis is a primary concern of the deep tissue therapist. The body as a whole cannot become integrated until the process of relaxing the core is initiated.

The primary pelvic muscle group is the iliopsoas. The psoas is the major integration muscle for the entire body. It connects the spine to the thigh, and it contributes to determining the position of the pelvis. When the psoas is functioning properly, the body's movements come under the control of the core, giving increased power, grace, and stamina.

The area of the trunk joining the pelvis and the rib cage is known as the abdomen. The entire region is wrapped in muscles and fascial sheaths. The muscles of the abdomen are responsible for the movements of forward and lateral flexion as well as rotation of the trunk. These muscles attach along the ribs and the pelvic rim. They provide support and protection for the abdominal organs. The deepest muscle of the abdomen is the quadratus lumborum, which forms the back of the abdominal wall and contributes to extension and lateral flexion of the spine. The abdominal muscles work in conjunction with the back muscles to maintain pelvic alignment from above.

Correct alignment of the pelvis is crucial for maintaining the health and vitality of the abdominal organs. Poor posture compresses the organs and diminishes their efficiency. Sluggish or irregular function of the intestines is a major problem and affects a high percentage of the population. The factors contributing to intestinal dysfunction include poor diet, lack of exercise, inadequate intake of water, and lack of tone and balance of the abdominal muscles. Proper intestinal activity is encouraged by deep tissue massage.

■ MUSCULOSKELETAL ANATOMY AND FUNCTION

The Pelvis

The pelvis is made up of three pairs of bones: the ilia, the ischia, and the pubic bones. The ilium bones brace the sacrum, which is situated in the center of the back of the pelvis. The articulation of the ilium and the sacrum is called the sacroiliac joint. The ilia flare in the back in a fan shape. They taper as they curve around to the front, fusing with the pubic bones. The pubic bones join in the front of the pelvis at the pubic symphysis, a moveable joint with a disk between the two bones. The ilia and pubic bones join with the ischia. The acetabulum is a cavity that is formed where the three pelvic bones join. It consists of equal portions of the ilium, pubic bone, and ischium. This arrangement allows equal forces from all three bones in the pelvis to pass to the hip joint. (See Essential Anatomy Box 9-3 for a summary of muscles, bones, and landmarks.)

The sacrum is the keystone for the human skeleton. Weight from the upper body accumulates at the sacrum, then passes from the sacroiliac joints across the ilia to the hip joints and, when a person is standing, from there to the heads of the femora. In a seated position, the weight is transferred to the ischial tuberosities, which are ring-shaped projections at the base of the ischia. This balanced weight transfer depends on soft tissue interaction to keep the joints aligned. The sacrum is subject to a variety of displacements, including slight rotation and posterior deviation, but the most common aberration by far is anterior displacement.

Weight pressing on the sacrum tends to shift the upper portion forward, causing it to become displaced below the fifth lumbar vertebra. This tendency is counteracted by strong ligaments that wrap the sacrum and prevent it from sliding. The attachment of the **piriformis** muscle to the front side of the sacrum also contributes to its stability. When the sacrum shifts, it causes irritation and pain in the sacroiliac joints, and it disrupts the sequence of weight transfer through the lower body. The piriformis muscles become contracted as they attempt to stabilize the sacrum and pass this tightness to the other lateral rotator muscles. During massage work, the therapist should never press down hard on a client's sacrum, because this will cause it to slide anteriorly, creating the problems described above.

The base of the pelvis is a diaphragm composed of muscles and ligaments, known as the pelvic floor. The principal muscle is the levator ani, which operates like a sling

---

BOX 9-3 ESSENTIAL ANATOMY　The Pelvic Routine

MUSCLES	BONES AND LANDMARKS
Psoas major and minor	Ilium
Iliacus	Iliac crest
Rectus abdominus	Ischium
Obliques—external and internal	Pubic symphysis
Gluteus maximus, medius, and minimus	Sacrum
Inguinal ligament	Sacroiliac joint
	Lesser trochanter of the femur

that supports the pelvic organs above it. It attaches to the inner surfaces of the pubic bones and ischia in the front, then runs posteriorly, around the genitals and anus, to attach in the back to the coccyx. The fascia that wraps this muscle is a continuation of the fascia of the inner thigh muscles, thus creating an essential bond between the pelvis and the inner thigh. The degree of tightness in the inner thighs affects the condition of the internal pelvic structures. When the pelvic floor is constricted, it pulls the bones of the pelvic bowl closer together, creating both compression and restriction of function in the pelvic region. For women, childbirth is much easier when the pelvic floor is able to relax. Impact injuries to the coccyx have a major effect on the tone of the levator ani muscle.

The iliopsoas is made up of three muscles, the **iliacus**, **psoas major**, ● and **psoas minor**, with each having a slightly different purpose (Fig. 9-22E). The psoas major muscle attaches to the bodies of the 12th thoracic vertebra and the five lumbar vertebrae. It passes over the pelvis like a sling and inserts on the lesser trochanter on the inside of the femur.

When the hip joints are stable, the psoas major flexes the trunk on the legs, as in the action of a sit-up. In this capacity, the psoas works in conjunction with the rectus abdominis muscle. Flexion of the spine should be initiated by the psoas, because it is positioned closer to the spine. It is then reinforced by the action of the abdominal muscles. In disorganized movement patterns, the rectus abdominus muscle does most of the work while the psoas remains inactive.

The range of influence of the psoas major muscle is extensive. The origin of the psoas on the 12 thoracic vertebra is very close to the attachments of the crura of the diaphragm. Inadequate functioning of the psoas can influence the position and action of the diaphragm, thus affecting respiration. The psoas also affects autonomic function in that the lumbar plexus passes through it. The nerves of this plexus control the abdominal viscera. Therefore, the general health and well-being of the body is tied to the condition of the psoas.

The psoas minor has its origin at the 12th thoracic vertebra and inserts on the ilium bone. It connects the spine with the pelvis, and it assists in flexion of the trunk and lumbar spine.

The iliacus muscle originates on the iliac crest and the anterior surface of the ilium. It joins the psoas major in its insertion on the lesser trochanter of the femur. The iliacus connects the pelvis with the legs, giving increased power to hip flexion movements, like running and kicking. These three muscles, acting as a group, provide force and stability to the body's central core.

The Abdomen

The muscles of the abdomen are the **rectus abdominus**, **external obliques**, ● **internal obliques**, and **transverse abdominus**. In addition to providing support for the abdominal contents, they are important accessory breathing muscles. As they collectively contract during exhalation, they push the diaphragm back up into position for inhalation. (See Essential Anatomy Box 9-4 for a summary of muscles, bones, and landmarks.)

The rectus abdominus forms the most superficial layer of the abdominal wall and connects the rib cage to the pelvis at the pubic bone (Fig. 9-22A). When it contracts, it draws the base of the pelvis upward, causing the top of the pelvis to tip posteriorly. In this action, it is the antagonist to the psoas major when a person is standing. In the standing position, when the psoas major contracts, it pulls the lumbar spine forward, causing the top of the pelvis to tilt anteriorly. The balancing action of the rectus abdominus and psoas muscles as an agonist–antagonist pair is essential for proper alignment and coordinated movement of the body as a whole.

The external obliques, acting together, also flex the spine (Fig. 9-22B). Unilaterally, they laterally flex the trunk and cause rotation to the opposite side. The fibers of the external obliques angle toward the midline, matching the direction of the external intercostal muscles.

The internal obliques duplicate the actions of the external obliques, except that when acting unilaterally, they rotate the trunk to the same side (i.e., the right internal oblique rotates the trunk to the right, and the left internal oblique rotates the trunk to the left). The fibers of the internal obliques angle away from the midline, matching the direction of the internal intercostal muscles (Fig. 9-22C).

The transverse abdominus is the deepest of these three muscles. Its fibers run in a horizontal direction (Fig. 9-22D). It acts to compress the abdominal contents. Its strong contraction causes regurgitation.

The **quadratus lumborum** forms the posterior wall of the abdomen (Fig. 9-22F) and is situated behind the psoas muscle. The quadratus lumborum consists of three sections, which have their origin on the inner lip of the iliac crest and the iliolumbar ligaments. The insertions are on the lower border of the 12th rib and the transverse processes of the first four lumbar vertebrae. The muscle is wrapped in thoracolumbar fascia.

The quadratus lumborum is a strong stabilizer of the lumbar spine. It prevents excessive lateral bending to the opposite side. Acting bilaterally, the quadratus lumborum extends the spine, and when overly contracted, it contributes to increased lordosis. Unilaterally, the muscle assists in lateral flexion to the same side. The quadratus lumborum is known as "the hip hiker." In a standing position, if the upper border of one of the iliac crests is higher than the upper border of the other, the quadratus lumborum on that side will be shortened.

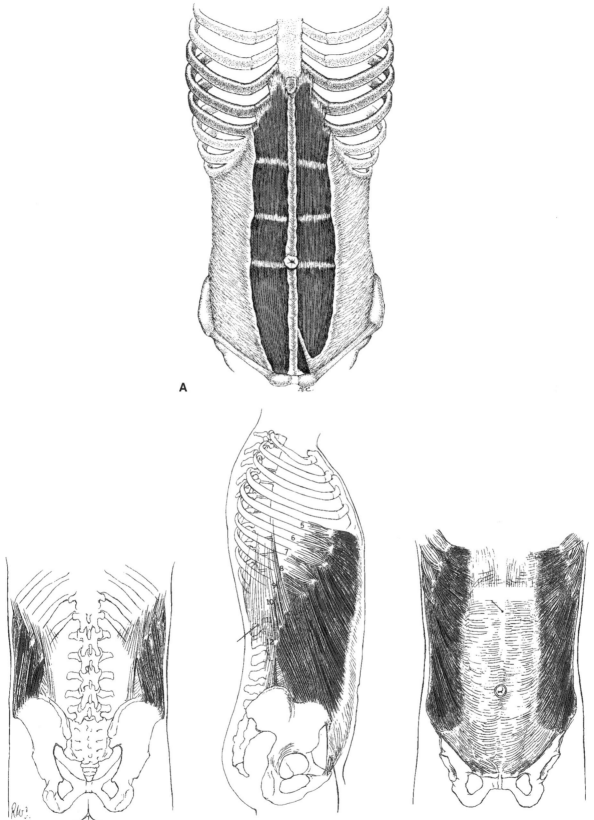

FIGURE 9-22 A. Rectus abdominus. (Reprinted with permission. MediClip image copyright © 2003 Lippincott Williams & Wilkins. All rights reserved.) **B.** External obliques. (Reprinted with permission from Kendall FP, McCreary EK, Provance PG. Muscle: testing and function with posture and pain, 4th edition. Philadelphia, PA: Lippincott Williams & Wilkins, 1993.)

Linea alba

Fascia transversalis

Rectus abdominis

D   **Posterior view**   **Lateral view**   **Anterior view**

FIGURE 9-22 *(continued)* **C.** Internal obliques. (Reprinted with permission from Kendall FP, McCreary EK, Provance PG. Muscle: testing and function with posture and pain, 4th edition. Philadelphia, PA: Lippincott Williams & Wilkins, 1993.) **D.** Transverse abdominus. (Reprinted with permission from Kendall FP, McCreary EK, Provance PG. Muscle: testing and function with posture and pain, 4th edition. Philadelphia, PA: Lippincott Williams & Wilkins, 1993.)

Psoas minor

Psoas major

Iliacus

David Rini

L₁
L₂
L₃
L₄

E

F

FIGURE 9-22 *(continued)* **E.** The iliopsoas group. **F.** Quadratus lumborum. (Reprinted with permission. MediClip image copyright © 2003 Lippincott Williams & Wilkins. All rights reserved.)

BOX 9-4 ESSENTIAL ANATOMY The Abdominal Routines

MUSCLES
Rectus abdominus
External obliques
Internal obliques
Transverse abdominus
BONES AND LANDMARKS
Costal cartilage
Ilium
Anterior superior iliac spine (ASIS)

Pubic bone
Inguinal ligament
Small intestine
Areas of the colon—ascending, transverse, descending
Ileocecal valve
Appendix
Hepatic and splenic flexures
Sigmoid colon and rectum
Aorta

■ CONDITIONS

1. *Anterior Pelvic Tilt.* This is a forward tipping of the ilium that creates an increased lumbar curve and often a protrusion of the abdomen. If the pelvis is visualized as a bowl that is filled with water, the water would be spilling in front of the person. The iliopsoas and the rectus femoris on both sides will be shortened, causing compression of the vertebral disks and strain on the soft tissues of the low back.

2. *Posterior Pelvic Tilt.* This is a backward tipping of the ilium. It causes the buttocks to appear tucked under and is often accompanied by contraction in the gluteal muscles, a tight rectus abdominus, and shortened hamstrings. The erector spinae muscles will be pulled downward, and the lumbar curve will be diminished, which will affect the transfer of weight through the spine.

3. *"Short leg."* This is a general term, describing a lateral tilt of the pelvis, presumably because one leg is shorter than the other, causing the pelvis to lean toward the short side. In most cases, however, the unevenness of the pelvis is caused by spinal curves or twists. The shortened side is often indicative of a tight psoas and quadratus lumborum muscle.

    Differences in length between the right and left psoas can also lead to pelvic rotation. The pelvis will be pulled forward and down on the side of the shortened psoas.

4. *Sciatica.* This is an irritation or inflammation of the sciatic nerve, which exits the spinal cord at L4–S3 and runs down the back of the leg. Compression and/or misalignment of the lumbar spine and sacrum can be responsible for the condition. In this case, the pathway of pain usually extends down the back of the leg and sometimes even to the ankle.

    In some cases, the source of irritation is at the site of the piriformis muscle at the back of the hip, under which the sciatic nerve passes. (In some people, the sciatic nerve passes *through* the piriformis.) If tightness in the piriformis is the source of the irritation, the pain is usually localized at the hip and back of the thigh.

5. *Psoas Strain.* The psoas muscle is difficult to pull, but it may become strained from extreme stretching motions of the trunk and groin, as in a jump initiated from a crouched position. This kind of injury is common in basketball players reaching for the hoop and in volleyball players. To test for psoas impairment, have the client sit on the edge of the table, with the feet hanging toward the floor. Place your hand on the thigh of the side you are checking, and have the client try to lift the thigh as you resist. If the psoas is injured, the client will experience pain in the groin area.

6. *Premenstrual Syndrome and Menstrual Cramps.* Premenstrual syndrome occurs several days before menstruation. It can induce irritability, mood changes, pain in the pelvic region, headache, and water retention, among other symptoms. A hormonal factor is suspected in premenstrual syndrome. Deep tissue massage has a beneficial effect on both of these conditions.[1] The relaxation of the pelvic muscles helps to diminish tension and takes pressure off the abdominal organs.

7. *Pelvic Inflammatory Disease.* This is caused by a bacterial infection, which can involve the vagina, uterus, fallopian tubes, and broad ligaments. It is a painful condition that requires medical treatment. This condition is a contraindication to massage therapy.

8. *Abuse Issues.* It is not uncommon for both male and female clients to have experienced sexual abuse, either as children or adults. As a result, they may be afraid of having their pelvic area touched. In fact, this work can be sensitive for anyone to receive because of the societal taboos imposed on the pelvic region, as result of our attitudes about sex and the eliminative functions. As a therapist, always approach this work sensitively, and respect the client's limitations. It may take time for the client to come to terms fully with all the issues lodged in the pelvic area. Be patient and nurturing, and allow healing to unfold at its own pace.

    Abdominal massage should be introduced slowly to a client who has a history of abuse or concerns about having the abdominal area touched. It may take several sessions before the client is comfortable with work being done on that area. Initial contact with the abdomen may consist of gentle contact; such as simply holding the hands there while the client relaxes. Keeping the abdomen covered with a drape while touching it often adds to the client's sense of safety. This contact may be included in several sessions before full abdominal massage is attempted. Never perform abdominal work without the client's willingness and permission.

9. *Constipation.* The back-up of waste matter in the intestinal tract is one of the major causes of toxic build-up in the body, which allows disease conditions to develop.[2] Several factors contribute to constipation; these include poor diet, lack of abdominal tone, and inadequate intake of water. Deep tissue massage is very helpful in breaking down impacted fecal matter that is adhered to the intestinal walls so that it may move through the colon and be eliminated properly.

10. *Ileocecal Valve Dysfunction.* The ileocecal valve is a one-way valve located at the junction of the small and large intestines. This valve prevents the back-up of feces from the colon into the sterile environment of the small intestine. When this valve becomes weakened and breaks down, the waste material can enter the small intestine, creating a toxic environment that eventually makes its way to other organs via the bloodstream.[3] Lack of abdominal tone and support around the valve during elimination is one of the primary causes of its weakening. Learning to eliminate from a

BOX 9-5 INDICATIONS/CONTRAINDICATIONS Conditions Affecting Abdominal Massage

INDICATIONS	CONTRAINDICATIONS
Constipation	Diverticulitis
Low back pain	Severe hypertension
Colitis	Pregnancy
Distended belly	Severe illness
Poor digestion	Recent surgery
Gas	Skin rash
Stomach ache	Recent heavy meal
Menstrual cramps	Ulcer

squatting position is beneficial for maintaining the integrity of the ileocecal valve.

11. *Diverticulitis.* This is an inflammatory condition of the colon. Diverticula are tiny pouches in the colon wall that are filled with fecal matter. They are created by pressure from straining to push feces through the colon. When these sacs of waste material become inflamed, they cause pain. This condition is a contraindication to massage work.

12. *Colitis.* This is an inflammation of the colon. Although its cause is unknown, episodes can be exacerbated by psychological factors, such as stress, worry, and anxiety. It is often accompanied by spasms of the colon muscles. Light massage on the abdomen may be beneficial between flare-ups.

13. *Prolapsed Bowel.* This is a collapse of the transverse colon that is caused by the build-up of feces. The increased weight pulls the colon downward, resulting in pressure on the bladder, which may cause retention of urine. In women, there may also be pressure on the fallopian tubes or the ovaries; in men, there may be pressure on the prostate gland.[4]

14. *Pot Belly.* Excess weight in the abdominal region has many negative effects. The displacement of weight puts excessive pressure on the low back and moves the abdominal organs out of position, inhibiting their proper function. Increased intra-abdominal pressure pushes the diaphragm upward, inhibiting full breathing and putting pressure on the heart. A distended, bloated belly is often the result of a build-up of feces and the resultant stagnant gases. Maintaining strong abdominal muscles contributes to proper alignment of the torso and helps to reduce pot belly conditions.

Please refer to Indications/Contraindications Boxes 9-5 and 9-6 for further indications and contraindications for massage of the abdomen and pelvis.

■ POSTURAL EVALUATION

The Pelvis: Front View

1. Check the level of the iliac crests. Are they on the same horizontal line?
2. Look for rotation of the pelvis. If one ASIS is more prominent than the other, it indicates that side of the pelvis is rotated forward.

BOX 9-6 INDICATIONS/CONTRAINDICATIONS Conditions Affecting Pelvic Massage

INDICATIONS	CONTRAINDICATIONS
Low back pain	Pelvic inflammatory disease
Menstrual cramps	Recent surgery
Postural distortions	Broken bones
Limping gait	Inflammation of the sacroiliac joint
Immobile pelvis	Inflammation of the sciatic nerve
Lack of flexibility	Hernia
Jaw tension	

The pelvis is the body's structural center. All parts of the body come into equilibrium when balanced around the pelvis. Muscles function with their maximum efficiency in this alignment, and neuromuscular patterns generate smooth, flowing, stress-free movement. The pelvis acts as the focal point of the body, much like the hub does for a wheel. Feeling and acting from this centered place means that we are operating freely, from an instinctual level. It means we are not having to control movements and impulses but, rather, are surrendering to the natural grace of the body and consciousness.

Few of us, however, function at this level of balance. For the most part, we feel our identity and initiate our actions from a place farther up in the body. The emphasis placed on intellectual processes draws most people's awareness up toward the head. Muscular initiation of movement tends to occur more from the chest and thoracic region of the spine. This not only strains the muscles that are responsible for breathing but also disconnects us from the more powerful and effective muscles of motion that originate in the hips and thighs.

These core muscles correspond with our more instinctive nature. When living out of our core, we are more prone to incorporate feeling and intuition into our bodily experience. A more complete integration of all the modes of cognition becomes available to us, and we begin to reclaim our full stature as human beings.

The pelvis houses the organs of reproduction and elimination. Culturally, we are not comfortable with these functions. Many societal constraints and restrictions are placed on both. Children are often trained to control defecation at too young an age, before the muscles of the pelvis have developed sufficiently to operate in this capacity. As a result, a young child, in a vain attempt to stop elimination, will squeeze the sphincters and the muscles around them with a great deal of effort, creating a high degree of constriction in the pelvic floor and inner thighs.[5] This forms the basis of a potentially lifelong pattern of associating the maintaining of control with tightening the pelvic floor and inner thighs. In adults, this pattern can also be seen in rigidly contracted gluteal muscles.

Sexual issues are another area in which conflict between natural impulses and societal dictates creates inhibition in the pelvic structures. The sexual drive is a potent force, and many moral codes define how and where it is to be expressed. Many people withdraw from or suppress this energy by clamping down on the muscles of the pelvis, inner thigh, and/or low back. The psychiatrist Wilhelm Reich theorized that most conditions of neurosis result from the conflict imposed by the suppression of the sexual urge along with other expressions of the primary life force.[6]

The pelvis is designed to swing freely between the hip joints and the lumbar spine. This capability can be severely limited by chronic muscular contractions in and around the pelvic region. Voluntary muscle action is controlled by the nervous system, which is ultimately under the jurisdiction of the mind. Therefore, our mental attitudes and beliefs play an important part in determining our body posture. Because of the extent of muscular interaction in determining pelvic positioning, we have a tremendous capacity to distort pelvic placement and movement through our responses to the issues associated with this body segment. Observation of a person's core may reveal much about their beliefs regarding control and surrender as well as their attitudes about sex.[7] Some typical examples of pelvic misalignment to which sexual suppression contributes are the anterior tilt of the pelvic bowl, tucking under of the hips, and constriction across the lumbar muscles. All of these denote some form of muscular imbalance that inhibits complete mobility of the pelvis. Clients who are interested in pursuing this subject further may be referred to a psychologist who has studied a Reichian-based approach to psychotherapy, such as bioenergetics.

The abdomen is a cylinder of soft tissue covering the viscera. Having no bony protection, this area is commonly perceived as being vulnerable and weak. A feeling of apprehension is often associated with touching this body segment, partly because of a common revulsion over anything associated with the "guts."

The image of the tight, washboard abdomen is considered to be a desirable one by most people. We are enticed by TV commercials and videos extolling the virtues of a trim, tight midsection. By overly tightening the abdominal muscles, we effectively restrict our feelings, creating a shield of armor around our perceived vulnerabilities in an attempt to protect ourselves from our emotions.

A truly balanced abdomen has a slightly rounded contour. It is supple and toned, not cinched in tight. Neither is it flaccid and weak, allowing the abdomen to protrude and disorganizing the alignment of the lumbar spine and rib cage.

When the muscles of the pelvis and abdomen are working in conjunction with each other to maintain the integrity of the trunk, the ability to experience emotions, process them, and take appropriate action (or not) according to the dictates of the moment is enhanced. Balance in the midsection is reflective of a quality of poise and integrity that allows one to experience fully the kinesthetic unity of the body without getting caught up in distorted perceptions that manifest as chronic tightness and postural aberrations.

TABLE 9–2	Body Reading for the Pelvis	
Conditions	**Muscles That May Be Shortened**
Anterior tilt—the iliac crests are tipped forward	Iliopsoas Rectus femoris Erector spinae Quadratus lumborum
Posterior tilt—the iliac crests are tipped backward	Rectus abdominus Gluteus maximus Lateral rotators Hamstrings
Lateral tilt—one iliac crest is higher than the other	Gluteus medius Quadratus lumborum Abductors on high side Adductors on low side

3. Is there space between the rib cage and the iliac crests, or does the waist area seem compressed, forming bulges at the sides (i.e., love handles)?
4. When the client's knees are flexed, do they align over the feet properly? Incorrect tracking of the knees over the feet will affect psoas function.
5. Does the pelvis seem too large or too small for the rest of the body?

The Pelvis: Side View

1. Observe the direction and degree of pelvic tilt, if any.
2. From a standing position, can the pelvis swing forward and backward freely? If not, in which motion is it restricted?

Please refer to Table 9-2 for a list of variations in pelvic alignment and possible muscles involved.

The Abdominal Region

1. Check the position of the lower ribs.
   - Squeezed together, pulling downward?
   - Spread apart, lifted, protruding?
2. General shape of the abdomen.
   - Tight, withdrawn, held in?
   - Distended?
   - Lower belly larger, which may indicate a constipated condition?
   - Upper belly larger, which may indicate build-up of gases from the intestines?
3. Describe the distribution of fat content.
4. Does the belly move with the breath?

Please refer to Table 9-3 for a list of common tension patterns found in the abdominal region and possible muscles involved.

TABLE 9–3	Body Reading for the Abdomen	
Conditions	**Muscles That May Be Shortened**
Distended belly—overall bloating accompanied by anterior tilt of the pelvis	Quadratus lumborum Iliopsoas group Rectus femoris Erector spinae
Tight midsection—rectus abdominus is overly defined, lower ribs are pulled in and down; rigid abdominal wall	Rectus abdominus Transverse abdominus Hamstrings
"Bladder belt"—upper abdominal area is distended; lower area is pulled in, as if wearing a tight belt	Obliques Pelvic floor muscles

■ EXERCISES AND SELF-TREATMENT

Pelvis

Pelvic Opening (Integrates Muscular Action in the Pelvis and Low Back Regions)

Preparation

Sit on the edge of a chair, with both feet flat on the floor, or sit in a cross-legged position on the floor. Do each movement slowly and consciously. The purpose of the exercise is to increase awareness of the pelvic region (Fig. 9-23).

Execution

• Roll the pelvis posteriorly, rounding the low back and taking your weight off the ischial tuberosities (Fig. 9-23A). Let your chin drop forward naturally. Return the pelvis to the vertical position, and repeat a few more times.

• Roll the pelvis anteriorly, arching the low back slightly (Fig. 9-23B). Return to the upright position, and repeat several more times.

• Combine the two movements above, creating a fluid, forward and backward, rocking motion of the pelvis. Rest briefly afterward, and note any changes in your level of awareness in the pelvic region.

• Beginning with your weight distributed evenly over the base of the pelvis, shift slightly to the right, increasing the weight on the right ischial tuberosity. Keep the left hip on the chair or floor. Return to the center position, and repeat the shift to the right several more times.

• Beginning with your weight distributed evenly over the base of the pelvis, shift slightly to the left, increasing the weight on the left ischial tuberosity. Keep the right hip on the chair or floor. Return to the center position, and repeat the shift to the left several more times.

• Combine the previous two movements, rocking your weight from side to side several times. Rest briefly afterward, noting any changes in your level of awareness in the pelvic region.

David Rini

DAR

A   **B**

FIGURE 9-23 A. Tilting the pelvis posteriorly. **B.** Tilting the pelvis anteriorly.

FIGURE 9-24 Sit-down exercise to strengthen rectus abdominus.

Abdomen

Sit-Downs (Strengthens Rectus Abdominus, External and Internal Obliques, and Transverse Abdominus)

Preparation
Sitting on the floor, bring your knees to your chest, with both feet remaining on the floor. Place your hands under the thighs just above the knees.

Execution
Exhaling, pull in your abdomen, and tuck your pelvis under as you roll down the back slightly (Fig. 9-24). Hold for a few seconds as you breathe normally, Then, exhale strongly, and roll down the back a little farther. Continue to roll toward the floor in small increments. If your back begins to hurt or the abdominal muscles cannot support the rolling motion any further, lie down on your back and rest.

Abdominal Stretch (Stretches Rectus Abdominus, External and Internal Obliques, and Transverse Abdominus)

Lying on your back on the floor, extend your arms overhead. Exhaling, press the low back to the floor as you reach the arms behind you, until you feel a stretch in the abdominal muscles (Fig. 9-25). Hold for 20 seconds. Slightly arching the back increases the stretch. Laterally flex the trunk to the right by reaching both arms slightly to the right. Hold for 20 seconds. Laterally flex the trunk to the left by reaching both arms slightly to the left. Hold for 20 seconds.

FIGURE 9-25 Stretch for rectus abdominus.

The subject is a 27-year-old man named Eric, who is an actor. Eric is in good physical health. He enjoys reading about and becoming involved in activities that contribute to his health and self-improvement. He participates in yoga and dance classes regularly, and he tries to maintain a low-fat diet. Eric enjoys outdoor activities like bicycling and hiking. He has been receiving a series of deep tissue therapy sessions as part of his health and high-level wellness regimen. This case describes the session that focused on his hip flexors.

Eric has a well-balanced musculature overall. His anterior thigh and gluteal muscles, however, appear to be overdeveloped in relation to the rest of his body. He exhibits an anterior pelvic tilt and slight pelvic rotation, with the left iliac crest drawn both forward and downward. Observing his walking pattern reveals that he initiates thigh movements primarily with the rectus femoris muscles. This is apparent on observation because instead of allowing his thighs to swing from a mobile pelvis when he walks, he lifts his knees toward his chest and remains rigid in the pelvic region.

Eric complains that his thighs become very sore after dance classes and after hiking. He also gets winded sooner than he feels he should during strenuous activities, and he sometimes experiences cramping (a "stitch") under his rib cage. At irregular intervals, he experiences pain in his low back, more concentrated on the left side, near the sacrum.

Eric provides an example of someone who does not move from his core. His rectus femoris muscles overwork during hip flexion movements, and his psoas muscles are underactive. Eric has gained fairly good control of his body, but his movements are not as fluid as they could be if initiated from the pelvic center. His poor stamina reflects the lack of coordinated action between the extrinsic and intrinsic muscles. This is the fourth session dealing with the core; the abdominal and thigh muscles have been worked on previously. Getting Eric more in touch with the iliopsoas complex will likely provide the missing key for him in understanding how to control his body movements properly.

The rectus femoris muscles were fairly sore. Elongation strokes along the fibers were performed extremely slowly, giving time for Eric to relax and the muscle to lengthen. At least 10 minutes were spent on each rectus femoris muscle, allowing it to soften and lengthen fully. The attachment of the rectus femoris on the anterior inferior iliac spine was particularly sensitive. Initially, the client experienced extreme ticklishness when the attachment was contacted. After being directed to focus on slowing his breathing and to relax into the sensations, however, the ticklishness transformed into extreme pain.

The pressure was adjusted to a tolerable level and maintained without any movement until the client reported a considerable diminishing of the sensation. At that point, the therapist began a cross fiber motion on the tendon to complete the release of the rectus femoris.

After warming up the abdominal region, the border of the iliacus was contacted along the rim of the ilium. Surprisingly little discomfort was experienced there. The muscle responded well to the strokes, and it softened considerably. After placing his fingers in the left lower quadrant of the abdominal cavity in the proper location to palpate the psoas, the therapist had the client flex his left thigh to contract the muscle fibers. It was difficult to locate the psoas initially, but when the muscle was finally palpated, the fibers felt extremely taut, like a thin cord. This was an unusual occurrence, because the psoas is a thick, cylindrically shaped muscle. It obviously was extremely contracted, appearing to be frozen in position. The therapist very gradually moved the fingers up the length of the muscle, parallel to the bodies of the lumbar vertebrae. The client was not experiencing much sensation other than awareness of the presence of the fingers deep in his abdomen. At the level of L_3 vertebra, however, he experienced a sharp pain as the therapist rolled across a tight knot of fibers. The pain was radiating into Eric's low back, near the sacrum. This was exactly the area where he had reported experiencing intermittent low back pain. The point was held until Eric reported an almost complete disappearance of the pain in his low back.

After the psoas muscles were worked on both sides, the client expressed feeling a wonderful sense of freedom, almost euphoria. He said he felt much more of a sense of being in his body. He felt light and open in his legs and feet, and he was actually aware of his spinal column, an experience he had never had before. It is not uncommon for clients to have a renewed burst of self-awareness after receiving psoas work. It is often the most profound deep tissue session they experience.

Topics for Discussion

1. How would you teach a client to attain greater awareness and function of the psoas muscles?
2. Describe the ideal walking pattern of a person who initiates thigh movements primarily from the psoas muscles.
3. A client's left psoas muscle is stronger than the right psoas. How is the client's pelvic alignment affected by this situation?
4. What is the relationship of the psoas and rectus abdominus muscles in reference to the pelvis when a person is in a standing position?
5. Which exercises stretch the psoas muscles?

■ ABDOMINAL MUSCLES ROUTINE

Objectives

- To elongate the portion of the trunk that connects the thorax and pelvis
- To release the attachments of the trunk muscles along the pelvis and the lower ribs
- To separate the abdominal muscles so that each may function optimally
- To release shortness in the quadratus lumborum muscle, which can contribute to low back pain and misalignment of the pelvis

Energy

POSITION

- The client is lying supine on the table, with a bolster under the knees.
- The therapist is standing at the side of the table next to the client's waist.

POLARITY

Place the left palm (negative pole) on the abdomen (positive pole). Slide the right palm (positive pole) underneath the client's back to contact the lumbar spine (negative pole). Your palms should be aligned to each other vertically through the client's trunk. Keep your hands relaxed, allowing them to mold to the contours of the client's body and to be moved by the motions generated by the client's breathing action. During this polarity hold, you should project feelings of trust and nurturing, allowing the client to become accustomed to being touched in the abdominal region. Hold for at least 1 minute.

SHIATSU

Slide the fingers of both hands under the client's back, palpating the lateral edge of the erector spinae in the lumbar region with your fingertips. Straighten the fingers, allowing the weight of the client's trunk to rest on your fingertips. Repeat on the other side of the back. The outer branch of the bladder channel runs along the lateral border of the erector spinae. This move helps to relax tightness in the muscles of the low back, allowing the lumbar spine to decompress.

Swedish/Cross Fiber

1. Perform circular effleurage on the abdomen.
2. Perform two-handed pétrissage on both sides of the torso, between the rib cage and pelvis.

3. Perform circular friction around the abdomen in a clockwise direction.
4. Perform fingertip raking across the abdominal muscles.

Connective Tissue

Place your right palm on the abdomen, over the navel area. Place your left palm on top of your right hand. Begin to make a slow, clockwise spiraling motion, moving the skin over the underlying tissues. Do not glide over the skin. Gradually increase the size of the spiral, stretching the skin and fascia to their maximum degree.

Deep Tissue/Neuromuscular Therapy

SEQUENCE

1. Abdominal muscle attachments on the iliac crest
2. Inferior border of the costal cartilage of the ribs
3. Abdominal muscle attachments on the ribs 🔘
4. Rectus abdominus 🔘
5. Obliques—external and internal
6. Transverse abdominus
7. Quadratus lumborum 🔘
   a. 12th rib attachment—tendon
   b. Iliac crest attachment—tendon
   c. Belly—muscle fibers

Trigger point patterns in the abdominal muscles are not as predictable as those in other muscle groups. Characteristically, the referred pain from these trigger points is mistaken for visceral pain. Trigger points in these muscles often cause pain bilaterally.

Check all muscle attachments thoroughly, feeling for strings and lumps that are frequently found around trigger points. The origin of the rectus abdominus at the pubic symphysis often harbors trigger points, as does its insertion along the inferior border of the rib cage, just lateral to the xiphoid process.

1. Abdominal Muscle Attachments on the Iliac Crest (External and Internal Obliques and Transverse Abdominus)

Strokes
- Stand at the side of the table, and face the upper border of the client's iliac crest. Placing one or both thumbs on the upper border of the iliac crest, apply short, side to side strokes against the inner edge of the bone.
- Continue around the pelvis as far as your hand can reach.

2. Inferior Border of the Costal Cartilage of Ribs 7–10 (Transverse Abdominus)

Strokes

- Placing the thumbs just lateral to the xiphoid process, apply short, side to side strokes along the inferior border of the rib cage to the tip of rib 11.

3. Abdominal Muscle Attachments on the Ribs

See Figure 9-26 for muscle attachments on the ribs.

Rectus Abdominus

Strokes

- Place your fingers on the costal cartilages of ribs 5–7, next to the xiphoid process.
- Using short, up and down and side to side strokes with your fingertips, release the muscular attachments.

External Obliques

Strokes

- The attachments for this muscle are on the lower eight ribs, interweaving with the serratus anterior. Place your fingers on rib 5, near the sternum. Perform short, up and down and side to side strokes on the rib.
- Continue to work the attachments on each rib, in succession. On each rib, slide your fingers a little further laterally to make contact with the muscle insertion. Use the border of the serratus anterior for a guideline.

Internal Obliques

Strokes

- The muscle attaches on the costal cartilages of ribs 8–10. Place your fingers or thumbs along the lower portion of rib 8, just lateral to the rectus abdominus. Apply short, side to side and up and down strokes on the attachment.
- Moving slightly lateral, slide down to rib 9. Repeat the same strokes on the attachment, then repeat once more on the rib 10 attachment.

4. Rectus Abdominus

Origin: Medial tendon from the pubic symphysis, lateral tendon from the crest of the pubis.

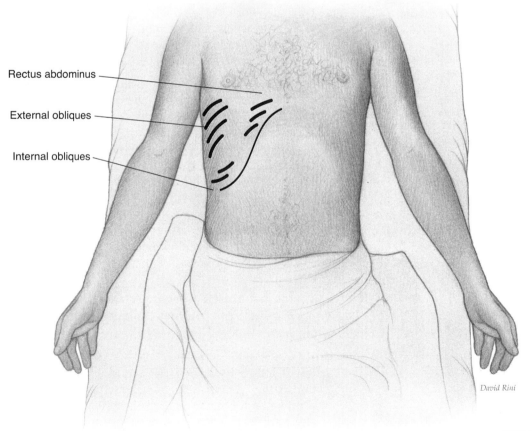

Rectus abdominus

External obliques

Internal obliques

David Rini

FIGURE 9-26 Abdominal muscle attachments on the ribs.

Insertion: Costal cartilages of ribs 5–7, xiphoid process.

Action: Flexion of the spine, posterior tilt of the pelvis; compresses abdominal contents.

Strokes

- Place your fingers next to the midline of the upper abdomen, just below the rib cage.
- Using a spreading technique, slide your fingers across the fibers of the muscle (Fig. 9-27). Pause and work on abnormalities in the muscle tissue with side to side strokes. Release trigger points as they are found. Continue, working in strips, down the rectus abdominus. Be sure to palpate the tendinous sheath between each section of the muscle.

⚠ **Avoid pressure on the linea alba, which is the fascial sheath running down the midline of the rectus abdominus that joins its right and left halves. The aorta runs down the center of the trunk directly beneath this area. If you feel a strong pulse under your fingers when massaging the rectus abdominus, immediately move off it.**

- Place your thumb or fingers along the upper border of the pubic symphysis. Using short, side to side strokes, contact the attachment of the rectus abdominus.

Note: Be sure that the client is comfortable with this procedure before attempting it. Describe the move to the client first, and get his or her permission to perform it.

5. External and Internal Obliques

Obliquus Externus Abdominis

Origin: Ribs 4–12, interdigitating with the serratus anterior.

Insertion: Anterior part of the iliac crest, abdominal aponeurosis.

Action: Flexion of the trunk (bilaterally), lateral flexion of the trunk and rotation of the trunk (unilaterally), support and compression of abdominal viscera; assists in forced exhalation.

Obliquus Internus Abdominus

Origin: Thoracolumbar fascia, lateral two-thirds of the inguinal ligament, anterior two-thirds of the iliac crest.

Insertion: Cartilages of ribs 9–12, abdominal aponeurosis to the linea alba.

Action: Flexion of the trunk (bilaterally), lateral flexion of the trunk and rotation of the trunk (unilaterally), support and compression of abdominal viscera; assists in exhalation.

Strokes

- Begin lateral to the border of the rectus abdominus. Do a spreading stroke, with your fingers across the direction of the fibers, as described above. Remember that the fibers of the external obliquus angle on a lateral diagonal, so cross fiber strokes on the muscle are performed on a medial diagonal perpendicular to the fibers (Fig. 9-28A). The fibers of the internal obliquus

FIGURE 9-27 Cross fiber technique on the rectus abdominus.

DAR

A

DAR

B

FIGURE 9-28 A. Cross fiber technique on external obliques. **B.** Direction of cross fiber strokes on internal obliques.

angle on a medial diagonal, so cross fiber strokes on the muscle are performed on a lateral diagonal that is perpendicular to the fibers (Fig. 9-28*B*).

• Continue outward to the lateral border of the latissimus dorsi on the side of the body. Cover the muscles

thoroughly, pausing at tender areas and working in detail on tissues that feel aberrant. It is important to visualize the muscle you are working on under your fingers to be able to palpate it effectively, because the abdominal muscles overlap each other.

FIGURE 9-29 Cross fiber technique on the transverse abdominus.

6. Transverse Abdominus

Origin: Lateral third of the inguinal ligament, anterior two-thirds of the lip of the iliac crest, thoracolumbar fascia, costal cartilages of ribs 7–12.
Insertion: Abdominal aponeurosis to the linea alba.
Action: Compresses the abdomen, assists in forced exhalation.

Strokes
- Place your fingers next to the lateral border of the rectus abdominus, facing in a superior direction. Apply short, up and down strokes across the muscle fibers, covering the area between the base of the rib cage and the iliac crest thoroughly (Fig. 9-29).

FIGURE 9-30 Contacting the lateral border of the quadratus lumborum.

David Rini

FIGURE 9-31 Stretch for the quadratus lumborum and obliques.

7. Quadratus Lumborum

Origin: Inner lip of the iliac crest, iliolumbar ligament.

Insertion: Lower border of the 12th rib, transverse process of L1–L4 vertebrae.

Action: Extension of the lumbar spine (bilaterally), lateral flexion of the spine (unilaterally), fixation and depression of the 12th rib.

Trigger points in the superficial layer of the muscle are located in the lateral section, with one near the attachment on the 12th rib and the other near the attachment on the iliac crest. Pain from the 12th rib attachment point is referred along the iliac crest and gluteus medius region. The referral zone for the iliac crest attachment point is to the greater trochanter and outer thigh area.

Two trigger points in the deeper layer are found near the transverse process of L3 and between the transverse processes of L4 and L5. The trigger point at L3 refers pain to the sacroiliac joints and across the upper sacral region. The second trigger point lower down refers pain to the lower gluteal area.

Position

- Place the client in side posture. Place a bolster between the knees and a small support under the side of the head.

A bolster may also be placed between the side of the client's waist and the table. Have the client stretch the topmost arm overhead.

- The therapist stands behind the client.

Strokes

- Place your front hand on the client's hip for support. Using the heel of your back hand, do deep, circular friction on the muscles from the 12th rib to the iliac crest.
- Slide your thumbs upward, along the lateral border of the erector spinae, until the 12th rib is felt. Using the thumbs or a knuckle, do short, side to side strokes across the underside of the rib to the spine. It is likely that knotted areas and trigger points will be found here.
- Turn to face the iliac crest. Apply short, side to side strokes along the superior border of the iliac crest with the knuckle or thumbs, pausing at tender points.
- Standing behind the client's waist, place both palms on the side of the torso with the thumbs pointed downward toward the spine. Finding the edge of the erector spinae, slide the thumbs slightly anterior, and press downward toward the transverse processes of the spine (Fig. 9-30). Be careful not to push into the tips of the bones. Perform short, up and down and side to side

FIGURE 9-32 Stretch for the rectus abdominus.

strokes along the quadratus lumborum. Work between the 12th rib and the iliac crest.

STRETCH

1. *Quadratus Lumborum and Obliques.* The client is lying in side posture and slides to the edge of the table near the therapist. The bottom leg is flexed at the knee. The top leg is straight, and the uppermost arm is stretched overhead, grasping the end of the table. Place one hand on the client's uppermost arm and the other hand on the client's top leg.

   The straightened top leg is positioned behind the bottom leg so that it can hang off the side of the table. As you push down on the top arm, press the leg toward the floor until a stretch is felt in the quadratus lumborum (Fig. 9-31).
2. *Rectus Abdominus.* The client is lying supine and slides the heels toward the hips, keeping the feet flat on the table and with both knees flexed. The arms are stretched overhead, reaching toward the head of the table (Fig. 9-32). If further stretch is required, a bolster may be slid under the client's back.

ACCESSORY WORK

1. This work should be done in conjunction with the pelvic session.
2. The solar plexus reflex point is located on the sole of the left foot slightly inferior to the bases of the metatarsal bones of the first through third toes (Fig. 9-33). Pressing this point will bring relaxation to the upper abdominal region.
3. The reflex zone for the lumbar spine is along the medial side of the instep on both feet, in the space be-

tween the first cuneiform bone and the calcaneus. Press this point to help relieve low back stress and pain.

CLOSING

Sitting at the foot of the table, lightly hold the heels of the client's feet in your hands for 30 to 60 seconds. Remove your hands slowly to complete the session.

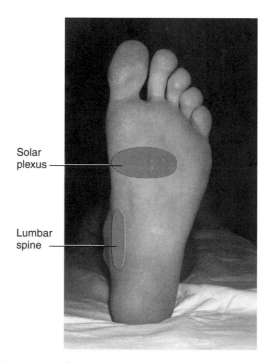

Solar plexus

Lumbar spine

FIGURE 9-33 Reflex zones on the foot to accompany an abdomen session.

■ LATERAL THIGH/INNER THIGH/ INTESTINES ROUTINE

Objectives

- To balance the muscular action of the inner and outer thighs
- To release uneven pulls on the pelvis coming from thigh muscles that attach on it
- To improve the function of the intestines
- To further open the abdominal cavity

Energy

POSITION

- The client is in side posture, with a small pillow under the head. The leg lying against the table is slightly flexed. The top leg is flexed 90°, with a bolster placed under the knee.
- The therapist is standing behind the client's hip.

POLARITY

Place the palm of your top hand on the client's hip and your bottom hand on the side of the knee. Breathe deeply and rhythmically, envisioning the client's thigh area relaxing between your two hands. Hold for at least 30 seconds.

SHIATSU

1. *Top Leg.* Using your forearm, perform shiatsu compression movements along the side of the hip, from the iliac crest to the greater trochanter (Fig. 9-34). Both you and the client should exhale each time you lean your forearm into the hip. Continue the compression movements down the side of the leg to the knee. The gallbladder channel traverses this area.
2. *Bottom Leg.* Using your palm or the tiger's mouth position of the hand (the webbing between the thumb and index finger), perform shiatsu compression movements on the inner thigh, from the pelvis to the knee (Fig. 9-35).

Deep Tissue/Neuromuscular Therapy

SEQUENCE

Lateral Thigh

1. Vastus lateralis
2. Iliotibial tract
3. Tensor fascia latae

FIGURE 9-34 Forearm compression down the side of the hip.

DAR

FIGURE 9-35 Tiger's mouth position on the inner thigh.

Inner Thigh

1. Pes anserinus
2. Adductor muscles—adductor magnus, brevis and longus; pectineus, and gracilis

Intestines

1. Large intestine
2. Small intestine

▮ LATERAL THIGH

Swedish/Cross Fiber

POSITION

• The therapist moves to the front side of the table and faces the client's top leg.
1. Perform effleurage strokes on the top leg from the knee to the iliac crest.
2. Perform circular friction with the heel of your hand from the knee to the iliac crest.

Connective Tissue

MYOFASCIAL SPREADING

Place the heels of your hands on the midline of the thigh at the knee. Stroke outward with both hands, spreading the tissues in opposite directions. Continue, working in strips, to the iliac crest.

Deep Tissue/Neuromuscular Therapy

POSITION

• The client remains in side posture.
• The therapist stands at the front side of the table and faces the client's flexed thigh.

1. Vastus Lateralis

Origin: Intertrochanteric line, greater trochanter, gluteal tuberosity, lateral lip of the linea aspera, lateral intermuscular septum.
Insertion: Lateral border of the patella, patellar ligament to the tibial tuberosity.
Action: Extension of leg at the knee joint.

 Along the anterior portion, a group of trigger points may be found at midthigh level that refer pain along the length of the muscle. The majority of trigger points form along the lateral aspect of the muscle. They may be spaced just above the knee, in the middle of the thigh, and at the attachment on the upper femur.

Trigger points in the superficial fibers will fire more locally. Trigger points in the deeper layers shoot pain throughout the muscle and down to the side of the knee.

FIGURE 9-36 Deep tissue strokes on the vastus lateralis and iliotibial tract.

Strokes
- Perform elongation strokes with the forearm or knuckles along the lateral thigh in the space between the rectus femoris and iliotibial tract. Pause to treat trigger points (**A** in Fig. 9-36).
- Perform elongation strokes with an elbow or the thumbs along the distal half of the lateral thigh, in the space between the iliotibial tract and biceps femoris (**C** in Fig. 9-36).

- Pause to treat trigger points.

2. Iliotibial Tract

Strokes
- With your thumbs or elbow, press a line of points along the iliotibial tract, from the knee to the greater trochanter (**B** in Fig. 9-36).

FIGURE 9-37 Position for contacting the tensor fascia latae.

3. Tensor Fascia Latae

Origin: Anterior part of the outer lip of the iliac crest, ASIS.
Insertion: Iliotibial tract.
Action: Flexion, abduction, medial rotation of the hip.

 Trigger points in this muscle usually refer pain along the iliotibial tract.

Strokes
- Standing behind the client at the level of the hip, place your elbow on the anterior surface of the hip. Apply short, up and down and side to side strokes along the fibers of the muscle, between the iliac crest and greater trochanter (Fig. 9-37).
- Pause to treat trigger points.

■ INNER THIGH

Swedish/Cross Fiber

POSITION

- The client remains in the same position as above.
- The therapist works on the inner thigh muscles of the leg that is against the table.

1. Perform effleurage strokes from the knee to the pelvis.
2. Perform circular friction on the muscle attachments at the knee.
3. Perform cross fiber fingertip raking on the adductor muscles.

Connective Tissue

MYOFASCIAL SPREADING

Standing at the front side of the table and facing the client's bottom leg, place the fingertips of both hands along the fibers of the adductor muscles, slightly above knee level. Using the spreading technique, slowly glide the fingers in a posterior direction, perpendicular to the direction of the fibers. Continue, working in strips, to the pelvis.

Deep Tissue/Neuromuscular Therapy

POSITION

- The client remains in side posture.
- The therapist stands at the front of the table and faces the inner thigh of the client's leg, which lies against the table.

1. Pes Anserinus (Attachment Points of Sartorius, Gracilis, and Semitendinosus)

Location: on the medial side of the proximal end of the tibia.

Strokes
- Press down on the insertion points on the bone with your thumbs or fingers. Move slowly up and down and side to side.
- Hold tender points.

2. Adductor Muscles

Adductor Magnus
Origin: Inferior ramus of the pubis, inferior ramus of the ischium, inferior and lateral part of the ischial tuberosity.
Insertion: Linea aspera of the femur.
Action: Hip adduction; assists in hip extension and lateral rotation.

 The trigger points in this muscle will probably be found in the middle portion. They project pain deep into the groin and pelvic region.

Adductor Brevis
Origin: Inferior ramus of the pubis.
Insertion: Proximal third of the medial lip of the linea aspera, distal pectineal line.
Action: Hip adduction.

Adductor Longus
Origin: Anterior part of the pubis.
Insertion: Middle third of the medial lip of the linea aspera.
Action: Hip adduction; assists in lateral rotation when the hip is in extension.

 Trigger points in these muscles are frequently located near their attachment on the pubis. Pain is referred to the upper medial thigh and into the groin region. Trigger points in the section of the muscles closer to the femur attachment will shoot pain down to the knee and perhaps over the upper tibia.

Gracilis
Origin: Inferior ramus of the pubis near the symphysis.
Insertion: Medial surface of the shaft of the tibia below the tibial condyle.
Action: Hip adduction, knee flexion; assists in medial rotation of the knee when the leg is flexed.

 There may be a trigger point found halfway up the length of the muscle and another found three-quarters of the way up to the pubis. Pain from these trigger points can be intense and burning, traveling along the entire muscle.

Pectineus
Origin: Pectineal line on the superior ramus of the pubis.
Insertion: Femur from the lesser trochanter to the linea aspera.
Action: Hip adduction; assists in hip flexion.

 The common trigger point is palpated on the attachment of the muscle on the pubis. It sends pain deep into the groin.

DAR

FIGURE 9-38 Direction of strokes on the adductor muscles.

Strokes
- Place the fingertips of both hands along the fibers of the adductor muscles, as in the connective tissue technique above. Use short, up and down and side to side strokes on the muscle bellies to release adherent fibers and locate trigger points (Fig. 9-38).

David Rini

FIGURE 9-39 Contacting the adductor muscle attachments on the pubis.

- Find the borders of the muscles with your fingers. Slide in between the muscles, and move the fingers up and down along the borders to separate the muscles from each other. Work from the knee to the pelvis.

⚠ **Avoid any pressure in the femoral triangle, which is located in the upper third of the medial thigh. It is bounded medially by the sartorius, laterally by the adductor longus, and superiorly by the inguinal ligament. The femoral nerve, artery, and vein pass through this area.**

- Place your fingers or the broad side of the thumb against the pubis, and move slowly side to side across the bone to contact the adductor muscle attachments on the pelvis (Fig. 9-39).

Note: Obtain the client's permission before performing this stroke.

STRETCH

1. Tensor Fascia Latae

Position
- The client is lying in side posture, with the leg to be stretched positioned on top.
- Standing behind the client, take hold of the ankle of his or her top leg. Abduct the leg, medially rotate the thigh by letting the knee drop somewhat toward the bottom leg, and extend the thigh until a stretch is felt on the front of the hip at the location of the tensor fascia latae (Fig. 9-40).

FIGURE 9-40 Stretch for the tensor fascia latae.

FIGURE 9-41 Stretch for the adductor muscles.

2. Adductors

Position

- The client is lying supine on the table, with both legs extended.
- The therapist stands at the foot of the table. Holding the client's ankle, laterally rotate the leg slightly, and move the leg into abduction, keeping it straight, until the client feels a stretch in the adductor muscles (Fig. 9-41).

■ INTESTINES

Swedish/Cross Fiber

POSITION

- The client is lying supine on the table with a bolster under the knees. Female clients are covered with a separate chest drape.
- The therapist is standing at the side of the table at the level of the client's waist.
1. Perform circular effleurage on the abdomen.
2. Perform cross fiber fingertip raking on the abdominal muscles (Fig. 9-42).

Connective Tissue

Placing the right palm on the abdomen over the navel and the left palm over the right hand, begin an outward spiraling, clockwise motion, stretching the fascia of the abdomen.

Deep Tissue/Neuromuscular Therapy

POSITION

- The client remains supine with a bolster under the knees.
- The therapist is standing at the side of the table on the left side of the client's abdomen.

1. Large Intestine

Strokes
- Reach across the table, and place your fingers lateral to the ascending colon, on the right side of the client's abdomen (Fig. 9-43). Gently draw the fingers inward, against the edge of the large intestine, without gliding over the skin. Continue tracing the border of the colon with your fingers, pulling it away from the outer edge of the abdomen until you reach the midline of the

FIGURE 9-42 Cross fiber fingertip raking on the rectus abdominus.

FIGURE 9-43 Contacting the lateral border of the large intestine.

body. Walk around to the right side of the table, and continue pulling the fingers inward, along the border of the large intestine, until you reach the left ASIS.

- Beginning at the ileocecal valve, do slow, circular fingertip friction over the large intestine, tracing its entire length around the abdominal cavity (Fig. 9-44).
- Repeat the same path as above, doing short, up and down and side to side strokes with your fingers over the large intestine. Spend extra time on impacted areas.

 Pay close attention when applying pressure over the intestines. Never push against resistance. Elicit client feedback often, and move very slowly.

2. Small Intestine

Strokes

- Cupping your palm, curve and spread the fingers. Place your fingertips on the abdomen, over the small intestine. Press down, and circle the fingers, palpating the small intestine (Fig. 9-45).
- Work thoroughly, spending time on impacted areas.

ACCESSORY WORK, INTESTINES

Reflex Points on the Feet

See Figure 9-46 for an illustration of the reflex zone of the large intestine.

David Rini

FIGURE 9-45 Massaging the small intestine.

1. *Ileocecal Valve Point.* This point is located on the heel line on the lateral side of the right foot. Support the heel of the client's right foot with your right hand as you press the ileocecal valve point with your left thumb.
2. *Intestinal Reflex Zone.* To locate this zone, divide the sole of the foot into quarters, excluding the toes. The intestinal zone is located in the third quadrant, just above the heel line. To cover the area thoroughly, begin

FIGURE 9-44 Sequence of deep tissue strokes on the large intestine.

Ileocecal valve

FIGURE 9-46 Reflex zone for the large intestine.

at the ileocecal point on the right foot. Press on the point with the pad of your left thumb. Move the thumb slightly forward, and press on the next point (approximately one-sixteenth of an inch in front of the first point). The thumb hinges slightly from the joint of the first phalanx.

Continue to move with the thumb tip across the foot in a horizontal direction toward the medial side, covering all points. To access the next strip of points, begin again on the lateral edge of the foot, above the first horizontal line. Repeat the sequence until the entire zone is covered. Switch hands, and repeat the entire sequence, with the exception of the ileocecal point, on the left foot.

CLOSING

Sitting at the foot of the table, lightly hold the heels of the client's feet in your hands for 30 to 60 seconds. Remove your hands slowly to complete the session.

■ ANTERIOR THIGH/ILIOPSOAS ROUTINE

Objectives

- To release and lengthen the quadriceps muscles
- To help correct anterior tilt of the pelvis
- To complete the opening and balancing of the pelvic region
- To achieve more efficient movement patterns, originating from the core muscles

Energy

POSITION

The client is lying supine, with the leg to be worked on fully extended. A bolster may be placed under the knee of the other leg, if desired.
The therapist is standing at the side of the table and is facing the client's pelvis.

POLARITY

The palm of the superior hand contacts the ASIS. The palm of the inferior hand rests on the knee. Envision the thigh lengthening and the tissues reorganizing themselves along the vertical axis running along the center of the thigh. Be sensitive to any subtle movements occurring in the thigh, and let your hands softly follow them. Hold for 30 to 60 seconds.

SHIATSU

With the palms or fists, compress the thigh from the hip to the knee. These compression movements stimulate the

stomach and spleen channels, running approximately along the lateral and medial borders of the rectus femoris muscle.

Swedish/Cross Fiber

1. Perform effleurage strokes on the anterior thigh and knee.
2. Perform kneading strokes on the anterior thigh muscles.
3. Perform friction strokes on the anterior thigh and knee.
4. Apply cross fiber strokes to the quadriceps muscles using the broad side of the thumb and/or the heel of the hand.

Connective Tissue

MYOFASCIAL SPREADING

Place the heels of the hand on the midline of the thigh, just above the patella. Slowly draw the hands apart, spreading the tissues. Continue, working in horizontal strips, to the hip.

Deep Tissue/Neuromuscular Therapy

SEQUENCE

1. Patellar ligament
2. Quadriceps (vastus lateralis, rectus femoris, vastus intermedius, and vastus medialis)
3. Abdominal warm-up
4. Iliacus
5. Psoas

1. Patellar Ligament

Strokes
- Place your thumbs on the tibial tuberosity below the patella. Do short, up and down and side to side strokes on the ligament (Fig. 9-47D).

2. Quadriceps (Vastus Lateralis, Rectus Femoris, Vastus Intermedius, and Vastus Medialis)

Vastus Lateralis
Origin: Intertrochanteric line, greater trochanter, gluteal tuberosity, lateral lip of the linea aspera, lateral intermuscular septum.
Insertion: Lateral border of the patella, patellar ligament to the tibial tuberosity.
Action: Extension of leg at the knee joint.

Along the anterior portion, a group of trigger points may be found at midthigh level that refers pain along the length of the muscle. The majority of trigger points form along the lateral aspect of the muscle. They may be spaced just above the knee, in the middle of the thigh, and at the attachment on the upper femur.

Trigger points in the superficial fibers will fire more locally. Trigger points in the deeper layers shoot pain throughout the muscle and down to the side of the knee.

Rectus Femoris

Origin: Anterior head—AIIS. Posterior head—groove of the ilium above the acetabulum.

Insertion: Patella and tibial tuberosity via the patellar ligament.

Action: Extension of the leg at the knee joint, flexion of the thigh at the hip joint.

 The most commonly occurring trigger point in this muscle is found just below its attachment on the AIIS. It refers pain to the knee area.

Vastus Intermedius

Origin: Anterior and lateral surfaces of the upper two-thirds of the shaft of the femur, lower part of the lateral intermuscular septum.

Insertion: Deep aspect of the quadriceps tendon, patella, and tibial tuberosity via the patellar ligament.

Action: Extension of the leg at the knee.

 Trigger points in this muscle are difficult to palpate because of its position deep to the rectus femoris. These trigger points tend to develop in clusters rather than singly. The pain referral zone is most concentrated at midthigh level but may extend down over the knee or to the upper thigh, depending on the location of the trigger point.

Vastus Medialis

Origin: Lower half of the intertrochanteric line, medial lip of the linea aspera, medial intermuscular septum, medial supracondylar line.

Insertion: Medial border of the patella, tibial tuberosity via the patellar ligament.

Action: Extension of the leg at the knee.

The most frequently occurring trigger point is located in the lower, thick fibers on the medial thigh, slightly above the knee. Pain may be exhibited along the medial side of the muscle. A second trigger point may form about halfway up the thigh. Left untreated, these trigger points may cause a weakening in the quadriceps and bouts of buckling of the knee when the person is walking.

Strokes

- Using the forearm or knuckles, perform elongation strokes from the knee to the AIIS. Cover the area thoroughly between the sartorius muscle and the iliotibial tract (**A** in Fig. 9-47).

FIGURE 9-47 Sequence of deep tissue strokes on the quadriceps.

- With the thumbs or elbow, trace the lateral and medial borders of the rectus femoris muscle, from the patella to the AIIS (**B** in Fig. 9-47).
- Using the thumbs or elbow, thoroughly work small sections of the muscles with up and down and side to side strokes (**C** in Fig. 9-47).

3. Abdominal Warm-Up

Position

- The client is lying supine, with a bolster placed under both knees.
- The therapist is standing at the side of the table next to the client's waist.

1. Perform circular effleurage on the abdomen.
2. Wave stroke—Place the heels of both hands against the border of the rectus abdominus muscle on the side of the body you are standing next to, with your fingers curled around the opposite edge of the muscle (Fig. 9-48). Gently push against the abdomen with

FIGURE 9-48 Beginning hand position for the wave stroke.

the heels of the hands, creating a bulge in front of your palms. With your fingers, reach across to the opposite side of the wave, and pull the abdominal tissue back toward you. Repeat several times, creating a fluid, continuous motion.

3. Using the heel of the hand, apply circular friction around the abdomen in a clockwise direction.

4. Iliacus

Origin: Superior two-thirds of the iliac fossa, inner lip of the iliac crest, anterior sacroiliac and iliolumbar ligaments.
Insertion: Lesser trochanter of the femur.
Action: Hip flexion, trunk flexion, hip external rotation (in conjunction with the psoas).

> A trigger point in the iliacus is frequently found in the upper portion of the muscle, slightly superior to the ASIS.

Strokes

• Place your fingers against the inner border of the iliac crest, just above the ASIS (Fig. 9-49). Allow your fingers to melt into the tissues, as if being drawn into quicksand.

• Apply short, side to side strokes with your fingers, sinking further into the muscle. Pause at areas of resistance and/or tenderness.

> **Remain above the ASIS at all times. Avoid putting pressure on the inguinal ligament, which attaches to the ASIS and the pubis.**

5. Psoas Major

Origin: Inferior borders of transverse processes of the L1–L5 vertebrae, bodies and intervertebral disks of the T12–L5 vertebrae.

FIGURE 9-49 Contacting the iliacus on the inner rim of the tubercle of the iliac crest.

Insertion: Lesser trochanter of the femur.
Action: Hip flexion with origin fixed, trunk flexion with insertion fixed (in conjunction with the iliacus), external hip rotation, flexion of the lumbar spine (bilaterally), lateral flexion of the lumbar spine to the same side (unilaterally).

> The psoas major may manifest an active trigger point at the level of L3. The pain pattern for the iliopsoas complex is along the side of the lumbar spine and into the sacral and buttock region. Pain may also be felt in the groin and down the front of the thigh.

When pressed, these trigger points usually refer pain to the back of the body. If the trigger points are on one side only, the pain zone is more vertical, along the lumbar spine. If the trigger points are bilateral, pain may shoot in a horizontal pattern across the low back.

Strokes

• Place the fingers of both hands against the border of the rectus abdominus muscle. Point your fingers slightly inward, toward the spine, and reach under the edge of the rectus abdominus (Fig. 9-50). Allow your fingers to sink into the tissues. Pause at resistance and/or tenderness, and wait for the musculature to soften.

• Perform short, side to side strokes with your fingers, sinking further toward the psoas.

FIGURE 9-50 Contacting the psoas, starting with fingertips along the border of the rectus abdominus.

Note: Check to be sure that you are on the psoas by having the client lift the knee a few inches to contract the muscle. You should be able to feel the muscle contracting under your fingers.

- While maintaining pressure on the psoas, have the client flex the knee and straighten the leg, aiming the foot toward the ceiling, and then lower the straight leg to the table to alternately shorten and lengthen the muscle. Repeat a few times, moving your fingers along the length of the psoas.
- With the client's leg flexed, slide your arm under the client's knee, and lift the leg off the table. The fingers of your other hand remain in contact with the psoas. Adduct the client's thigh to access the lateral portion of the psoas. Abduct the thigh to reach the medial fibers of the muscle next to the spine (Fig. 9-51).

STRETCH

The client slides toward the end of the table so that the hips are against the edge of the table. The client then lies back on the table and holds the flexed knee of the non-stretched leg to his or her chest. The leg to be stretched is hanging off the end of the table, with the knee flexed.

Place one hand over the client's hands that are holding the flexed knee. Assist in pressing the client's thigh toward his or her chest as your other hand holds the thigh on the stretched side slightly above the knee. Press the thigh toward the floor (Fig. 9-52). This stretches the psoas muscle.

To stretch the rectus femoris, the client remains in the same position as above. Kneel down, and hold the ankle of the leg to be stretched. Slowly bring the heel in the direction of the table as the client tucks the hips under. A stretch should be felt in the belly of the rectus femoris muscle.

FIGURE 9-51 Position for releasing the psoas with the client's leg flexed.

DAR

FIGURE 9-52 Stretch for the psoas.

David Rini

FIGURE 9-53 Reflex zone for the pelvis on the heel.

ACCESSORY WORK

1. This session may be balanced with deep tissue work on the erector spinae, quadratus lumborum, gluteals, and hamstrings.
2. The muscles around the temporomandibular joint reflex to the pelvis and psoas. They should also be contacted to balance the upper pole of the body with the pelvis.
3. On the foot, the heel is the reflex area corresponding to the pelvis. Points in the heel region on the sole of the foot may be pressed with the thumb tip. The therapist may then hold the foot around the metatarsal region with one hand while the other hand cups the heel (Fig. 9-53). With the fingers of the hand supporting the heel, the therapist may reach around to the side of the foot to press points below the malleolus. Switching hand positions allows the therapist to work on the other side of the heel.

CLOSING

Sitting at the foot of the table, lightly hold the heels of the client's feet in your hands for 30 to 60 seconds. Remove your hands slowly to complete the session.

REFERENCES

1. Hernandez-Reif M, Martinez A, Field T, Quintino O, Hart S, Burman I. Premenstrual syndrome symptoms are relieved by massage therapy. J Psychosom Obstet Gynaecol 2000; 21: 9–15.
2. Jensen B. Constipation. In: Dr. Jensen's guide to better bowel care: a complete program for tissue cleansing through bowel management. New York, NY: Avery, 1999: 46.
3. Williams DG. The ileocecal valve syndrome. In: Weinberger S. Healing within: the complete colon health guide. Larkspur, CA: Healing Within Products, 1996.
4. Jensen B. Prolapse of the transverse colon. In: Dr. Jensen's guide to better bowel care: a complete program for tissue cleansing through bowel management. New York, NY: Avery, 1999: 78.
5. Heller J, Henkin WA. Bodywise: an introduction to Hellerwork for regaining flexibility and well-being. Berkeley, CA: North Atlantic Books, 2004.
6. Reich W. The function of the orgasm. Volume 1 of the discovery of orgone. New York, NY: Farrar, Straus, and Giroux, 1986.
7. The pelvis. In: Dychtwald K. Bodymind. New York, NY: Jeremy P Tarcher, reissue edition, 1986.

Chapter 10

Balancing the Upper Pole

■ GENERAL CONCEPTS

The neck defines the area around the cervical vertebrae. Although it is often considered to be a separate body unit, the neck is actually the upper portion of the spine. Posturally, it serves the important function of balancing the head over the shoulders. The neck also serves as a transitional segment, creating both space and integration between these two body parts. The adult head usually weighs between 13 and 15 pounds. Strong muscles and ligaments, anchored to the neck and shoulder girdle, are required to support it.

Releasing contracted neck muscles and repositioning the head are important elements of deep tissue release work. The neck serves as a barometer of tension throughout the body. Imbalances in lower portions of the body are reflected in compensating displacements of the head, neck, and shoulders. In this series, neck and head work comes after the abdomen and pelvis sessions, because these two body segments counterbalance each other. If one of these segments is off-center, the other must adjust its position to maintain full-body integrity and balance.

Correct positioning of the head on the neck is crucial to proper alignment throughout the body. When the bones are stacked evenly over each other, weight transfer from the head to the feet occurs efficiently. If the head is properly poised over the atlas, the body carries a feeling of vertical lift. This sensation is the consequence of muscle balance and the body's proper relationship to gravity. The head should not tilt to either side nor forward or backward.

The cranium and spine protect the brain and the spinal cord. Misalignment of these bones can induce pressure and restriction on the nerves that pass through the spinal cord, thus inhibiting the function of the nervous system.

Proper alignment of the head can occur only if the condyles of the atlas, on which the head sits, are on the horizontal plane. The cervical vertebrae will be displaced to the degree that the head deviates from this position, and muscles will be called into action to prevent the head from sliding further off-center. Balance of the head can be checked by noting if the two ears are on the horizontal plane. From a side view, a vertical line should pass from the center of the ear through the center of the shoulder.

The deepest layer of neck muscles, the intervertebral muscles, serve as scaffolding for the vertebrae, and they are responsible for stabilizing and moving the cervical vertebrae. More superficial muscles, notably the sternocleidomastoid (SCM), levator scapulae, and trapezius, serve to connect the head to the shoulder girdle. When the head–neck relationship is off, the more superficial muscles that connect the head to the shoulder girdle tend to take over the job of stabilizing the head and the cervical spine. This situation occurs because the deeper, intrinsic muscles have become more or less frozen in their effort to constantly brace the vertebrae against further misalignment. This imbalance of muscle action results in diminished movement in the neck and a sensation of tension. When the superficial muscles are overworked, they appear ropy, with prominent tendons.

Patterns of chronic muscular contraction diminish the flow of fluids to the neck muscles and into the brain. Muscle tissues that receive inadequate nutrition through the blood and lymph become very dysfunctional. As the tissues atrophy, the neck area shortens further, compressing vertebrae and restricting nerves. Some types of headache are the result of this lack of circulation to the neck and head. Over time, reduction of fluid flow can lead to deposits in the arteries and diminished oxygen to the brain. Some signs of senility may be a result of lack of oxygen to brain cells.[1]

■ MUSCULOSKELETAL ANATOMY AND FUNCTION

The Neck

The cervical spine consists of seven vertebrae. The first two vertebrae (C1 and C2) are uniquely designed to allow support and movement of the head. The other five vertebrae (C3–C7) are similar to those of the thoracic and the lumbar spine, except that their bodies are smaller, with thinner disks between them. This design favors greater mobility in the cervical spine. Lateral bending of the vertebrae, however, is limited by the rectangular shape of the bodies and the short, broad, transverse processes that block further lateral movement after they make contact with each other. (See Essential Anatomy Box 10-1 for a summary of muscles, bones, and landmarks.)

As a group, the posterior neck muscles are responsible for extension when acting bilaterally and for lateral flexion and rotation when acting unilaterally. Muscles acting on the head alternate with those acting on the cervical spine throughout the muscle layers of the posterior neck.

The most superficial muscle, the **trapezius**, extends the head, as does the **splenius capitis** in the intermediate layer. The two other muscles in the intermediate layer, the **splenius cervicis** and the **levator scapula**, extend the cervical spine (Fig. 10-1A). In the first layer of deep muscles, the **longissimus capitis** and the **semispinalis capitis** are capital (head) extensors. The transversospinalis mus-

cles, which link the vertebrae, are cervical extensors. They are the **semispinalis**, **multifidus**, and **rotatores**. The deepest-lying muscles, the **suboccipitals**, extend the head. This alternating of actions throughout the layers provides additional strength and support to neck and head movements.

To varying degrees, all the posterior neck muscles are subject to strain. Trauma to the neck and head occurs easily because of their rather fragile design. Trigger points that develop in these muscles often refer into the head or shoulders and can be a major contributing factor in certain headache pain.

The **sternocleidomastoid** (or **SCM**) is the largest neck flexor. It has two branches, both originating on the mastoid process and inserting separately on the sternum and clavicle (Fig. 10-1B). This muscle serves several functions. When contracted bilaterally, the SCM flexes the neck and draws the head forward and downward toward the chin. Unilateral contraction produces lateral flexion of the head to the same side and rotation of the head to the opposite side. When the neck is in a straight-up or extended position and the head is still, the SCM elevates the sternum and clavicle, assisting inspiration.

The SCM also provides an important stabilizing function. It prevents hyperextension of the neck when the head is turned upward, and it resists strong, backward movement of the head during sudden body shifts, such as a backward fall. It aids the trapezius in maintaining a stable head position when the mandible is moving, as in talking and chewing. Active trigger points in the SCM most commonly are felt in the head rather than in the neck. They can also be responsible for feelings of disequilibrium when standing or moving.

BOX 10-1 ESSENTIAL ANATOMY The Neck Routines

MUSCLES	BONES AND LANDMARKS
Upper trapezius	Cervical vertebrae
Splenius capitis, splenius cervicis, and levator scapula	Occipital ridge
Longissimus capitis and semispinalis capitis	Clavicle
The transversospinal muscles—semispinalis, multifidus, and rotatores	Sternum
The suboccipital muscles	Mastoid process
Platysma	Styloid process
Sternocleidomastoid	Mandible
Scalenes	Digastric fossa
Suprahyoid muscles—digastric, stylohyoid, and mylohyoid	Hyoid
Infrahyoid muscles—omohyoid, sternohyoid, and sternothyroid	Greater horns of hyoid
Prevertebral muscles—longus capitis and longus colli	Lesser horn of hyoid
	Trachea

A

Semispinalis capitis

Splenius capitus

Splenius cervicis

Longissimus capitis

DAR

C

Longus capitis

Middle scalene

Anterior scalene

Posterior scalene

Middle scalene

Posterior scalene

Longus colli

DAR

B

Sternocleidomastoid

Hyoid bone

Trapezius

Omohyoid (lower belly)

DAR

Diagastric (posterior belly)

Stylohyoid

Diagastric (anterior belly)

Suprahyoid muscles

Geniohyoid

Thyrohyoid

Omohyoid (upper belly)

Infrahyoid muscles

Sternohyoid

Sternothyroid

FIGURE 10-1 A. Posterior neck muscles, deep layer. **B.** Hyoid muscles, with sternocleidomastoid and trapezius. **C.** Prevertebral muscles.

The **scalenes** have three divisions: anterior, medial, and posterior (Fig. 10-1C). They all originate on the transverse processes of the cervical vertebrae. The anterior and middle scalenes insert on the first rib. The posterior scalene muscle inserts on the second rib.

When contracting unilaterally, all three scalenes contribute to lateral flexion of the cervical spine, particularly the posterior scalene, because of its almost vertical position along the side of the neck. The anterior and middle scalenes are positioned at a forward oblique angle to the cervical spine. When they contract bilaterally, they increase the curve in the neck. They are opposed in this action by the **longus colli** and **longus capitism,** which straighten the cervical spine. All three scalenes aid in respiration by lifting the first two ribs during forced inspiration.

The space formed between the anterior and middle scalenes is known as the thoracic outlet. The brachial plexus (composed of spinal nerves C5–C8 and T1) and the subclavian artery emerge from this opening, then pass through the space between the clavicle and the first rib. The spinal nerves merge into cords to become the median, radial, and ulnar nerves, which continue down the arm to the hand and fingers.

The hyoid bone is a horseshoe-shaped bone that is located on the front of the neck, between the mandible and the larynx. It does not articulate with any other bone; rather, it is suspended in place by a series of muscles and a ligament. The main purpose of the hyoid is to provide an attachment for muscles that control movements of the tongue. It also assists in cervical flexion.

The muscles that attach above the hyoid are called the suprahyoid muscles (Fig. 10-1B). They are the **digastric, hyoglossus, geniohyoid, mylohyoid,** and **stylohyoid**. The muscles that originate below the hyoid, on the sternum, clavicle, and scapula, are called the infrahyoid muscles, and they are the **sternohyoid, thyrohyoid,** and **omohyoid**. Restrictions in the hyoid muscles can interfere with the mechanics of sound articulation in speech and with the function of swallowing. Trigger points in these muscles have led to chronic sore throats and diminished thyroid activity.

The longus colli and longus capitis are both located on the anterior side of the spinal column, deep to the trachea (Fig. 10-1C). The longus colli extends from the atlas to the body of the third thoracic vertebra. The longus capitis runs from the transverse processes of the C3–C6 vertebrae to the base of the occiput. The longus colli flexes the cervical spine, while the longus capitis flexes and stabilizes the head. Both muscles contribute to side-bending of the cervical spine.

Several structures are located in the anterior neck that need to be taken into consideration when performing massage in this area. The thyroid gland is located on the anterior surface of the trachea, from the level of the C5–T1 vertebrae. It is deep to the sternothyroid and sternohyoid muscles. The vertebral artery passes through the foramen of the transverse processes of the cervical vertebrae. The common carotid artery runs along the anterior border and posterior to the SCM muscle. Its pulse can be palpated by pressing lightly near the tips of the transverse processes of the cervical vertebrae. The internal jugular vein is located lateral to the common carotid artery. The vagus nerve lies posteriorly between the two.

The first cervical vertebra is called the atlas. It rests on the second cervical vertebra, called the axis. A small, peg-like projection on the axis, called the odontoid process (or dens), fits into the inside of the anterior arch of the atlas above it. It is held in place by a transverse ligament. The head and atlas can pivot around the dens, allowing for rotational movements. The atlas is the only vertebra capable of independent movement; all the other vertebrae move as a unit. This limits the range of motion at each joint of the spine, protecting the spinal cord from damage caused by excessive bending in one place.

The Cranium

The cranium consists of eight bones: the frontal, sphenoid, ethmoid, two temporals, two parietals, and the occipital. The head shares a design feature with the pelvis, in that it is not a massive singular structure but, rather, is a series of bones connected together to form a bowl, or basin. The cranium is filled with air spaces, called sinuses, to decrease its weight. The bones of the head are joined by sutures that are saw-toothed in shape and fit together like pieces of a jigsaw puzzle. They are supported by fascial tissues and require little muscular reinforcement. These sutures are pliable, allowing the cranium to shift subtly and absorb trauma that might otherwise injure the brain. (The perspective of moveable cranial joints is advocated by craniosacral practitioners. The classic anatomic view is that these sutures are immobile. For a complete explanation of craniosacral theory, refer to Upledger and Vredevoogd.[2]) Easing tension in the scalp helps to mobilize the sutures and retains their springiness. Reducing pressure between the cranial bones has been known to ease sinus congestion brought about by blockage in the small sinus drainage ducts.

The occipital bone is located at the posteroinferior portion of the skull. The spinal cord passes through a hole in its base, called the foramen magnum, and into the tunnel formed by the cervical vertebrae below. On either side of the foramen magnum are two oval, convex condyles, which fit into two corresponding, concave articular facets on the first cervical vertebra, or atlas. The atlas is ring-shaped; it does not have a central body, as the other vertebrae do. This design allows the spinal cord to pass through it freely.

The rounded surfaces of the articulations form an enarthrosis, which is a ball-and-socket type joint that can perform movements in all three planes.[3] The oval shape of the condyles, however, which are longer than they are wide, favor forward and backward motions, like those of a rocking chair. Because of its weight, the head tends to slide forward on the condyles. Many daily activities, such as reading, writing, and working at a computer, can lead to a forward tilting of the head. The posterior muscles of the neck have to work to prevent the head from sliding further forward in this position, leading to strain and possible trigger point formation. Attaining proper alignment of the head is a primary goal in reducing tension in the neck.

Several muscles play an important role in stabilizing the head on the atlas. These muscles are the multifidus, interspinalis, semispinalis capitis, and semispinalis cervicis. It is essential that these muscles do not become chronically contracted for the head to subtly adjust its position as needed to maintain equilibrium in the body and to prevent restriction of the arteries, veins, and nerves that pass into the head from the neck.

Maintaining the head in a horizontal balance over the atlas is important for many reasons. Chronically holding the head in altered positions affects the flow of blood, lymph, and spinal fluid, and it changes internal pressures. According to craniosacral theory, the cranium and spine form a hydraulic pump, the uninhibited operation of which forms the basic rhythm on which many of the metabolic processes of the body rely.[4] Any alterations in internal pressures affect this pumping system, which can potentially damage functions of the brain and nervous system.

■ CONDITIONS

1. *"Forward Head."* This is a commonly seen postural deviation, in which the head is held forward of proper alignment. It can be easily observed by having the subject stand in profile next to a plumb line. The earlobe will be forward of the plumb. Holding the head forward of the center of gravity proportionally increases its weight. As stated previously, the head normally weighs about 15 pounds. A head that is held 3 inches forward of the vertical line of gravity, however, weighs approximately 30 pounds.[5] In this position, the cervical spine is compressed, setting the stage for disk problems. The thoracic curve is often exaggerated as well.

   This postural deviation can be caused by poor postural habits, like slumping while reading or watching a computer screen. Spinal conditions, such as osteoporosis, kyphosis, and degenerative arthritis, can also cause the head to be projected forward. If the cause is poor postural habits, a simple exercise can help to re-establish proper head position. The person should spend some time each day performing common activities with a small weight, such as a bean bag, balanced on top of the head; proper head positioning becomes mandatory to prevent the object from sliding off the head. Additional weight on top of the head also contributes to the feeling of heaviness when the head is held forward, thus reminding a person to maintain proper vertical alignment.

2. *"Military Neck."* This is the opposite deviation of forward head. In this posture, the cervical curve is diminished or absent, and the back of the neck appears elongated. The chin may be drawn downward, and a noticeable strain can often be seen in the tendons of the SCM muscles. The SCMs assist in capital and cervical flexion and are involved in maintaining this position along with the longus colli and longus capitis.

3. *Torticollis.* This condition is commonly referred to as "stiff neck." It is a twisting or a tilt of the head that is caused by spasms in the neck muscles. Torticollis can be brought about by some disease conditions, trauma to the neck area, or tension. When the cause is neck tension, some precipitating factors are sleeping in an awkward position, allowing the neck to become chilled, watching a sporting event that requires moving the head back and forth, leaning over a desk, and reading. The muscles most often involved are the levator scapula, the trapezius, and the posterior cervical muscles.

4. *Whiplash.* This is a general term referring to injuries to the tissues of the neck caused by rapid, front to back or side to side movements of the head. These movements cause the neck muscles to be hypercontracted and hyperstretched. Damage to the neck can consist of microscopic tears to the muscles and ligaments as well as damage to the other structures of the cervical region. A massage therapist should always be sure that a medical doctor has examined the client before attempting any massage work.

5. *Bulging Disks.* In the cervical region, bulging disks can manifest themselves in a number of ways. Irritated nerves can produce tingling down the arm all the way to the hand. Weakness may be present in the affected arm and hand. To check for disk involvement, have the client perform range-of-motion movements for the neck. If severe pain occurs in one direction of movement but not in the other, it is a good indicator of a disk problem. Clients exhibiting signs of disk problems should be referred to a medical doctor for evaluation.

6. *Ligament Tears.* Damage to neck ligaments can occur from injury or chronic misuse and from poor alignment of the head and neck, causing a weakening of the ligamentous tissue. This injury is characterized by pain, particularly during resisted head movements.

7. *Thoracic Outlet Syndrome.* This syndrome is caused by entrapment of the neurovascular bundle that passes through the space between the anterior and middle

BOX 10-2 INDICATIONS/CONTRAINDICATIONS Conditions Affecting Neck Massage

INDICATIONS	CONTRAINDICATIONS
Stiff neck	Severe trauma
Pain in neck/shoulders	Fever
Pain/numbness in arm	Skin disorders
Whiplash	Recent injury/surgery
Tension in throat	Severe hypertension
Postural deviations	

scalenes and the space between the clavicle and the first rib. Symptoms of nerve compression include pain and paresthesia (tingling) in the neck, shoulder, arm, hand, and fingers. Vascular compression may produce numbness, pain, cold, and fatigue in the shoulder and arm. The syndrome can be diagnosed by electromyographic measurements.

Causes of thoracic outlet syndrome include build-up of the fascial tissue around the scalenes, which decreases the size of the spaces that the nerves and blood vessels pass through. Rounded shoulders accompanied by kyphosis and an increased cervical curve lead to chronic shortness and fascial thickening in the scalenes. Restrictions in the breathing muscles, resulting in shallow upper chest breathing, also strain the scalenes. Treatment includes deep tissue massage to the scalenes, correction of faulty postural and breathing habits, and regular, slow stretching of the scalenes.

Please refer to Indications and Contraindications Box 10-2 for a list of further indications and contraindications affecting neck massage.

■ POSTURAL EVALUATION

Frontal View

1. Does the head appear to be resting on a horizontal base?
2. Are the two sides of the neck of equal length?
3. Does the head tilt or rotate to one side or to the other?
4. Assess the musculature of the neck.

- Are one or both of the SCM muscles prominent?
- Are the tendons of the SCM muscles at the manubrium prominent?
- Are there hollows above the clavicles? (Hollows denote shortness of the scalenes.)

the **mind body** *connection*

The neck serves as a channel linking the head with the rest of the body. Passageways in the neck function in the transfer of food, air, and nerve impulses. The neck is also responsible for balancing the head. The constant activity occurring through the neck makes it an area of transition. For having so many duties, it is a small, weak region, making it vulnerable to overuse and stress conditions.

Integration is a quality that is associated with the neck. It acts as a bridge between the intellect and the heart, or the emotions. In this role, the neck serves as a mediator. We often have a choice whether to process an internal impulse as a thought or as a feeling. The neck helps to determine the route the expression will take—to the thinking center in the head, or to the emotional center in the chest.

Constantly rerouting emotional experiences to the thinking facility diminishes their power and can serve as a form of repression or avoidance. This may be reflected in tension in the neck muscles. The opposite case, in which we indulge emotions rather than seek rational alternatives, can also be problematic. Exercising choice over how and when to express ourselves is a desirable state and helps to maintain an open, healthy condition of the neck and throat.

The neck is a vulnerable area that may lodge much repressed fear. Very likely, someone who has been attacked or raped was grabbed and held at the neck. Having that area, particularly the anterior neck region, touched may elicit feelings of fear, rage, or panic. The therapist should always check with a client before touching the anterior neck to ensure that the client is comfortable with receiving massage in this region.

If a client has experienced neck trauma and decides to proceed with the work, the therapist should move slowly and deliberately, allowing the client time to relax and to verbalize any feelings of discomfort. The client must always feel in control and know that he or she can have the massage stopped at any time, if desired.

TABLE 10–1	Body Reading for the Neck
Conditions	**Muscles That May Be Shortened**
Lateral tilt of the head	Sternocleidomastoid Scalenes Upper trapezius Levator scapula
Military neck	Sternocleidomastoid Longus capitis Longus colli
Forward head	Scalenes Splenius capitis Upper trapezius Semispinalis capitis

Side View

1. Are the centers of the earlobe, shoulder, hip, knee, and ankle aligned in a straight line?
2. Check the tilt of the head.
   - Forward?
   - Backward?
   - Neutral

3. Is there the appearance of vertical lift in the body, a sense of being led upward by the head?
4. Does the body appear to be compressed, with the head pushing down into the neck?

Refer to Table 10-1 for a list of common distortions of the neck and Table 10-2 for range of motion of the neck.

TABLE 10–2	Range of Motion (ROM) for the Neck
Action	**Muscles**
Flexion (ROM 45°)	Longus capitis Longus colli Scalenes Sternocleidomastoid
Extension (ROM 55°)	Splenius cervicis Splenius capitis Upper trapezius Semispinalis capitis Semispinalis cervicis
Lateral flexion (ROM 40°)	Longus colli Scalenes Sternocleidomastoid Splenius capitis Splenius cervicis Upper trapezius
Rotation same side (ROM 70°)	Longus colli Longus capitis Splenius cervicis Splenius capitis
Rotation opposite side (ROM 70°)	Scalenes Sternocleidomastoid Trapezius Semispinalis

■ EXERCISES AND SELF-TREATMENT

1. *Forward Flexion* (stretches the neck extensor muscles—splenius cervicis, splenius capitis, upper trapezius, semispinalis capitis, and semispinalis cervicis). Tilt your head forward, bringing your chin toward the chest. Place your hands on the back of the head, and gently press down until you feel a mild stretch in the back of the neck.
2. *Extension* (stretches the neck flexor muscles—longus capitis, longus colli, scalenes, and SCM). Slowly raise your head to look up toward the ceiling. Reach up from the back of the neck and the front to prevent compression of the cervical vertebrae. Draw your lower teeth up over the upper teeth to further stretch the anterior neck muscles.
3. *Lateral flexion* (stretches scalenes, SCM, splenius capitis, splenius cervicis, and upper trapezius).
   • Looking straight ahead, with your head upright, place your right hand on the left side of your head above the left ear. Slowly move your right ear toward the right shoulder. Press gently against the left side of your head to increase the feeling of stretch. Relax, and imagine breathing into the tight muscles on the left side of your neck.
   • Place your left hand on the right side of your head, above the right ear. Slowly move your left ear toward the left shoulder. Press gently against the right side of your head to increase the stretch. Relax, and imagine breathing into the tight muscles on the right side of your neck.
4. *Relaxation of the Neck and Head.* Lie on your back on the floor, with the knees flexed and both feet on the floor. As you breathe deeply, imagine that your head is a heavy bag filled with sand. Visualize the sand slowly flowing out of the bag from a small hole located just below the external occipital protuberance (EOP), emptying the interior of the head and neck of all stress and tightness. Rest in this position for several minutes.

■ NECK AND HEAD EXTENSORS ROUTINE

Objectives

• To lengthen the posterior neck
• To begin the process of repositioning the head on the cervical spine
• To relieve tightness in neck muscles, which may be contributing to neck or head pain
• To reduce muscular pulls on cervical vertebrae
• To assist the client in acquiring more effective neck and head alignment in everyday activities to help reduce stress factors

Energy

POSITION

• The client is in side posture. A small pad is placed under the side of the head; a bolster is positioned between the knees.
• The therapist is standing behind the table at the client's neck and head region.

POLARITY

The palm of one hand is placed lightly across the occipital ridge. The palm of the other hand contacts the C7 vertebra. Envision the neck lengthening as the cervical vertebrae decompress and the musculature of the neck relaxes. Maintain contact for at least 1 minute.

SHIATSU

Place one hand on the client's shoulder. Wrap your other hand around the posterior neck, just below the occipital ridge, with the thumb on one side of the trapezius and the fingers on the other. Slowly squeeze the neck, and hold for a few seconds (Fig. 10-2). Release, slide your hand to the middle of the neck, and repeat. Then, putting your hand at the base of the neck, squeeze again. This move helps to stimulate the points on the portion of the bladder channel that passes through the posterior neck

Swedish/Cross Fiber

1. Perform effleurage strokes from the acromion to the occipital ridge.

FIGURE 10-2 Shiatsu compression of the posterior neck.

The subject is a 20-year-old woman named Chloe, who is a college student. Chloe is not a regular massage client. She schedules appointments sporadically, usually during high-stress periods in her life. Her reason for seeking deep tissue therapy at this time is that for the past week, she has been experiencing severe pain in her posterior neck. It radiates down her upper back to the level of the T12 vertebra and up to the occiput. She is experiencing pain in the temporal region of her head, which she feels is being generated by the tight muscles in her neck. It is difficult for her to study, because the act of leaning forward at a desk to read causes shooting pains to radiate to the top of her head and throughout the posterior neck and upper back.

Chloe has been involved in several car accidents over the last 5 years. She has never been seriously injured, but she has experienced whiplash to varying degrees as a result of each accident. She has received medical treatment for neck injuries sustained from these accidents and currently visits a chiropractor twice a month.

Although she has a history of neck injuries, Chloe feels that the source of the pain is as much psychological as it is physical. The pain is always much worse during times of high stress. In addition to studying for exams, she is experiencing relationship problems that have her concerned to the point that she is not sleeping well at night. She often wakes in the morning with a stiff, painful neck.

The focus of this session will be deep tissue work on the posterior and anterior neck, the muscles of the upper back (particularly the trapezius), and the cranium. Some work will also be done on the jaw muscles, along with stimulation of spinal reflex points on the feet.

With the client lying in a prone position, the layers of posterior neck muscles were meticulously worked, from superficial to deep. As expected, the muscles were very tender. Trigger points were discovered along the borders of the upper trapezius that radiated pain to the anterior portion of the temporal muscle, where she frequently experiences headache pain. A significant softening of the region was noted following the completion of deep tissue therapy on the neck. The entire upper back was massaged, with careful attention paid to the entire trapezius.

Immediately after the client turned supine, the occipital release procedure was applied. When the therapist initially placed the fingers under her occipital ridge, Chloe reported feeling a throbbing pain near the top of her head. This pain was triggered by pressure to the fibers of the upper portion of splenius capitis, between the borders of the trapezius and SCM. Chloe was willing to stay with the sensation, however, so the therapist continued to apply the occipital release technique. During approximately the first 30 seconds of the procedure, Chloe's head was held suspended, away from the palms of the therapist's hands, because of constrictions in the neck muscles. After about 1 minute of holding, her head began to sink toward the therapist's palms. Within another minute of holding, the back of her head was resting in the therapist's palms, and she was smiling broadly. She reported that the pain at the top of her head was completely gone and that her head felt light and free.

Massage to the cranium and facial muscles was followed by deep tissue therapy to the SCM, scalenes, and prevertebral muscles. All these muscles were tender and elicited much radiated pain, particularly the attachments to the scalenes on the anterior side of the transverse processes of the cervical vertebrae. Swedish and cross fiber strokes were applied to the pectoralis major to balance the work done on the upper and midback. The session was completed with foot massage accompanied by reflexology and polarity.

After the session, the client reported feeling "like a new person." She said it felt as if someone had lifted her head off her shoulders. Because of the extreme tenderness in some of the neck muscles and the high incidence of radiating pain that was uncovered, Chloe decided to schedule another massage for the following week. She was shown neck stretches to perform whenever she began to feel strain in her neck muscles. The benefits of purchasing a portable editor's desk or bookstand to use when studying so that she does not have to flex her neck and head was discussed. She also agreed to consider using a smaller pillow when she sleeps so that her head is not elevated so much, causing her neck to remain flexed all night.

Topics for Discussion

1. Why is examination by a medical doctor crucial before massage therapy is applied to a client who has experienced a neck injury?
2. Describe the head and neck displacements characterized by the "forward head" and "military neck" positions. Which muscles are likely to be shortened in each of these patterns?
3. Name all the muscles that are directly affected by the occipital release procedure.
4. Create a self-care program to aid a client who regularly experiences tension headaches.
5. Why is it advantageous to perform some neck work at the beginning of every massage session?

2. Perform one-handed pétrissage:
   • From the shoulder to the base of the neck
   • From the base of the neck to the occiput
3. Perform fingertip raking across the posterior neck, working in horizontal strips, from the C7 vertebra to the occiput.

Connective Tissue

Reaching across the posterior neck, place the fingers of one hand just posterior to the transverse processes of the cervical spine on the opposite side from where you are standing. Allow your fingers to sink into the tissues. As the tissues melt under your touch, let your fingers glide toward you, to the sides of the spinous processes of the cervical spine (Fig. 10-3).

Deep Tissue/Neuromuscular Therapy

SEQUENCE

1. Superficial layer—upper trapezius
2. Intermediate layer—splenius capitis, splenius cervicis, and levator scapula
3. Deep layer—longissimus capitis and semispinalis capitis
   a. Transversospinal muscles—semispinalis, multifidus, and rotatores
   b. Suboccipital muscles—obliquus capitis superior, obliquus capitis inferior, rectus capitis posterior major, and rectus capitis posterior minor

1. Superficial Layer

Upper Trapezius
Origin: Medial third of the superior nuchal line and EOP, ligamentum nuchae and spinal processes of C1–C5 vertebrae.
Insertion: Lateral third of the clavicle.
Action: Elevation and upward rotation of the scapula, capital extension.

Trigger points in this muscle frequently are responsible for tension headaches that may be felt at the temple, behind the eye, and sometimes, at the mastoid process and down the posterior neck. Trigger points are located in the fibers slightly behind the border of the muscle, near where it attaches on the lateral portion of the clavicle. They are best palpated by squeezing the edge of the muscle between the thumb and fingers.

Strokes
• Wrap your hand around the base of the neck, as in the shiatsu procedure above, with the thumb pad at the border of the trapezius. Using the thumb pad, stroke posteriorly, from the border of the trapezius to the spinous process of the C7 vertebra (Fig. 10-4).
• Sliding your thumb a half-inch superior, repeat the stroke. Continue, working in strips, to the occipital ridge.
• Using the thumbs, apply up and down and side to side strokes to the attachment of the upper trapezius on the superior nuchal line on the occiput.

FIGURE 10-3 Connective tissue release of the posterior neck.

FIGURE 10-4 Deep tissue stroking on the upper trapezius, from C7 to the occiput.

2. Intermediate Layer

Splenius Capitis

Origin: Ligamentum nuchae from the C3–C7 vertebrae, spinous processes of the C7–T4 vertebrae.

Insertion: Mastoid process of the temporal bone, lateral third of the superior nuchal line of the occiput.

Action: Extension of the head, lateral flexion of the head to the same side.

> A trigger point may be found in the upper portion of the muscle, on the occiput, in the space between the trapezius and SCM. It refers pain to the highest point on the head on the same side as the trigger point.

Strokes

- Using your thumb pad, stroke at an oblique angle from the spinous processes of C3 and C4 to the mastoid process. Repeat the stroke, beginning at the C5 vertebra. Continue, working in strips, to T3 (Fig. 10-5).
- Roll your thumb across the fibers of the muscle, and feel for taut bands. Check for trigger points.

Splenius Cervicis

Origin: Spinous processes of the T3–T6 vertebrae.

Insertion: Transverse processes of the C1–C3 vertebrae (varies).

Action: Extension of the cervical spine, rotation of the cervical spine to the same side, flexion of the cervical spine to the same side.

> A commonly experienced trigger point can be palpated near the transverse process of C3. It refers pain to the eye on the same side. In some cases, treatment of this trigger point may relieve blurred vision in that eye.

FIGURE 10-5 Deep tissue strokes on the splenius capitis.

FIGURE 10-6 Working the attachments of the splenius cervicis and levator scapula, from C2-C4.

Strokes

- With your fingertips, find the posterior aspects of the transverse processes of the C2–C4 vertebrae. Perform short, up and down strokes (Fig. 10-6).
- Pause at tender points and hold.

3. Deep Layer

> Three areas of trigger point activity form in the line of the lamina groove:

- The first one is found at the level of C4 and C5. Pain can be referred up to the suboccipital area and also down to the upper vertebral border of the scapula.
- The second area of trigger point activity is located at the level of C2. The pain referral zone is around the occiput and upward toward the top of the head.
- The third location of trigger points is right below the occipital ridge at the attachment point of semispinalis capitis. The pain pattern forms a band around the head, with the most severe sensation felt at the temple and forehead over the eye.

Longissimus Capitis

Origin: Transverse processes of the T1–T5 vertebrae, articular processes of the C4–C7 vertebrae.

Insertion: Posterior margin of the mastoid process of the temporal bone.

Action: Extension of the head, lateral flexion and rotation of the head to the same side.

FIGURE 10-7 Deep tissue strokes on the longissimus capitis and semispinalis capitis, from C7 to the occiput.

Semispinalis Capitis

Origin: Transverse processes of the T1–T7 vertebrae (varies), articular processes of the C4–C6 vertebrae.
Insertion: Occiput between the superior and inferior nuchal lines.
Action: Extension and lateral flexion of the head.

Strokes
- With your thumb, perform combination stroking (up and down and side to side), working in small sections in the space between the spinous processes and the transverse processes of the cervical vertebrae. Begin at the level of the C7 vertebra, and continue to the occiput (Fig. 10-7). Treat trigger points when you find them.
- Work on the attachments of the muscles on the occiput using the combination strokes:
- Longissimus capitis—posterior margin of the mastoid process.
- Semispinalis capitis—the space between the superior and inferior nuchal lines.

Transversospinal Muscles (Semispinalis, Multifidus, and Rotatores)

Origin (Semispinalis cervicis, multifidi, and rotators): Transverse processes of cervical vertebrae.
Insertion: Semispinalis cervicis—spinous processes of the C2–C5 vertebrae. **Multifidi**—spinous processes of two to four vertebrae above the origin. **Rotatores**—base of spinous process of the next highest vertebra.

Strokes
- With your thumb, perform the combination stroke in the lamina groove of the cervical spine, from C7 to the occiput (Fig. 10-8). Working in small sections, pay attention to soft tissue dysfunction at the deepest level, next to the bone. Treat trigger points as you find them.

Suboccipital Muscles (Obliquus Capitis Superior, Obliquus Capitis Inferior, Rectus Capitis Posterior Major, and Rectus Capitis Posterior Minor)

Obliquus Capitis Superior
Origin: Transverse process and superior surface of the atlas.
Insertion: Occiput between the superior and inferior nuchal lines (lateral to semispinalis capitis).
Action: Extension of the head of the atlas, lateral flexion to the same side.

Obliquus Capitis Inferior
Origin: Apex of the spinous process of the atlas.
Insertion: Inferior and dorsal part of the transverse process of the atlas.
Action: Extension of the head, lateral flexion to the same side.

Rectus Capitis Posterior Major
Origin: Spinous process of the axis.
Insertion: Lateral part of the inferior nuchal line of the occiput.
Action: Extension of the head, rotation of the head to the same side, lateral flexion of the head to the same side.

Rectus Capitis Posterior Minor
Origin: Tubercle on posterior arch of atlas.
Insertion: Medial part of inferior nuchal line of occiput.
Action: Extension of head, lateral flexion of head to same side.

Strokes
- Standing at the head of the table, cup your palm over the back of the cranium, hooking your fingers under the occipital ridge. Allow them to sink in as far as the client's tissues will allow without discomfort (Fig. 10-9A). Do slow, up and down and side to side strokes.

FIGURE 10-8 Deep tissue strokes on the transversospinalis muscles.

A   B

FIGURE 10-9 A. Using the fingertips to release the suboccipital muscles. **B.** Deep tissue thumb strokes to release the suboccipital muscles.

- Standing at the side of the table and facing the client's head, place the thumbs on the occipital ridge, next to the EOP. The thumbs should be in a horizontal position, one above the other (Fig. 10-9 B). Roll the thumbs alternately upward along the base of the cranium and slightly below, on the neck, at the level of C1 and C2.

STRETCH

The client sits upright, on the edge of the table. Sitting or standing behind the client, place one palm on the shoulder and the other palm on the same side of the head, above the ear. Laterally flex the head while stabilizing the shoulder (Fig. 10-10). Have the client slowly rotate the head to bring the chin toward the chest. Pause, and maintain the stretch where tightness and/or tenderness are experienced. Be careful not to overstretch the neck in this position. Direct the client to imagine breathing into the muscles being stretched as they relax and lengthen.

ACCESSORY WORK

1. Work on neck and head extensors in conjunction with the neck and head flexors to balance the musculature of the cervical region.
2. Jaw work should accompany the neck session, because imbalance is almost always reflected in both segments simultaneously.
3. Work on the feet synchronizes the upper and lower poles of the body and grounds the client after neck and head massage.

CLOSING

Sitting at the foot of the table, lightly hold the heels of the client's feet in your hands for 30 to 60 seconds. Remove your hands slowly to complete the session.

■ NECK AND HEAD FLEXORS ROUTINE

Objectives

- To elongate the muscles of the anterior neck
- To balance the anterior neck muscles with the posterior neck muscles
- To continue the process of balancing the head on the cervical spine
- To relieve painful conditions caused by shortened flexor muscles
- To reduce uneven pulls on the hyoid bone

Energy

POSITION

- The client is lying supine on the table.
- The therapist is sitting at the head of the table.

POLARITY

The therapist holds the client's head by placing his or her right palm (positive pole) across the client's occipital ridge (negative pole) and the left palm (negative pole) across the forehead (positive pole) (Fig. 10-11). This head

FIGURE 10-10 Stretch for posterior neck muscles.

FIGURE 10-11 Polarity balancing head hold.

FIGURE 10-12 Contacting conception vessel 22 point.

hold is very relaxing. It is sometimes referred to as the "brain drain" because of its effectiveness in easing excessive mental activity. The position is held for at least 1 minute.

SHIATSU

Press the **conception vessel** 22 point, which is located in the notch at the base of the throat, just above the sternum (Fig. 10-12). This point helps to open the throat passage and to relieve sore throat and other inflammatory conditions of the throat and chest.

> ⚠️ **Keep your finger on the superior edge of the manubrium. Do not press into the soft tissues above it, because nerves and blood vessels are close to the surface here.**

Swedish/Cross Fiber

1. Perform effleurage strokes down the sides of the neck.
2. Apply circular fingertip friction along both sides of the neck.
3. Perform thumb sweeping on the side of the neck, stroking each side individually.

Connective Tissue

Holding the client's head in one hand, rotate it slightly to the side. Place the fingers of your other hand along the anterior border of the SCM. Allow your finger pads to sink into the muscle. As the tissues yield, let your fingers

slowly glide in a posterior direction. Repeat along the length of the neck.

Deep Tissue/Neuromuscular Therapy

SEQUENCE

1. Platysma
2. SCM
3. Scalenes
4. Suprahyoid muscles—digastric, stylohyoid, and mylohyoid
5. Infrahyoid muscles—omohyoid, sternohyoid, and sternothyroid
6. Prevertebral muscles—longus capitis and longus colli

1. Platysma

Origin: Fascia covering the upper portion of the chest.
Insertion: Mandible, subcutaneous fascia, and muscles of the chin and jaw.
Action: Depresses lower lip and draws it backward, lifts skin of the chest.

> Ⓧ **Active trigger points in this muscle are usually found where it covers the SCM. These trigger points may be palpated best by sifting the platysma between the thumb and fingers. The trigger points refer to the area of the mandible. The sensation of pain is superficial, as if originating in the skin over the jaw.**

Strokes
• Place the fingers of one hand on the mandible, just below the corner of the mouth. Perform a slow elongation stroke, following the fibers of the muscle, down the neck, over the clavicle, and onto the upper chest (Fig. 10-13).

FIGURE 10-13 Direction of deep tissue stroking on the platysma.

2. Sternocleidomastoid

Origin: Sternal head—sternum, ventral surface of the manubrium. **Clavicular head**—superior and anterior surface of the medial third of the clavicle.

Insertion: Mastoid process of the temporal bone, lateral half of the superior nuchal line of the occiput.

Action: Flexion of the cervical spine (both muscles), lateral flexion of the cervical spine to the same side, rotation of the head to the opposite side, capital extension (posterior fibers); lifts the sternum in forced inhalation.

 Trigger points may be found almost anywhere along the length of the sternal and clavicular branches of the muscle.

Sternal Division

 A trigger point in the lower portion of the muscle refers pain downward, over the upper part of the sternum.

Trigger points in the middle section tend to shoot pain across the cheek area, around the eye orbit, into the eye, and sometimes, into the external part of the ear canal. Trigger points along the medial border of the middle SCM refer pain into the throat and the back of the tongue, creating the sensation of a sore throat. Trigger points in the upper section refer pain to the occipital ridge and the top of the head.

Eye problems, such as blurred vision and an inability to control eye muscles fully, can be an associated autonomic response to trigger points in the sternal division of the SCM.

Clavicular Division

 Trigger points in the middle section refer pain to the forehead.
Dizziness can be an associated autonomic response to trigger points in the clavicular division, particularly after the SCM muscle has been stretched.

Strokes

- Holding the client's head in one hand, rotate the head slightly. Place your thumb pad on the mastoid process. Using the broad side of the thumb, perform an elongation stroke along the fibers of the SCM, ending at the sternum.
- With the thumb or index finger, apply cross fiber strokes to the SCM attachment on the sternum. Glide your thumb along the top edge of the clavicle to the clavicular attachment of the SCM, and apply cross fiber strokes to it.
- Grasp the SCM muscle between your fingers and thumbs, and sift the muscle fibers thoroughly, searching for trigger point activity (Fig. 10-14). Begin near the insertion on the mastoid process, and continue down to the origins on the sternum and clavicle.

FIGURE 10-14 Sifting the sternocleidomastoid.

3. Scalenes

Scalenus Anterior

Origin: Transverse processes of the C3–C6 vertebrae.

Insertion: Scalene tubercle on the inner border of the first rib.

Action: Flexion of cervical spine, elevation of the first rib on inhalation, rotation of the cervical spine to the opposite side, lateral flexion of the cervical spine to the same side.

Scalenus Medius

Origin: Transverse processes of the C2–C7 vertebrae.

Insertion: Superior surface of the first rib.

Action: Flexion of the cervical spine (weak), elevation of the first rib on inhalation, lateral flexion of the cervical spine to the same side, cervical spine rotation to the opposite side.

Scalenus Posterior

Origin: Transverse processes of the C4–C6 vertebrae (variable).

Insertion: Outer surface of the second rib.

Action: Cervical flexion (weak), elevation of the second rib on inhalation, lateral flexion of the cervical spine (assists), cervical spine rotation to the opposite side.

 The order of frequency of trigger point activity in the scalene muscles is from anterior to medial to posterior. Trigger points in the three scalenes may refer pain to the chest, the upper arm and shoulder, and in the back of the body, to the medial border of the scapula. Trigger points in these muscles often form secondarily to trigger points in the SCM, so it is important to check both muscles together.

FIGURE 10-15 Contacting the scalene attachments on the transverse processes of C3–C6.

Strokes

- With your fingers, find the posterior border of the SCM. Moving it slightly anterior and avoiding the jugular vein, gently press your fingers down on the front portion of the transverse processes of the cervical vertebrae (Fig. 10-15). Hold tender points.
- Using the broad side of your thumb, perform an elongation stroke in the triangle formed by the posterior border of the SCM and the anterior border of the upper trapezius (Fig. 10-16). Move, in an inferior direction, to the clavicle (**A** in Fig. 10-16). Then, with your fingers, stroke across the direction of the muscle fibers of the medial scalene, seeking taut bands of tissue (**B** in Fig. 10-16). Pause to treat trigger points.

⚠ Do not apply deep pressure in the posterior triangle area, because the subclavian artery and vein are located here. Light, cross fiber strokes are sufficient to relax the scalene muscles.

- With your index finger, reach under the superior edge of the clavicle, toward the scalene attachments on the first and second ribs (**C** in Fig. 10-16). Apply cross fiber strokes to the attachments. Keep your finger against the inside surface of the clavicle to avoid pressing on nerves.

4. Suprahyoid Muscles (Digastric, Mylohyoid, and Stylohyoid)

Digastric

Origin: Posterior belly—mastoid notch on the temporal bone. **Anterior belly**—inner side of the inferior border of the mandible near the symphysis.

Insertion: Intermediate tendon and to hyoid bone via a fibrous sling.

Action: Mandibular depression, elevation of the hyoid bone during swallowing, anterior belly draws the hyoid forward, posterior belly draws the hyoid backward.

 A trigger point may be found in the digastric muscle near its attachment on the mandible, just under the chin. It refers to the lower front teeth and the alveolar ridge below them.

Strokes

- *Digastric and Mylohyoid Attachments on the Mandible.* Place the pad of your index finger on the underside of the mandible near the center, at the digastric fossa. Slowly stroke across the inside border of the bone, to the angle of the mandible (Fig. 10-17).

FIGURE 10-16 Sequence of deep tissue strokes on the scalenes.

FIGURE 10-17 Working the digastric and mylohyoid attachments on the inside border of the mandible.

FIGURE 10-18 Direction of deep tissue strokes on the bellies of the digastric (**A**) and mylohyoid and stylohyoid (**B**).

- *Belly of Digastric.* Beginning with your index finger at the digastric fossa of the mandible, stroke along the fibers of the muscle on the underside of the chin, to the fibrous loop on the superior border of the hyoid (Fig. 10-18).

Mylohyoid
Origin: Mylohyoid line (from symphysis to molars) on the inside surface of the mandible.
Insertion: Hyoid bone.
Action: Raises the hyoid bone and the tongue for swallowing.

Stylohyoid
Origin: Styloid process of the temporal bone.
Insertion: Hyoid bone.
Action: Hyoid bone drawn upward and backward; assists in opening the mouth; possible participation in mastication and speech.

Strokes
- *Belly of Mylohyoid and Stylohyoid.* Place your fingers at the inferior border of the mandible. Stroke in an inferior direction from the mandible to the hyoid bone (see Fig. 10-18). Repeat the stroke, starting more laterally on the mandible and covering the entire surface area of the muscles. Feel for taut bands, and hold at tender points. This stroke moves across the fibers of the muscles rather than parallel to them.

Note: The mylohyoid muscle forms the floor of the mouth.

⚠ **Be careful to avoid moving off the mylohyoid muscle fibers on the lateral side, because the submandibular gland is located here.**

- *Attachments on the Hyoid Bone.* To locate the hyoid bone, slide the fingers of one hand downward from the infe-

FIGURE 10-19 Palpating the superior border of the hyoid bone.

rior border of the mandible until they touch the superior border of the hyoid bone (Fig. 10-19). To stabilize the hyoid, keep the index finger on the superior border of the bone while placing your thumb on the tip of the greater horn of the hyoid on one side and your middle finger on the tip of the greater horn on the other. To relax the muscles that attach to the hyoid bone, remove your index finger from the superior border. Maintaining the hold on the ends of the bone, slowly shift the hyoid from side to side. To work the suprahyoid muscle attachments, place the index finger of your other hand on the superior border of the hyoid while you continue to hold on to the ends of the bone (Fig. 10-20). Move

FIGURE 10-20 Hand position for contacting muscle attachments on the hyoid bone.

your finger across the edge of the bone, getting client feedback about tenderness. Pay special attention to the fibrous loop on the lesser horn of the hyoid that connects the digastric muscle to the bone.

 The hyoid bone is fragile. Do not squeeze it tightly or apply strong pressure.

5. Infrahyoid Muscles

Strokes
- Still stabilizing the hyoid with one hand, place the index finger of your other hand on the body of the hyoid, and slowly stroke side to side. Hold sensitive points.
- Slide your finger down slightly, and stroke side to side on the inferior border of the hyoid.
- Slide the pad of your index finger onto the inner surface of the clavicle, and stroke side to side on the medial end to contact the attachment of the sternohyoid.

6. Prevertebral Muscles (Longus Capitis and Longus Colli)

Longus Capitis
Origin: Transverse processes of the C3–C6 vertebrae.
Insertion: Inferior basilar part of the occiput (anterior to the foramen magnum).
Action: Capital flexion, rotation of the head to the same side.

Longus Colli
Superior Oblique Part
Origin: Transverse processes of the C3–C5 vertebrae.
Insertion: Tubercle of the anterior arch of the atlas.

Inferior Oblique Part
Origin: Anterior bodies of the T1–T3 vertebrae (variable).
Insertion: Transverse processes of the C5–C6 vertebrae.

Vertical Portion
Origin: Anterior bodies of the C5–C7 and T1–T3 vertebrae.
Insertion: Anterior bodies of the C2–C4 vertebrae.
Action of all three parts: Cervical flexion (weak), cervical rotation to opposite side (inferior oblique), lateral flexion (superior and inferior oblique).

Strokes
- Place the fingers of both hands lengthwise along the borders of the trachea. Slowly and lightly slide the fingers medial, under the trachea, toward the anterior bodies of the cervical vertebrae (Fig. 10-21).

 Do not press on the top of the trachea so that the thyroid gland can be avoided. Move slowly and sensitively in this area, because the vertebral artery runs parallel to the trachea. If you feel a pulse as you slide under the trachea, lift your fingers slightly, and move them more medial to take pressure off the artery.

FIGURE 10-21 Contacting the prevertebral muscles underneath the trachea.

- Slowly move the fingers of one hand at a time up and down and side to side along the prevertebral muscles, feeling for knots and taut bands. Work each side individually. Get client feedback about tenderness. Hold trigger points.

Note: A cough reflex may be encountered at the base of the neck, near the sternal attachment of the SCM.

STRETCH

The client sits upright, on the edge of the table. Sitting or standing behind the client, place one palm on the shoulder and the other palm on the same side of the head, above the ear.

Laterally flex the head while stabilizing the shoulder. Slowly turn the client's head toward extension (Fig. 10-22). Move in small increments, pausing to hold as the various muscle groups just worked on are stretched.

ACCESSORY WORK

1. *Occipital Release.* Sitting at the head of the table, slide your fingers under the client's occipital ridge. Let them sink into the tissues under the base of the cranium. Hold for 1 or 2 minutes.
2. *Reflex Zone.* The reflex zone on the foot that corresponds to the neck is the shaft of the big toe. With your thumb and index finger, hold the sides of the big toe near the base (Fig. 10-23). Glide the fingers up and down in small movements. Repeat on the other foot. Press and hold tender points.

CLOSING

Sitting at the foot of the table, lightly hold the heels of the client's feet in your hands for 30 to 60 seconds. Remove your hands slowly to complete the session.

FIGURE 10-22 Stretch for the anterior neck muscles.

FIGURE 10-23 Contacting the neck reflex zone on the big toe.

The Facial Muscles and Temporomandibular Joint

■ GENERAL CONCEPTS

Probably more than any other part of the body, the head and face tend to define a person's identity. Many people have the image of themselves as a head carrying around the body like baggage. When asked the question, "Where do you feel yourself to reside in your body?" the majority of people will answer, "In my head." One of the greatest benefits of deep tissue bodywork is the reconnection of the head with the rest of the body.

In our society, the values most appreciated are those associated with the head. In the workplace, people are generally judged and valued more for their mental abilities than for their physical prowess. Most occupations rely on mental and sensory acuity for success and advancement. Partly because of these factors, the head and face readily accumulate stress. Headaches related to tension are common and often debilitating. Massage to the scalp and facial muscles has a relaxing, rejuvenating quality that does much to counteract the effects of strain on the face.

The temporomandibular joint (TMJ) of the jaw is one of the most frequently used joints in the body. Its movement accompanies talking and eating, two of the most common functions in which we engage. Therefore, the muscles that control the TMJ need to have strength and quite a bit of stamina. These muscles are subject to stress and dysfunction because of overuse and emotional factors. Tightening the jaw by clenching the teeth is a frequent response to tension and is often done unconsciously, even while a person is asleep. Chronically shortened jaw muscles can generate painful trigger points and misalign the TMJ.

Dysfunction of the TMJ is becoming recognized as a major problem that is often misdiagnosed and untreated. In addition to muscle overuse and fatigue, other causes of TMJ disorder include trauma to the jaw, keeping the mouth open for long periods of time (as during a dental examination), and loss of teeth.

Many symptons of TMJ disorder are possible. Pain may occur around the joint itself, in the jaw muscles, and in or above the ears. Dizziness is also common. Referred pain patterns may be perceived as toothache or neck pain. It may be difficult to open or close the mouth, and a clicking sound may be heard. Dysfunction of the TMJ may affect the position of the facial and cranial bones. They can become compressed, resulting in ringing in the ears, vision disorders, headaches, and/or chronic sinus inflammation.

Often, a correspondence is found between tension areas in the jaw and the pelvis. The two are connected by a polarity relationship, being at both ends of the spinal column. The head and jaw represent the positive pole, and the pelvis acts as the negative pole. There is even a similarity in shape between the mandible and the pelvis. The balance of both poles helps to integrate the entire body.

■ MUSCULOSKELETAL ANATOMY AND FUNCTION

The TMJ is the articulation of the mandible with the temporal bone of the cranium. This joint is unique in the body in that the lower portion hangs from the upper portion, requiring muscular action to keep the jaw shut (Fig. 10-24).

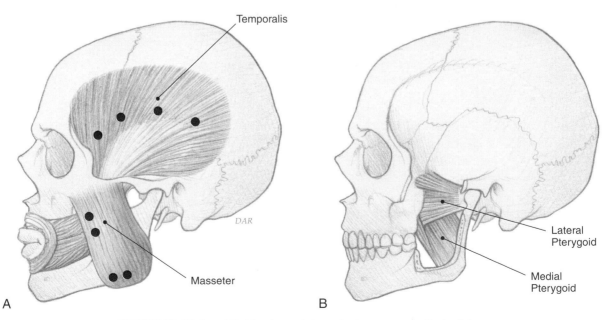

Temporalis

Masseter

DAR

Lateral Pterygoid

Medial Pterygoid

A   B

FIGURE 10-24 A and **B.** Muscles acting on the temporomandibular joint.

BOX 10-3 ESSENTIAL ANATOMY BOX

The Cranium and Facial Routines

MUSCLES
Temporalis
Occipitalis
Galea aponeurotica
Auricularis
Frontalis
Procerus
Orbicularis oculi
Masseter
Buccinator

BONES AND LANDMARKS
Occipital
Temporal
Parietal
Frontal
Orbital ridge
Maxilla
Mandible
Zygomatic arch

The joint consists of the convex-shaped mandibular condyle, the concave articular eminence of the temporal bone, and a disk between these bony surfaces. There actually are two joints, an upper and a lower portion. The articulation of the temporal bone and disk form the upper joint, while the mandible and disk form the lower joint. Complete opening and closing of the mouth is dependent on coordinated action of these two joints. (See Essential Anatomy Box 10-3 for a summary of muscles, bones, and landmarks of the cranium and face and Essential Anatomy Box 10-4 for those of the TMJ.)

The disk is irregularly shaped, being narrower in the center than at the two ends, causing its center to be concave at both the top and bottom surfaces. This allows a greater adaptability of fit against differently shaped bony surfaces. The disk is attached to the medial and lateral sides of the condyle of the mandible, allowing it to rotate around the condyle without sliding off. The anterior end of the disk is attached to both the joint capsule and the **lateral pterygoid** muscle. At the posterior end, the disk is

attached to two bands of fibers, called the bilaminar retrodiskal pad. The other end of the upper band attaches to the tympanic plate. It is composed of elastic fibers that stretch when the disk slides anteriorly and help to pull the disk back into position posteriorly when the jaw closes. The lower band is composed of inelastic fibers attached to the neck of the condyle. The function of this band is to prevent the disk from sliding too far forward.

The mandible is a U-shaped bone that articulates with the temporal bone on both ends. It is capable of depression and elevation (opening and closing the mouth), protrusion and retrusion (jutting the jaw forward and backward), and lateral deviation or sliding from side to side. The mandible can also move asymmetrically around its condyles, a motion that is used in chewing. The TMJ is frequently called into action during chewing, talking, and swallowing.

When the jaw first opens, the mandibular condyle rotates on the inferior surface of the disk, allowing between 11 and 25 mm of opening. To open the mouth further, the

BOX 10-4 ESSENTIAL ANATOMY The TMJ Routine

MUSCLES
Temporalis
Tendon of temporalis
Masseter
Lateral pterygoid
Medial pterygoid
Digastric

BONES AND LANDMARKS
Temporal
Sphenoid
Lateral pterygoid plate
Mandible
Ramus of mandible
Condyle of mandible
Coronoid process

disk and condyle unit glide anteriorly, along the articular eminence of the temporal bone. The normal vertical span of a fully open mouth is between 40 and 50 mm. To close the mouth, these actions occur in reversed order.

The muscles of the jaw, particularly the masseter, are very strong but, at the same time, are able to control small, precise movements. The articular surfaces of the joint are covered with fibrocartilage, which is resistant to damage and capable of quick healing.

Mandibular depression is accomplished primarily by the digastric muscle. The lower portion of the lateral pterygoid also assists in this action. Elevation of the mandible is performed by the **masseter**, **temporalis**, and **medial pterygoid** as well as the upper portion of the lateral pterygoid muscle.

Because of its prominent role in closing the jaw and chewing, the masseter is prone to dysfunction, including trigger point formation. Eating hard, chewy foods, such as gristly meat and bagels, causes the masseter to overwork. Biting down hard on ice or trying to hold things between the teeth can also be aggravating to this muscle. Emotional distress often is reflected in chronic contraction of the masseter, accompanied by gritting the teeth. Shortness in the masseter can be assessed by a person's inability to fully open the mouth vertically.

The temporalis assists the masseter in mandibular elevation. The posterior section of the muscle assists in retraction of the jaw and lateral deviation of the mandible to the same side. Dysfunction in this muscle as a result of trigger points may manifest as hypersensitivity in the muscle and tension headaches caused by referred pain patterns. Sometimes, pain in the upper incisor teeth originates from trigger points in the temporalis muscle.

The lateral pterygoid consists of two segments that work in opposition to each other. The upper portion, which is attached to the anterior end of the disk and to the condyle of the mandible, acts in unison with the temporalis and masseter to elevate the mandible. It also maintains traction on the disk when the jaw closes. When the upper lateral pterygoid becomes chronically short, it pulls the disk forward of the condyle as the jaw closes, causing a clicking sound and making the mouth difficult to close.

The lower portion of the lateral pterygoid acts to open the jaw, to protract the jaw when both sides of the muscle are contracting, and to pull the jaw to the opposite side when contracting unilaterally. Pain felt in the TMJ frequently comes from a shortened lateral pterygoid muscle.

■ CONDITIONS

1. *Bell's Palsy.* This is a partial facial paralysis involving cranial nerve VII, also known as the facial nerve. Symptoms may include a drooping mouth or eye and in some cases severe, one-sided facial distortion. Several factors, including viral diseases, cause the nerve to swell and become impinged. In some cases, onset of Bell's palsy is precipitated by an emotionally upsetting circumstance. Recovery usually takes several months. Massage treatments may help to relieve some of the stress accompanying the condition.

2. *Headaches.* There are many types and causes of headaches. Listed below are some of the more common types:

   a. *Tension.* Tension headaches are caused by chronic contraction or spasm of the muscles of the neck, causing a restriction of blood flow to the cranial region. Massage to the tight muscles will frequently bring relief.

   b. *Allergic.* Allergic headaches are brought on by the body's reaction to foods or environmental factors. They are usually characterized by a dull, aching sensation over the forehead and cheeks. Monosodium glutamate (MSG), caffeine, nitrites, and other additives frequently trigger allergic headaches. Some foods that contain common allergens include wines, cheeses, processed foods, pickled foods, and chocolate. The most effective treatment is to trace the allergy-producing food or foods and remove them from the diet.

   c. *Migraine.* A migraine headache is brought about by dilation of the extracranial blood vessels. It is characterized by sharp and debilitating pain on one side of the head, sometimes behind the eye. It may be accompanied by visual disturbances, such as seeing lights or ropes floating in front of the eyes, and possibly by vomiting. The headache may last from several hours to several days. Migraine headaches have many precipitating factors, including stress, exposure to bright light, and allergic reactions. Treatment consists of reversing blood flow out of the head by applying ice compresses to the forehead and/or occiput and immersing the hands and feet in warm water.

3. *Some Types of Hair Loss.* In some cases, a person loses hair as a result of tightness of the scalp muscles strangling hair follicles, which prevents them from receiving adequate nutrition. Deep tissue massage will increase circulation to the area and may restimulate hair growth.

4. *Sinus Congestion.* This may be relieved through a combination of heat, massage, and acupressure treatment to the appropriate areas of the face.

Please refer to Indications and Contraindications Boxes 10-5 and 10-6 for a list of other indications and contraindications for massage of the cranium, face, and TMJ.

BOX 10-5 INDICATIONS/CONTRAINDICATIONS　Conditions Affecting Cranial and Facial Massage

INDICATIONS	CONTRAINDICATIONS
Sinusitis	Recent trauma
Earache	Broken facial bones
Headache	Cranial fractures
Facial pain	Black eye or bruising
Fatigue	Sunburn
Tension	Recent dental surgery
Eye strain	

BOX 10-6 INDICATIONS/CONTRAINDICATIONS　Conditions Affecting TMJ Massage

INDICATIONS	CONTRAINDICATIONS
Headaches	Abscesses
Pain in teeth	Recent trauma
Facial pain	Broken facial bones
Earaches	Gum surgery
Sore throat	Serious illness
Bruxism (teeth grinding)	Fever

the mind body connection

The face projects our persona, or the part of us that we present to the world. A person's face is often the primary criterion used to assess his or her quality of character. We can frequently deduce a person's emotional state by interpreting his or her facial features.

The face can be thought of as the mask we take off to reveal ourselves or put on to hide what we are thinking or feeling. When the face is open and relaxed, it can reflect our inner state. It has been said that a person's soul can be seen through the eyes. In the same way, we can block or limit what we reveal about ourselves by holding the face frozen or in a fixed expression.

The conflict between the outer facade and the inner sensation is often a source of tension. It can be frightening and confrontational to have the face scrutinized and the muscles relaxed if a person is blocking access to his or her inner feelings through a fixed facial expression. Make-up and glasses are sometimes used as a means to shield the face, in an attempt to hide or protect the person inside.

It is fairly common to encounter people who do not want their faces massaged or even touched. Therefore, to avoid a possible adverse reaction, the therapist should ask permission before massaging a client's face.

The jaw is used in eating and speaking. The jaw and teeth are strong and capable of tearing and grinding. Animals frequently use the jaw and teeth as weapons, and we assert ourselves through the use of the jaw, claiming what we want through speech.

Tightness in the jaw muscles usually accompanies clamping down of the teeth and denotes a withholding of feeling or expression. A person who is contracting the jaw muscles might be blocking the communication of strong emotion. It is a common experience for many of us to "swallow my feelings" or "hold my tongue." This bottling up of expression can become chronic.

Bruxism, or grinding down the teeth by contracting the jaw muscles, is a condition that dentists deal with frequently. The release of tension in the jaw might be accompanied by a desire to speak out loud what one has been holding inside. Sometimes, just making sounds of different varieties can be very liberating. We tend to limit our vocal expression to words. Sounds like grunting, hissing, or screaming can release the more primal parts of our nature and, when expressed in an appropriate setting, can be very therapeutic.

TABLE 10–3	Body Reading for the Face	
Conditions		**Muscles**
Furrowed brow—lines on the forehead and/or between the eyebrows		Frontalis Temporalis Procerus
Constant frown—the corners of the lips are turned down		Platysma Digastric
Facial misalignment—asymmetry of the features and/or bone structure of the face		Treat the tight muscles that seem to be distorting the face Some imbalances may be permanent

■ EVALUATION OF THE FACIAL AREA

1. Observe the overall shape and contours of the head.
2. Check for symmetry in the face.
   - Imagine a vertical line dividing the face into right and left segments.
   - Compare the two sides.
3. Observe the eyes.
   - Are they the same size?
   - Are they on the same horizontal plane?
   - Where are they looking?
4. Make note of any lines of stress on the face.
   - Across the forehead?
   - Between the eyebrows?
   - Outside corners of the eyes and mouth?
5. Observe any muscular tension in the face and neck region.

Refer to Table 10-3 for a description of common tension manifestations in the facial area and the muscles involved.

■ EVALUATION OF THE TMJ

1. Have the client open and close his or her mouth a few times.
   - Observe the motion of the jaw. It should move symmetrically on both sides.
   - The bone at the TMJ junction should not jut out on either side when the mouth opens and closes.
   - Observe the alignment of the upper and lower teeth. The teeth should not shift laterally as the mouth opens and closes.
2. Place your fingers on both sides of the client's jaw, at the TMJ. Have the client slowly open and close the mouth a few times.
   - Feel for a smooth, gliding motion on both sides. Note any deviations.
   - Listen for any clicking or popping sounds.

Note: A number of injuries can displace the TMJ. These include blows to the jaw and whiplash injuries that cause the cervical spine and jaw to hyperextend. Biting down on hard food and overindulgence in chewing gum may also be culprits.

■ EXERCISES AND SELF-TREATMENT

1. *Eye Exercises.*
   - Slowly look straight up, toward the eyebrows, then down, toward the cheeks. Perform the movement three times. Close the eyelids, and rest for a few moments.
   - Slowly look across a horizontal path to the right corners of the eyes. Look across a horizontal path to the left corners of the eyes. Perform the movement three times. Close the eyelids, and rest for a few moments.
   - Look around the eye sockets in a clockwise direction, making a full circle. Begin by looking up, toward the eyebrows, and then continue around the eye orbit to the left. Perform the movement three times. Rest for a few moments, then trace three slow circles in a counterclockwise direction.
   - Lie down on your back. Rub both palms together vigorously to generate heat, then rest the palms over your closed eyes. Allow the warmth and energy to penetrate into the eyes and cheeks, and feel the entire area around the eyes relaxing. Rest, with the eyes closed, for several minutes.
2. *Facial Tension Release.* This exercise may be performed either sitting or lying down. As you inhale, expand the face by slowly making a look of surprise. Open the eyes very wide and the mouth as far as you can, and flare the nostrils. Hold for a few moments. Exhaling, pull all the features of the face toward the center by closing the eyes tight, draw the cheeks in, and pucker the mouth. Squeeze and hold for a few moments. Repeat both facial expressions two more times and then rest, allowing all the tension to flow out of the facial muscles.
3. *Jaw and Tongue Tension Release.*
   - Place the pads of both thumbs on the underside of your chin. Slowly begin to yawn as you press against

The subject is a 29-year-old woman named Rachel, who works as a part-time secretary. Her experience with massage therapy is limited. She has received several relaxation-style massages as gifts. She moved to the Southeast from the West Coast about 8 months ago, and since moving, she has been experiencing sinus headaches on a weekly basis, which she attributes to allergic reactions to the vegetation. She is also experiencing severe jaw pain and some restriction when opening her mouth wide. The jaw pain seems to be worse when she wakes in the morning. Rachel's dentist has informed her that she is clenching and grinding her teeth at night. She is going to be fitted with a night guard this week. The dentist also recommended that she receive massage therapy for the cranial and jaw muscles to reduce tension in those areas.

Rachel was asked if she had a history of TMJ dysfunction. She said that she did not, that her problems began after her move. She has never been struck in the face, and she has never suffered whiplash. About 5 years ago, however, as she was biting into an apple, her jaw momentarily stuck in an open position. It scared her quite a bit, but the mandible immediately slipped back into place. The incident has not recurred.

To evaluate movement of the jaw, Rachel was asked to slowly open and close her mouth as the therapist lightly held his fingers on her right and left TMJs. When her mouth reached about a 0.75-inch opening, the mandible slipped to the left, and a clicking sound was heard. When the mouth reached an opening of 1.25 inches, the client began to experience pain in the jaw muscles.

The session focused on the TMJ and related muscles. The neck massage was performed first, followed by the cranial massage. The temporalis muscles were sore, but the client said that pressure on the muscles felt good. Therefore, the therapist held points on both sides simultaneously for several seconds. After the entire cranial area was relaxed, the facial muscles were addressed. Focused attention was paid to the tendon of the temporalis muscle above the zygomatic bone. It was quite tender. The masseter muscles were bulky and unyielding to pressure. Circular friction strokes helped to relax the muscles. Numerous trigger points were found in the masseters.

The lateral pterygoids were the final muscles in the facial area to be massaged. Because the mandible pulled to the left, the right lateral pterygoid most likely was the more contracted. The therapist explained the intraoral procedures to the client and put on a latex glove. The left lateral pterygoid was massaged first, both to accustom the client to the protocol and to induce relaxation in the less-involved muscle before the more problematic right side was contacted. Even though both lateral pterygoid muscles had much tenderness, the client handled the procedure very well.

The procedure was done slowly to allow the client to breathe and relax throughout. The therapist removed his finger from inside the client's mouth several times during the procedure to allow her to relax and assimilate the release as well as to report her feelings toward the work. She said that, amazingly, when the therapist touched the lateral pterygoids, it triggered the pain in her sinus cavities that she had been attributing to allergies. Her eyes watered a little during the work, so she was given a tissue to wipe away the tears. She said the tears were not from pain or emotions but more of a reflexive reaction.

After the completion of the session, Rachel observed her face in a mirror. She noted that she looked like she had shed about 5 years of age in her face. She felt completely relaxed and elated at gaining some insight regarding her sinus pain as well as feeling pain relief in her jaw muscles. When her jaw movement was evaluated after the session, the click was minimal, and the mandible barely shifted. It was agreed that she should receive more TMJ work, along with deep tissue therapy to other areas of her body.

Rachel had a realization that much of her TMJ problem was a stress reaction to her moving to a new part of the country and starting her life over again. She also realized that she had been holding back from saying some important things to certain people in her life, and that the suppression of those feelings was contributing to her jaw pain. She greatly appreciated the support she was receiving through massage therapy and from her dentist. As part of a home care plan, she was taught deep abdominal breathing to incorporate as a stress reduction technique to help minimize nighttime teeth clenching.

Topics for Discussion

1. What are some common indications that a person may have a TMJ problem?
2. What suggestions to minimize aggravating TMJ discomfort could you offer to a client?
3. Explain to a client why his or her jaw clicks when opening or closing the mouth.
4. List several kinds of activities that may contribute to TMJ misalignment and pain.
5. Practice putting an apprehensive client at ease by fully explaining the purpose and methodology of intraoral procedures.

the underside of the chin with the thumbs, creating resistance to the opening of the mouth. Repeat a couple of times, and then rest the jaw muscles.

- With the mouth closed, circle your tongue in a clockwise direction over the upper and lower teeth. Repeat nine more times. Reverse the direction of the tongue circling, and complete 10 repetitions counterclockwise.

■ HEAD/FACE/JAW ROUTINE

Objectives

- To release tightness in the cranial muscles, which can be a major stress reliever
- To help alleviate aggravating factors in headaches and facial pain
- To reduce tension in muscles affecting the jaw and TMJ
- To reduce muscular stresses in the facial muscles

Energy

POSITION

- The client is lying supine on the table. A bolster may be placed under the knees for comfort.
- The therapist is sitting at the head of the table.

POLARITY

Place your right palm (positive pole) under the client's occipital ridge (negative pole) and your left palm (negative pole) across the client's forehead (positive pole). Imagine your hands drawing all the tension out of the head. Breathe deeply and relax fully as you maintain the contact. Hold for 1 to 2 minutes.

SHIATSU

Place your fingers on the sides of the client's head, above the ears. With your fingers curved and separated, press in against the cranium. Move your fingers to several different places on the sides of the head, and repeat. This move stimulates points on the gallbladder and triple heater channels.

Swedish/Cross Fiber

1. Perform circular friction with the fingertips on the scalp. Start from the back of the head, and work forward to the forehead.
2. Perform effleurage strokes with the fingertips across the forehead, cheeks, and chin.

3. Perform circular friction with the fingertips under the cheekbones and down the sides of the jaw.

Deep Tissue/Neuromuscular Therapy

SEQUENCE

1. Cranium—temporalis, occipitalis, and galea aponeurotica
2. Facial muscles—frontalis, procerus, and orbicularis oculi
3. Jaw—tendon of temporalis, masseter, and lateral pterygoid

1. Cranium

Temporalis
Origin: Temporal fossa, temporal fascia.
Insertion: Coronoid process and anterior border of the ramus of the mandible.
Action: Elevates the mandible, clenches the teeth; posterior fibers retract the mandible; assists in lateral grinding motion.

Several trigger points may form in this muscle. They usually occur in an arc around the section where the muscle fibers join the tendon. These trigger points often account for headache pain in the temple region and for pain around the eyes into the upper teeth.

The first trigger point, which is in the lower anterior portion of the muscle, refers pain along the supraorbital ridge and inferiorly into the upper front teeth. The second and third trigger point regions, which are in the middle lower portion of the muscle, send pain to the temple and into the maxillary teeth. The fourth section of trigger point formation, which is in the posterior aspect of the muscle, has a referral zone located behind and above the trigger point.

Strokes
- Place your fingertips or thumb on the side of the client's head, slightly above the ear (Fig. 10-25). To stabilize the head, put the palm of your other hand against the temporalis muscle on the other side.
- Move up and down and side to side, working on small sections of the muscle, and feel for stringy fibers and points of tenderness. Cover the entire muscle, and treat trigger points as you find them. Repeat on the other side.

Occipitalis
Origin: Lateral two-thirds of the superior nuchal line on the occipital bone, mastoid process on the temporal bone.
Insertion: Galea aponeurotica.

FIGURE 10-25 Hand position for releasing the temporalis.

Action: Draws back the scalp, helps the frontalis to raise the eyebrows and wrinkle the forehead.

> **Trigger points in this muscle are common culprits in the formation of headaches that shoot pain over the top of the head and into the eye.**

Strokes
- From the EOP, slide your fingers laterally, along the superior nuchal line to the mastoid process part of the temporal bone.
- Move your fingers up and down and side to side, working on small sections of the muscle (Fig. 10-26). Feel for taut bands and points of tenderness, and treat trigger points as you find them. Both sides may be worked simultaneously, or each side may be worked separately.

FIGURE 10-26 Palpating the occipitalis above the superior nuchal line.

Galea Aponeurotica (Tendinous Sheet Connecting the Occipitalis and Frontalis)
Strokes
- Positioning the fingers of both hands above the occipitalis muscles, move the scalp up and down, working in small sections and sliding it over the cranium. Pay attention to sections of tissue that are immobile. Hold tender points until they become less sensitive.
- Continue, moving up over the top of the head to the frontalis. Be thorough, and cover the galea aponeurotica completely.

2. Facial Muscles

Frontalis
Origin: Fascia of the facial muscles above the nose and eyes and the skin.
Insertion: Galea aponeurotica.
Action: Along with the occipitalis, draws the scalp back, raises the eyebrows, and wrinkles the forehead; working alone, raises the eyebrow on the same side.

> **A trigger point may be found about halfway between the eyebrow and the hairline, toward the midline of the forehead. It refers pain over the forehead on the same side that the trigger point is located.**

Strokes
- Place the fingers of both hands on the front portion of the scalp, above the hairline. Move the fingers up and down and side to side, working in small sections, over the fibers of the muscle (Fig. 10-27). Feel for taut, stringy fibers and for painful, stuck areas.
- Continue the stroke in an inferior direction, covering the entire forehead to the eyebrows.

Procerus
Origin: Nasal bone and nasal cartilage.
Insertion: Skin of the forehead between the eyebrows.
Action: Wrinkles the skin between the eyebrows, draws the medial part of the eyebrows downward.

DAR

FIGURE 10-27 Releasing the frontalis muscle.

Strokes
- Place your thumbs horizontally and parallel to each other on the bridge of the nose, in the space between the eyebrows (Fig. 10-28).
- Alternately roll the thumbs over each other, in the direction of the forehead, in a small, continuous motion

but without moving them off the space between the eyebrows.

Orbicularis Oculi
Origin: Nasal part of the frontal bone, frontal process in front of the lacrimal groove of the maxilla.
Insertion: All around the orbit of the eye, blends with the occipitofrontalis and corrugator, skin of the eyelid.
Action: Closes the eyelids gently or forcibly, draws the eyelids and lacrimal canals medially.

 Trigger points along the upper ridge of the eye socket may refer pain to the nose.

Strokes
- Place the pads of your index fingers against the medial side of the upper portion of the eye sockets (supraorbital ridge). Both sides may be worked simultaneously.
- Slowly trace the border of the bone with your finger to the lateral side of the upper part of the eye socket, pausing at areas of tenderness (Fig. 10-29). Repeat several times.

3. Jaw (Tendon of Temporalis, Masseter, and Lateral Pterygoid)

Tendon of Temporalis
Strokes
- Place your fingers or thumb slightly above the lateral portion of the superior border of the zygomatic process of the temporal bone.
- Pressing your fingers against the tendon, slowly move side to side, and feel for taut bands and tender points. Having the client open the mouth stretches the tendinous fibers, making them easier to palpate.

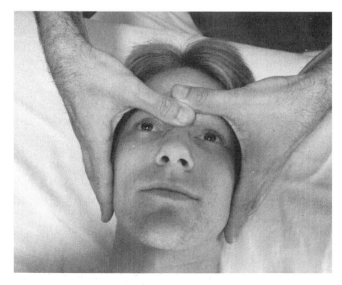

FIGURE 10-28 Deep tissue stroke on the procerus.

FIGURE 10-29 Pressing against the supraorbital ridge to release the orbicularis oculi muscles.

- With the client's mouth open, place your index finger in the space between the zygomatic bone and the coronoid process. Stroke side to side across the tendon.
- Stroke side to side on the top edge of the coronoid process. Pause and hold on points of tenderness (Fig. 10-30).

Procedures and Precautions for Performing Intraoral Techniques

1. Check local ordinances to ascertain whether performing intraoral procedures is legal where you practice massage therapy.
2. Obtain the client's permission before attempting this work. Although every precaution is taken to maintain the client's comfort and prevent pain, the act of contacting interior jaw muscles can be intense and may generate an emotional response. The client should be informed of this possibility before he or she gives consent to receive the work.
3. Always describe the procedure to your client beforehand. Explain how releasing the masseter and, especially, the lateral pterygoid muscles can alleviate many of the symptoms of TMJ syndrome and relax the jaw area in general. To ease any feelings of apprehension, explain where your fingers will be placed inside of the mouth and which muscles will be addressed. Showing clients an illustration of the jaw muscles may be helpful in furthering their understanding of the procedure.
4. Do the necessary preparatory work before performing intraoral techniques. These procedures are the final ones described in this book. All the sessions learned beforehand have led to this culmination point. It is not necessary to have completed all the deep tissue sessions on a client to perform these procedures, but the client's body should be in a fairly relaxed and healthy state before attempting this work. Intraoral massage procedures are always preceded by massage of the neck, cranial, and facial muscles.

David Rini

FIGURE 10-30 Contacting the insertion of the temporalis on the superior edge of the coronoid process.

5. The therapist always wears a latex glove or finger cot when performing intraoral techniques. These items may be purchased at massage or medical supply stores. Rinse away any powder on the latex surface with water before putting your finger in the client's mouth. The latex should always be moistened before placing your finger against the tissues inside the mouth. This can be accomplished by dabbing your finger on the client's tongue to coat the working surface of the glove with a layer of saliva. Dry latex can stick to the delicate tissues inside the mouth and cause minor abrasions.
6. Communication with the client is extremely important throughout the procedure; however, it may be difficult for the client to speak with your finger in his or her mouth. A system of finger signals may be incorporated to allow the client to communicate his or her reactions to the work. For instance, explain to the client that raising the thumb means more pressure can be applied. Forming a circle with the thumb and index finger means the pressure is adequate and comfortable. Turning the thumb down means the pressure is too intense and needs to be reduced. Raising the entire hand signals that the client needs to have the work halted immediately and the therapist's finger removed from the mouth. The therapist should remind the client of the meaning of each signal while performing the procedure so that the client does not forget or become confused.
7. The approach to treating the internal jaw muscles is very gentle. The tissues are contacted only to the point of mild resistance and then held without applying any further pressure until a softening of the muscles is sensed. Proceed slowly, maintaining your full attention on where your finger is placed, the response of the tissues, and the client's reaction to what is occurring.

Masseter

Origin: Superficial part—zygomatic process of the maxilla, maxillary process, and inferior border of the arch of the zygomatic bone. **Intermediate part**—inner surface of the anterior two-thirds of the zygomatic arch. **Deep part**—posterior one-third of the zygomatic arch.

Insertion: Superficial part—angle and lower half of the lateral surface of the ramus of the mandible. **Intermediate part**—central part of the ramus of the mandible. **Deep part**—superior half of the ramus and coronoid process of the mandible.

Action: Elevates the mandible.

 Trigger points in the superficial and deeper layers of this muscle have different referral zones. These layers are best distinguished using the sifting technique.

Trigger points in the superficial layer send pain to the lower jaw, maxilla, molars, and gums. Trigger points along the anterior border, in the upper portion, refer to

the maxilla, upper molars, and the gums around them. Pain coming from these trigger points often is misinterpreted by the client as inflammation of the sinus cavities.

Trigger points along the base of the mandible send pain in an arc across the temple and eyebrow.

The deeper layer trigger points can send pain into the cheek, around the lateral pterygoid, and sometimes, into the ear, which is perceived as a ringing sensation.

Strokes

- Place your fingers or thumbs on the anterior fibers of the muscle at the inferior border of the zygomatic arch (Fig. 10-31). Do an elongation stroke downward, to the base of the mandible. Press both sides simultaneously.

⚠️ **Avoid pressing on the most posterior fibers of the muscle, because the parotid gland covers them.**

- Have the client open the mouth to stretch the masseter. Place your thumbs or index fingers on the anterior borders of the masseter, at the origin. Press in and up, toward the zygomatic bone, and hold for a minimum of 10 seconds. This is an excellent tension release point. Continue to stroke along the border, inferiorly, to the base of the mandible.

Note: The remaining strokes are performed inside the client's mouth and require the therapist to wear a latex glove or finger cot.

- Sift the muscle by squeezing the fibers between your thumb and index finger, one of which is placed on the cheek and the other inside the mouth (Fig. 10-32). As you roll the fibers, check for trigger points.

Lateral Pterygoid

Origin: **Superior head**—lateral surface of the greater wing of the sphenoid. **Inferior head**—lateral surface of the lateral pterygoid plate of the mandible.

Insertion: Condylar neck of the mandible, anterior margin of the articular capsule and disk of the TMJ.

Action: Aids opening the mouth by protracting the mandibular condyle and disk of the TMJ joint forward while the mandibular head rotates on the disk; protracts the jaw, bringing the lower teeth forward of the upper teeth; acting on the same side with the medial pterygoid, causes the mandible and jaw to rotate to the opposite side (chewing motion).

Trigger points in this muscle are a major source of TMJ pain. They can also refer to the maxillary sinus.

David Rini

FIGURE 10-31 Palpating the anterior border of the masseter muscle.

FIGURE 10-32 Sifting the fibers of the masseter.

Strokes

- Have the client open the mouth slightly. Slide the pad of your index finger along the upper gum, fitting it into the pocket formed between the inside surface of the mandible and the lateral pterygoid plate on the sphenoid bone, behind the back upper molars.
- Press inward and upward, along the roof of the cheek and aiming the finger toward the condylar neck of the mandible, where the lateral pterygoid inserts (Fig. 10-33).

Move slowly, because extremely painful trigger points may be encountered.

STRETCH

The client places both thumbs under the center of the chin. The client then yawns, pressing up against the base of the chin to apply resistance to the downward movement of the mandible (Fig. 10-34). This stretch helps to relieve tension in the muscles of the jaw.

ACCESSORY WORK

1. Posterior and anterior neck work should accompany any work done on the jaw.
2. The pelvis is a reflex zone for the jaw. Simultaneously contacting tender points in both areas often brings relief of pain and balance to the body.
3. Working on the feet completes a session focusing on the cranium.

CLOSING

Sitting at the foot of the table, lightly hold the heels of the client's feet in your hands for 30 to 60 seconds. Remove your hands slowly to complete the session.

FIGURE 10-33 Palpating the lateral pterygoid.

FIGURE 10-34 Tension release exercise for the temporomandibular joint muscles.

REFERENCES

1. Rolf IP. Rolfing: re-establishing the natural alignment and structural integrity of the human body for health and well-being. Rochester, VT: Healing Arts Press, 1989: 238.

2. Upledger J, Vredevoogd J. Craniosacral theory. Seattle, WA: Eastland Press, 1983.

3. Kapandji IA. The physiology of the joints. 2nd edition. New York, NY: Churchill Livingstone, 1974; 3: 180.

4. Upledger JD. Your inner physician and you: craniosacral therapy and somatoemotional release. 2nd edition. Berkeley, CA: North Atlantic Books, 1997.

5. Cailliet R. Soft tissue pain and disability. 3rd edition. Philadelphia, PA: FA Davis, 1996: 154.

APPENDIX

American Massage Therapy Association Code of Ethics[1]

This Code of Ethics is a summary statement of the standards by which massage therapists agree to conduct their practices and is a declaration of the general principles of acceptable, ethical, professional behavior.

Massage therapists shall:

1. Demonstrate commitment to provide the highest quality massage therapy/bodywork to those who seek their professional service.
2. Acknowledge the inherent worth and individuality of each person by not discriminating or behaving in any prejudicial manner with clients and/or colleagues.
3. Demonstrate professional excellence through regular self-assessment of strengths, limitations, and effectiveness by continued education and training.
4. Acknowledge the confidential nature of the professional relationship with clients and respect each client's right to privacy.
5. Conduct all business and professional activities within their scope of practice, the law of the land, and project a professional image.
6. Refrain from engaging in any sexual conduct or sexual activities involving their clients.
7. Accept responsibility to do no harm to the physical, mental, and emotional well-being of self, clients, and associates.

---

[1] Reprinted with permission. Copyright © 2005, American Massage Therapy Association, 500 Davis St., Evanston, IL 60201. All rights reserved. For information joining AMTA, call 847-864-0123.

Glossary

acetylcholine—a common neurotransmitter that, when it attaches to a cell membrane, makes it highly permeable to sodium.

ATP—adenosine triphosphate. A compound that stores and releases energy in cells.

brachial plexus—the network of nerves that supply the arm, forearm, and hand. It is made up of lower cervical and upper dorsal spinal nerves.

cervicis—neck.

chakra—a Sanskrit word meaning "wheel." The chakras are seven subtle energy centers located along the spine that correspond in location to the major endocrine glands. They are responsible for governing functions on the physical, mental, and emotional levels.

collagen—a protein fiber found in connective tissue, cartilage, and bone.

conception vessel—one of the two central meridians, along with the governing vessel. It runs up the front of the body, from the perineum to the brain. It regulates all the yin channels in the body.

core—the central region of the body, encompassing the abdomen and pelvis.

dorsiflexion—movement of the foot upward, toward the knee.

effleurage—a variety of massage strokes used in Swedish massage, incorporating a gliding motion and following the contours of the body, utilizing the hands, knuckles, or forearms.

elastin—a mucoprotein fiber that is elastic in nature. It is found in pliable structures of the body, including connective tissue, ligaments, and tendons.

enarthrosis—a ball and socket joint.

endorphin—an opiate polypeptide produced in the brain that binds to opiate receptor sites, thus raising the threshold for pain perception.

enkephalin—an opiate polypeptide produced in the brain that binds to opiate receptor sites and acts as a pain analgesic.

eversion—a turning of the foot away from the midline of the body.

external occipital protuberance (EOP)—a prominence at the center of the outer surface of the squama of the occipital bone that gives attachment to the ligamentum nuchae.

facilitated nerve pathways—routes developed within the neural structures from areas of hyperirritation to other segments of the musculoskeletal system.

fibrils—minute fibers located in the sarcoplasm of muscle fibers.

fingertip raking—a cross fiber stroke executed with the finger pads of one hand. The fingers stroke back and forth, perpendicular to the direction the muscle fibers are running, while remaining in contact with the skin.

Golgi tendon organ—a nerve receptor located in muscle tendons that senses tension, or stretching.

hara—a Japanese word that refers to the core of the body, the abdominal-pelvic cavity, where the life force is concentrated.

inversion—a turning of the foot toward the midline of the body.

lumborum—referring to the region of the back between the 12th ribs and the iliac crests of the pelvis.

meridians—also known as channels. Meridians are energetic pathways often associated with the organs. Meridians distribute qi throughout the body.

mucopolysaccharide—polysaccharides that chemically bond with water. They are thick, gelatinous substances that form intercellular ground substance. They are also found in synovial fluids and mucous secretions.

muscle spindles—also called intrafusal fibers. Spindles are a specialized type of muscle fiber arranged in bundles within the larger muscle fibers. They register changes in the length of muscle fibers.

muscle splinting—increased tonus in muscle tissue surrounding injury to provide protection by limiting movement.

pétrissage—a variety of massage strokes used in Swedish massage that incorporate squeezing, kneading motions of skin and muscle to relax muscle tissue and increase the flow of blood and lymph.

phasic—a term applied to the muscles primarily responsible for movement of the body through space.

plantar flexion—turning the toes under, resulting in pointing the foot.

pronation—a rotational movement. A pronated foot is rotated so that the plantar surface faces in a lateral, or outward, direction. In standing, the medial arch is collapsed, placing more weight on the medial side of the foot.

qi—a Chinese word referring to the vital life force.

qi gong—exercises designed to cultivate or enhance the level of qi in the body.

referred pain zone—a site within the myofascial tissues that registers pain, numbness, weakness, or paresthesia from a stimulus originating in another area.

reflex arcs—nerve feedback loops operating through the spinal cord that link the sensory and motor systems. They monitor and direct muscle actions, mostly at an unconscious level.

sarcomere—the contractile unit of skeletal muscle.

shingles—a Swedish massage stroke. It is a variety of effleurage that utilizes an overlapping movement of the hands, in which one hand continuously replaces the other.

soft fist—a hand position used in shiatsu. It is a modification of a fist, with the distal phalanges of the fingers held in an extended position instead of tucked in against the palm.

sternocleidomastoid (SCM)—the largest neck flexor.

stress-tension-pain cycle—A self-perpetuating, dysfunctional cycle in which increased demand on the body/mind system causes a condition of stress, heightening the activity of the sympathetic nervous system. This leads to increased muscular tension, which diminishes the ability of the muscles to eliminate waste materials from the cells, resulting in stimulation of nociceptive nerve receptors and increased pain perception.

temporomandibular joint (TMJ)—articulation of the mandible with the temporal bone of the cranium.

thoracis—the chest region.

thumb sweep—a cross fiber stroke done with the broad side of the thumb. The thumb rolls back and forth across the muscle to release adherent fibers and spread the fascia.

tiger's mouth—a hand position incorporated in shiatsu in which pressure is exerted on a limb with one or both hands, using the webbing between the thumb and index finger.

tonic—a term referring to muscles with the primary function of supporting the body in static positions (i.e., postural muscles).

two-joint muscle—a muscle that crosses two joints, influencing the actions of both.

valgus—a condition of the lower extremity in which the bones deviate laterally from the longitudinal axis. Also called bow-legged.

varus—a condition of the lower extremity in which the bones deviate medially from the longitudinal axis. Also known as knock-kneed.

yang—the primary energetic movement of expansion or dispersion. Its qualities include light, heat, action, and dryness.

yin—the primary energetic movement of contraction or congealing. Its qualities include dark, cold, stillness, and dampness.

yoga—an ancient self-development system from India, with several branches that emphasize meditation, postures, breathing, service, devotion, and knowledge.

Bibliography

Agur AMR, Lee MJ. Grant's atlas of anatomy. 10th edition. Baltimore, MD: Lippincott Williams & Wilkins, 1999.

Calais-Germain B. Anatomy of movement. Seattle, WA: Eastland Press, 1993.

Chaitow L. Muscle energy techniques. New York, NY: Churchill Livingstone, 1996.

Chapman CF. Medical dictionary for the nonprofessional. Woodbury, NY: Barron's Education Series, Inc., 1984.

Clemente CD. Anatomy: a regional atlas of the human body. Baltimore, MD: Urban and Schwarzenberg, 1987.

Dychtwald K. Bodymind. Los Angeles, CA: Jeremy Tarcher, Inc., 1977.

Fahey BW. The power of balance: a Rolfing view of health. Portland, OR: Metamorphous Press, 1989.

Finando D, Finando F. Informed touch: a clinician's guide to the evaluation and treatment of myofascial disorders. Rochester, NY: Healing Arts Press, 1999.

Fritz S. Mosby's fundamentals of therapeutic massage. St. Louis, MO: Mosby–Year Book, Inc., 1995.

Gillanders A. The joy of reflexology: healing techniques for the hands and feet to reduce stress and reclaim health. Boston, MA: Little, Brown and Company, 1995.

Heller J, Henkin WA. Bodywise: regaining your natural flexibility and vitality for maximum well-being. New York, NY: Jeremy P. Tarcher, Inc., 1986.

Kurtz R, Hector D. The body reveals: what your body says about you. New York, NY: Harper & Row, 1977.

McCellan S, Monte T. Integrative acupressure: a hands-on guide to balancing the body's structure and energy for health and healing. New York, NY: The Berkeley Publishing Group, 1998.

McIntosh N. The educated heart: professional guidelines for massage therapists, bodyworkers, and movement teachers. Memphis, TN: Decatur Bainbridge Press, 1999.

Menkin D. Transformation through bodywork: using touch therapies for inner peace. Santa Fe, NM: Bear & Company, 1996.

Norking CC, Levangie PK. Joint structure and function: a comprehensive analysis. 2nd edition. Philadelphia, PA: F.A. Davis Company, 1992.

Oatis, C. Kinesiology: the mechanics and pathomechanics of human movement. Philadelphia, PA: Lippincott Williams & Wilkins, 2004.

Olsen A, McHose C. Body stories: a guide to experiential anatomy. Barrytown, NY: Station Hill Press, 1991.

Peters, LM. Manual muscle testing: a visual guide. Atlanta, GA: Susan Hunter Publishing, 1986.

Rolf IP. Rolfing: the integration of human structures. New York, NY: Harper and Row, 1977.

Scheumann DW. Deep tissue therapy student training guide. Atlanta, GA: Atlanta School of Massage Press, 1994.

Stedman's medical dictionary for the health professions and nursing. 5th edition. Philadelphia, PA: Lippincott, Williams & Wilkins, 2005.

Sweigard L. Human movement potential: its ideokinetic facilitation. New York, NY: Dodd, Mead, and Company, 1975.

Thomas CL, ed. Taber's cyclopedic medical dictionary. Philadelphia, PA: F.A. Davis Company, 1989.

Todd ME. The thinking body. Brooklyn, NY: Dance Horizons, Inc., 1972.

Travell JG, Simmons DG. Myofascial pain and dysfunction: the trigger point manual, Volumes 1 and 2. Baltimore, MD: Williams and Wilkins, 1983, 1992.

Travis JW, Regina SR. Wellness workbook. 2nd edition. Berkeley, CA: Ten Speed Press, 1988.

Zemach-Bersin D, Zemach-Bersin K, Reese M. Relaxercise: the easy new way to health and vitality. New York, NY: Harper Collins, 1990.

Index

Page numbers in *italics* denote figures; those followed by a "t" denote tables; and those followed by a "b" denote boxes